Diffusion Weighted and Diffusion Tensor Imaging

A Clinical Guide

Claudia da Costa Leite, MD, PhD
Associate Professor
Department of Radiology
University of São Paulo
São Paulo, Brazil
Associate Professor
Department of Radiology
School of Medicine
University of North Carolina at Chapel Hill
Chapel Hill, North Carolina

Mauricio Castillo, MD, FACR
Professor of Radiology
Chief, Division of Neuroradiology
School of Medicine
University of North Carolina at Chapel Hill
Chapel Hill, North Carolina

Thieme
New York • Stuttgart • Delhi • Rio de Janeiro

Executive Editor: William Lamsback
Managing Editor: Elizabeth Palumbo
Director, Editorial Services: Mary Jo Casey
Editorial Assistant: Haley Paskalides
Production Editor: Sean Woznicki
International Production Director: Andreas Schabert
Vice President, Editorial and E-Product Development: Vera Spillner
International Marketing Director: Fiona Henderson
International Sales Director: Louisa Turrell
Director of Sales, North America: Mike Roseman
Senior Vice President and Chief Operating Officer: Sarah Vanderbilt
President: Brian D. Scanlan

Library of Congress Cataloging-in-Publication Data

Diffusion weighted and diffusion tensor imaging : a clinical guide / [edited by] Claudia da Costa Leite, Mauricio Castillo. – First edition.
   p. ; cm.
 Includes bibliographical references.
   ISBN 978-1-62623-021-7 – ISBN 978-1-62623-020-0 (electronic)
 I. Leite, Claudia da Costa, editor. II. Castillo, Mauricio, editor.
 [DNLM: 1. Diffusion Magnetic Resonance Imaging. 2. Brain Diseases–radiography. 3. Central Nervous System Diseases–radiography. WN 185]
 RC386.6.M34
 616.07'548–dc23   2015010815

© 2016 Thieme Medical Publishers, Inc.

Thieme Publishers New York
333 Seventh Avenue, New York, NY 10001 USA
+1 800 782 3488, customerservice@thieme.com

Thieme Publishers Stuttgart
Rüdigerstrasse 14, 70469 Stuttgart, Germany
+49 [0]711 8931 421, customerservice@thieme.de

Thieme Publishers Delhi
A-12, Second Floor, Sector-2, Noida-201301
Uttar Pradesh, India
+91 120 45 566 00, customerservice@thieme.in

Thieme Publishers Rio de Janeiro, Thieme Publicações Ltda.
Edifício Rodolpho de Paoli, 25º andar
Av. Nilo Peçanha, 50 – Sala 2508
Rio de Janeiro 20020-906 Brasil
+55 21 3172-2297 / +55 21 3172-1896

Cover design: Thieme Publishing Group
Typesetting by DiTech Process Solutions

Printed in China by Everbest Printing Co, Ltd   5 4 3 2 1

ISBN 978-1-62623-021-7

Also available as an e-book:
eISBN 978-1-62623-020-0

Important note: Medicine is an ever-changing science undergoing continual development. Research and clinical experience are continually expanding our knowledge, in particular our knowledge of proper treatment and drug therapy. Insofar as this book mentions any dosage or application, readers may rest assured that the authors, editors, and publishers have made every effort to ensure that such references are in accordance with **the state of knowledge at the time of production of the book.**

Nevertheless, this does not involve, imply, or express any guarantee or responsibility on the part of the publishers in respect to any dosage instructions and forms of applications stated in the book. **Every user is requested to examine carefully** the manufacturers' leaflets accompanying each drug and to check, if necessary in consultation with a physician or specialist, whether the dosage schedules mentioned therein or the contraindications stated by the manufacturers differ from the statements made in the present book. Such examination is particularly important with drugs that are either rarely used or have been newly released on the market. Every dosage schedule or every form of application used is entirely at the user's own risk and responsibility. The authors and publishers request every user to report to the publishers any discrepancies or inaccuracies noticed. If errors in this work are found after publication, errata will be posted at www.thieme.com on the product description page.

Some of the product names, patents, and registered designs referred to in this book are in fact registered trademarks or proprietary names even though specific reference to this fact is not always made in the text. Therefore, the appearance of a name without designation as proprietary is not to be construed as a representation by the publisher that it is in the public domain.

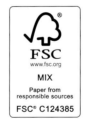

FSC
www.fsc.org
MIX
Paper from responsible sources
FSC® C124385

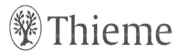

For my mother, my daughter Ana Beatriz, my son Gabriel, and my husband Ricardo

CCL

To Hortensia

MC

Contents

Foreword ix

Preface xi

Contributors xiii

1   Physics of Diffusion Weighted and Diffusion Tensor Imaging 1
    Maria Concepción Garcia Otaduy

2   Brain Edema: Pathophysiology 19
    Falgun H. Chokshi and Amit M. Saindane

3   Supratentorial White Matter Tracts and Their Organization 36
    Christopher P. Hess and Jason M. Johnson

4   Diffusion Weighted Imaging and Diffusion Tensor Imaging of the Brain
    during Early Brain Development: The First Two Years of Life 50
    Wei Gao, John H Gilmore, and Weili Lin

5   Diffusion Weighted and Diffusion Tensor Imaging in Aging 63
    Andrew Joseph Degnan and Lucien M. Levy

6   Diffusion Weighted Imaging in Vascular Pathology 79
    Sangam Kanekar and Chandan Misra

7   Diffusion Weighted Imaging in the Evaluation of Brain Tumors 99
    Fernanda C. Rueda-Lopes, Celso Hygino da Cruz Jr., and Emerson Leandro Gasparetto

8   Diffusion Weighted and Diffusion Tensor Imaging in Infectious Diseases 112
    Claudia da Costa Leite, Maria da Graça Morais Martin and Mauricio Castillo

9   Diffusion Weighted Imaging and Diffusion Tensor Imaging in Demyelination
    and Toxic Diseases 132
    Celi Santos Andrade, Carolina de Medeiros Rimkus, Claudia da Costa Leite, Alexander M. McKinney,
    and Leandro T. Lucato

10 Diffusion Weighted Imaging and Diffusion Tensor Imaging of White Matter
    Diseases In Children 154
    Julie H. Harreld and Zoltan Patay

11 Diffusion Imaging for the Assessment of Traumatic Brain Injury 170
    Michael L. Lipton

12 Diffusion Weighted Imaging in Hemorrhage 189
    Joana Ramalho and Mauricio Castillo

13   **Diffusion Weighted Imaging and Diffusion Tensor Imaging in Spine and Spinal Cord Diseases** 203

Majda M. Thurnher

14   **Diffusion Weighted Imaging and Diffusion Tensor Imaging in Head and Neck Diseases** 215

Eloisa M Santiago Gebrim, Regina Lucia Elia Gomes, Flavia K. Issa Cevasco, and Marcio Ricardo Taveira Garcia

15   **Future Applications of Diffusion Weighted Imaging: Diffusional Kurtosis and Other Nongaussian Diffusion Techniques** 239

Maria Gisele Matheus

Index 248

Foreword

Diffusion weighted imaging (DWI) has become an integral part of routine neuroimaging. It is virtually obtained in every brain magnetic resonance imaging (MRI) protocol and in a growing number of head and neck and spine protocols. It is fast and provides clinically relevant information for a variety of pathological conditions, including stroke, infection, and neoplastic processes.

Its counterpart, diffusion tensor imaging (DTI), is a powerful technique that has multiple potential applications, including neurosurgical guidance and the diagnosis of mild traumatic brain injury and psychiatric disorders. However, it is still under development and has yet to be fully translated from expert academic centers to the routine clinical practice.

This book, *Diffusion Weighted and Diffusion Tensor Imaging: A Clinical Guide*, edited by Drs. Claudia da Costa Leite and Mauricio Castillo, is a step in that direction. Its 15 chapters provide readers with all the information they will need to implement and interpret DWI and DTI studies. The chapters cover normal development, aging, and the most relevant pathologies, including trauma, white matter diseases, tumors, cerebrovascular disorders, and head and neck and spine disorders. The information is concisely presented, with key points and summaries for each chapter. The text is very easy to read, and the accompanying illustrations are of very high quality.

There is no doubt that radiologists interpreting neuroimaging studies should read this book and have it at the ready, not only for reference but also to refresh their memory about DWI and to learn ways to incorporate DTI in the care of their patients.

Max Wintermark, MD, MAS, MBA
Stanford University
Palo Alto, California

Preface

Diffusion weighted imaging (DWI) and diffusion tensor imaging (DTI) are magnetic resonance imaging (MRI) technologies that have been applied to research for some time. The translation of this research into clinical practice has increased in recent years to the point where the use of DWI is now routine in most if not all patients. Understanding the concepts and applications of DWI and DTI is necessary for their correct use and interpretation.

The introduction of MRI enabled easier diagnosis of white matter disease, and such capability was further improved with the advent of DWI and DTI. An increasing need to understand the organization and maturation of white matter, as well as to better characterize many diseases that affect it, has been in part successfully fulfilled with the use of DTI.

This book, *Diffusion weighted and Diffusion Tensor Imaging: A Clinical Guide*, comprises 15 chapters providing an overview of DWI and DTI focused on the practical clinical applications of these techniques for evaluations of the central nervous system and the head and neck.

The first chapter reviews the physics of DWI and DTI so readers can better understand the chapters that follow. Chapter 2 discusses the pathophysiology of brain edema, given that the first and most important use of DWI is to differentiate cytotoxic from vasogenic edema.

Chapter 3 describes the white matter tracts and their organizations, demonstrating DTI's capability to elegantly depict these structures. Understanding white matter tracts and their connections is the first step toward the development of the human connectome.

Considering that the characteristics of white matter differ throughout life, chapters 4 and 5 describe DWI and DTI features of white matter in different phases: during development and during aging. Knowledge of these differences is essential to differentiate normal from pathological states.

The chapters that follow focus on central nervous system pathologies for which DWI and DTI clearly have improved our ability to diagnose vascular diseases, tumors, infectious diseases, demyelinating and toxic diseases, white matter diseases in children, trauma, and hemorrhage. The goal is to present the main clinical applications of these techniques in these situations.

Besides the overview of the main applications of DWI and DTI in the brain, the book also reviews their applications in the spine and spinal cord and in the head and neck.

Ultimately this book discusses, albeit briefly, future applications of DWI and DTI, giving readers a glimpse of what is in store. We hope that you will enjoy this practical approach to DWI and DTI and find it useful for your day-to-day clinical practice. We are grateful to our contributors for sharing their knowledge with all of us.

Claudia da Costa Leite
Mauricio Castillo

Contributors

Celi Santos Andrade, MD, PhD
Post-doctoral Researcher
Department of Radiology
University of Alberta, Edmonton, Canada
Hospital das Clínicas, Faculdade de Medicina da
   Universidade de São Paulo
Centro de Diagnósticos Brasil
São Paulo, Brazil

Mauricio Castillo, MD, FACR
Professor of Radiology
Chief, Division of Neuroradiology
School of Medicine
University of North Carolina at Chapel Hill
Chapel Hill, North Carolina

Flavia K. Issa Cevasco, MD
Departament of Radiology
Universidade de São Paulo
São Paulo, Brazil

Falgun H. Chokshi, MD, MS
Director of Neuroradiology Services
Emory University Hospital Midtown
Assistant Professor
Department of Radiology and Imaging Sciences
Emory School of Medicine
Atlanta, Georgia

Celso Hygino da Cruz, Jr, MD
Department of Radiology,
Federal University of Rio de Janeiro
CDPI Clínica de Diagnóstico Por Imagem
Rio de Janeiro, Brazil

Andrew Joseph Degnan, MD, MPhil
Resident in Radiology
University of Pittsburgh Medical Center
Pittsburgh, Pennsylvania

Wei Gao, PhD
Assistant Professor
Department of Radiology
Biomedical Research Imaging Center
University of North Carolina at Chapel Hill
Chapel Hill, North Carolina

Marcio Ricardo Taveira Garcia, MD
Departament of Radiology
Universidade de São Paulo
São Paulo, Brazil

Emerson Leandro Gasparetto, MD, PhD
Department of Radiology
Federal University of Rio de Janeiro
Rio de Janeiro, Brazil

Eloisa M. Santiago Gebrim, MD
Department of Radiology
Universidade de São Paulo
São Paulo, Brazil

John H. Gilmore, MD
Thad and Alice Eure Distinguished Professor
Vice Chair for Research and Scientific Affairs
Director, Center for Excellence in Community Mental
   Health
Department of Psychiatry
University of North Carolina at Chapel Hill
Chapel Hill, North Carolina

Regina Lucia Elia Gomes, MD
Departament of Radiology
Universidade de São Paulo
São Paulo, Brazil

Julie H. Harreld, MD
Assistant Member
Department of Diagnostic Imaging
St. Jude Children's Research Hospital
Memphis, Tennessee

Christopher P. Hess, MD, PhD
Associate Professor of Radiology and Neurology
UCSF Department of Radiology and Neurology
University of California
San Francisco, California

Jason M. Johnson, MD
Assistant Professor
Diagonstic Radiology- Neuro Imaging
The University of Texas
MD Anderson Cancer Center
Houston, Texas

Sangam Kanekar, MD
Associate Professor
Division of Neuroradiology
Department of Radiology
Penn State Milton S Hershey Medical Center and
  College of Medicine
Hershey, Pennsylvania

Claudia da Costa Leite, MD, PhD
Associate Professor
Department of Radiology
University of São Paulo
São Paulo, Brazil
Associate Professor
Department of Radiology
School of Medicine
University of North Carolina at Chapel Hill
Chapel Hill, North Carolina

Lucien M. Levy, MD, PhD
Deceased
Professor of Radiology
Chief of Neuroradiology
The George Washington University School of
  Medicine
Washington DC

Weili Lin, PhD
Dixie Lee Boney Soo Distinguished Professor of
  Neurological Medicine and Director
Department of Radiology
Biomedical Research Imaging Center
University of North Carolina at Chapel Hill
Chapel Hill, North Carolina

Michael L. Lipton, MD, PhD, FACR
Professor of Radiology
Department of Radiology, Psychiatry and Behavioral
  Sciences
The Dominick P. Purpura Department of Neuroscience
Albert Einstein College of Medicine
The Gruss Magnetic Resonance Research Center
Department of Radiology
Montefiore Medical Center
Bronx, New York

Leandro T. Lucato, MD, PhD
Section Chief, Diagnostic Neuroradiology
Medical Director, Magnetic Resonance Center
Department of Radiology
Hospital das Clínicas, Faculdade de Medicina da
  Universidade de São Paulo
Centro de Diagnósticos Brasil
São Paulo, Brazil

Maria da Graça Morais Martin MD, PhD
Neuroradiologist
Instituto de Radiologia
Clinics Hospital, School of Medicine
University of São Paula
Hospital Sirio Libanês
São Paulo, Brazil

Maria Gisele Matheus, MD
Assistant Professor of Neuroradiology
Department of Radiology and Radiological Science
Medical University of South Carolina
Charleston, South Carolina

Alexander M. Mckinney, MD
Associate Professor
Vice Chair, Research
Neuroradiology Division Director
University of Minnesota
Minneapolis, Minnesota

Chandan Misra, MD
PGY-3 Resident
Penn State Hershey Radiology
Hershey, Pennsylvania

Maria Concepción Garcia Otaduy, PhD
Department of Radiology
Medical School of the University of São Paulo
Medical Physicist
Magnetic Resonance Department
Clinics Hospital of the University of São Paulo
São Paulo, Brazil

Zolton Patay, MD, PhD
Chief, Neuroradiology
Department of Diagnostic Imaging
St. Jude Children's Research Hospital
Memphis, Tennessee

Joana Ramalho, MD
Department of Neuroradiology
Centro Hospitalar Lisboa Central
Lisboa, Portugal
Division of Neuroradiology
University of North Carolina at Chapel Hill
Chapel Hill, North Carolina

Carolina de Medeiros Rimkus, MD, PhD
Post-doctoral Researcher
Department of Radiology
Vrije University Medical Center
Amsterdam, The Netherlands
Hospital das Clínicas, Faculdade de Medicina da
  Universidade de São Paulo
São Paulo, Brazil

Fernanda C. Rueda-Lopes, MD
Department of Radiology
Federal University of Rio de Janeiro
CDPI Clínica de Diagnóstico Por Imagem
Rio de Janeiro, Brazil

Amit M. Saindane, MD
Associate Professor
Department of Radiology and Imaging Sciences
Division of Neuroradiology
Director, Division of Neuroradiology
Radiology and Imaging Sciences
Emory University School of Medicine
Atlanta, Georgia

Majda M. Thurnher, MD
Professor of Radiology
Department of Biomedical Imaging and
  Image-guided Therapy
University Hospital Vienna
Medical University Vienna
Vienna, Austria

1 Physics of Diffusion Weighted and Diffusion Tensor Imaging

Maria Concepción Garcia Otaduy

Key Points

- Diffusion is a powerful diagnostic tool that measures water molecule displacement of the size order of cell structures (a few micrometers). Hence it is sensitive to microstructural changes in brain tissue, even before these changes can be detected by other types of magnetic resonance imaging (MRI).
- Water diffusion in the brain is relatively restricted, and, depending on the parameters of the diffusion pulse sequence, one can observe more or less of this restriction. The measured water diffusion coefficient depends on the (*b* values); thus the term *apparent diffusion coefficient* (ADC) is used.
- Water diffusion in the brain is anisotropic, meaning that it is facilitated parallel to myelin fibers and axons and restricted perpendicular to them. The tensor model is adopted to describe this diffusion anisotropy, and it allows one to quantify anisotropy parameters (related to white matter integrity) and to reconstruct the trajectory of white matter fibers (diffusion tractography).

1.1 Introduction

Diffusion weighted images (DWIs) provide tissue contrast related to the thermally driven random motion (Brownian motion) of water molecules in brain tissue. Water diffusion is heavily restricted by the brain tissue microstructure, and this restriction is higher when it occurs perpendicular to the white matter fibers (diffusion anisotropy). This restriction to water diffusion has two important consequences: First, any changes at the cytoarchitecture level will be reflected in the DWI, making this method extremely sensitive to pathological changes; and second, based on the orientation of the faster diffusion in a voxel, white matter trajectories can be reproduced. This is the principle behind diffusion tractography.

1.2 Diffusion Weighted Imaging

1.2.1 Brownian Motion

Due to thermal energy, water molecules in a liquid state are in constant motion, following a random pathway where the direction of the motion changes with the collisions of water molecules. This type of motion is called brownian motion, named after the botanist Robert Brown, who first described it in 1827 after observing the motion of pollen suspended in water. In 1906 Albert Einstein described this motion mathematically, introducing the idea of random walk and the self-diffusion coefficient *D*. In this random walk (▶ Fig. 1.1) it is impossible to predict the distance that a given water molecule will diffuse in a given time, but it is possible to obtain a statistical value on how a whole group of water molecules will diffuse. This value is the mean square displacement $<r^2>$, which reflects the mean of the gaussian distribution of displacements that water molecules accomplish in a given time period (see ▶ Fig. 1.1). As stated by the Einstein equation of diffusion in one dimension, $<r^2>$ increases with the diffusion time *t* (the observation time in the measurement), and the diffusion coefficient *D* is the proportionality constant, with a physical unit of mm²/s:

$$\langle r^2 \rangle = 2 \cdot D \cdot t \tag{1.1}$$

1.2.2 Stejskal and Tanner

In 1965 Stejskal and Tanner introduced the idea of measuring the diffusion coefficient of liquids by nuclear magnetic resonance (NMR) using pulsed gradients before and after the application of the 180-degree pulse in the spin-echo (SE) sequence (▶ Fig. 1.2). The first pulsed gradient causes a fast and controlled dephasing of the spins, afterward a 180-degree pulse is applied, which inverts all spins and initiates the process of spins rephasing for later formation of the echo. But, for the complete rephasing of the spins to occur, it is necessary to apply again exactly the same pulsed field gradient (with the same amplitude G and duration δ) that was applied before the 180-degree pulse, in order to compensate for the dephasing caused by the first pulsed gradient. If the spins do not change position relative to the applied field gradient during the time interval Δ, the time between the two pulsed field gradients, all spins will be correctly rephased and will contribute to the echo signal. However, most of the echo signal comes from water, which is in constant motion,

and from the Einstein equation we know that, after a given time Δ the $<r^2>$ will be nonzero. Hence the location of the water molecules relative to the applied pulsed gradient will change, and as a consequence water diffusing spins will not be correctly rephased and will not contribute to the signal of the echo. By measuring the signal intensity of the SE with (S) and without (S_0) the application of the pulsed field gradients the diffusion coefficient D can be calculated from the Stejskal and Tanner equation:

$$\frac{S}{S_0} = e^{xp - bD} \tag{1.2}$$

where b is known as the b factor of the diffusion acquisition and depends on the pulse sequence parameters as shown in the next equation,

$$b = \gamma^2 G^2 \delta^2 \left(\Delta - \frac{\delta}{3} \right) \tag{1.3}$$

with γ being the gyromagnetic ratio.

By increasing the b factor in the diffusion acquisition, more diffusion weight will be introduced in the images. When $b = 0$ (zero of diffusion weight) is applied, the result is basically a T2-weighted image, with high signal intensity for liquids (▶ Fig. 1.3a). When $b = 1,000 \, s/mm^2$ is applied we obtain a DWI, where higher diffusion is denoted by hypointensity (strong signal attenuation), and slower diffusion (restriction to diffusion) is denoted by high signal intensity (▶ Fig. 1.3b).

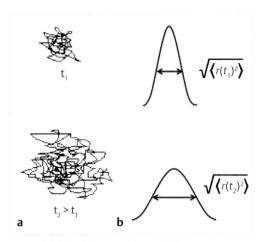

Fig. 1.1 (a) Example of random water molecule trajectories ("random walk") during diffusion (brownian motion) and (b) gaussian distribution of water molecule displacements characterized by the root mean square displacement as a function of time.

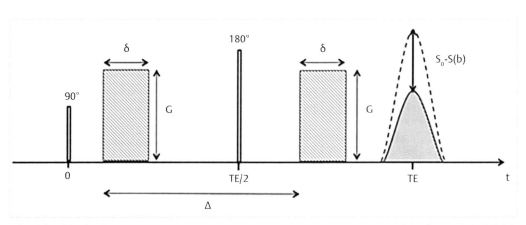

Fig. 1.2 Stejskal and Tanner pulse sequence for the measurement of diffusion. G, gradient amplitude; δ duration of the gradient pulse; Δ, interval between gradient pulses; TE, echo time. S0, signal without applying gradient pulses; S(b), signal after applying gradient pulses.

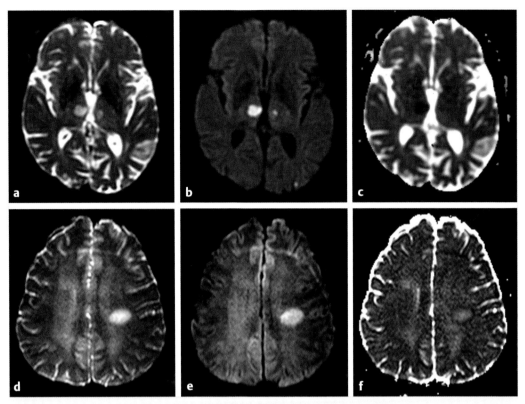

Fig. 1.3 (a) Non–diffusion weighted imaging (DWI) ($b = 0 \, s/mm^2$) of a stroke patient presenting two thalamic lesions. (b) DWI ($b = 1,000 \, s/mm^2$) with high signal intensity in both lesions. (c) Corresponding apparent diffusion coefficient (ADC) map confirming the restriction to diffusion in the lesions with a decrease in ADC. (d) Non-DWI ($b = 0 \, s/mm^2$) of another stroke patient with a left subacute lesion. (e) DWI ($b = 1,000 \, s/mm^2$) presenting high signal intensity in the lesion (T2 shine-through effect). (f) Corresponding ADC map showing that there is no restriction of diffusion, but rather an ADC increase in the lesion.

1.2.3 T2 Shine-through Effect and Apparent Diffusion Coefficcient Map

The interpretation of signal intensity in the DWI is not always straightforward. Sometimes the signal intensity may be high in both the non-DWI ($b = 0$) and the DWI ($b > 0$), independent of restriction to diffusion (▶ Fig. 1.3d,e). This is because DWIs are inherently also T2-weighted images because they are acquired with relatively long echo times (TEs) and long repetition times. In this case, the high signal intensity in the DWI may be due only to the T2 shine-through effect. To elucidate this question it is suggested to calculate the actual D for each voxel in the image as follows:

$$D = ADC = -\frac{\ln \frac{S_{b_2}}{S_{b_1}}}{(b_2 - b_1)} = -\frac{\ln \frac{S_b}{S_0}}{b} \tag{1.4}$$

where S_{b_1} and S_{b_2} are the signal intensities obtained with two different b values and $b_1 < b_2$. If we solve this equation for each voxel in the image, we obtain the so-called apparent diffusion coefficient (ADC) map (▶ Fig. 1.3c,f). In the ADC map, signal intensity directly reflects the ADC value, which is highest where there is free diffusion, like in the ventricular cerebrospinal fluid (CSF) with an ADC ≈ $3.2 \times 10^{-3} \, mm^2/s$, and lowest in regions of restricted diffusion, i.e. in the white matter with an ADC ≈ $0.7 \times 10^{-3} \, mm^2/s$. It is important to observe that, as indicated by the name of *apparent* diffusion coefficient, the calculated ADC in brain tissues depends on the choice of b_1 and b_2. Conventionally, in the brain the two b values chosen are 0 and $1,000 \, s/mm^2$, but different values can also be used. It is also possible to acquire images with more than two b values to obtain a better approximation of the ADC. In this case, the obtained signal intensity is fitted to an exponential function of b, derived from Equation (1.2):

$$S(b) = S_0 e^{-b \cdot ADC} \qquad (1.5)$$

However, it has been shown that, for calculation of the ADC, it is not efficient in terms of signal to noise ratio (SNR) to use more than two b values. Two b values are enough, and, ideally, for *in vivo* brain measurements the difference between them should be approximately 1,000 to 1,500 s/mm^2.[1]

1.2.4 Restriction of Water Diffusion in Brain Tissue

ADC as a Marker of Tissue Microstructure

Diffusion of water in biological tissues and in the brain is strongly restricted; water molecules constantly encounter barriers (e.g., cell membranes, myelin fibers, and axonal projections), which prevent the water from diffusing freely, such as it would in a glass of water. The water root mean square displacements that occur in the brain within the diffusion times used in conventional DWI are on the order of a few micrometers, which corresponds to the order of the size of cell structures. Hence the ADC measured in brain tissues reflects water motion restricted by these cell structures and is thus an extremely sensitive marker of tissue microstructure. For instance, it is possible to detect restriction in diffusion (decreased ADC) when there is an increase in cellular density caused by

tumor growth or with cellular swelling in cytotoxic edema. On the other hand, the increase of extracellular space caused by vasogenic edema, demyelination, or axonal loss, results in an increase of the observed ADC. Any biological or pathological change that causes changes in the tissue microstructure will be in principle detected by changes in the ADC, which renders the DWI technique very powerful.

Size of Tissue Compartments

The size of the tissue compartments where water can diffuse plays an important role in the resulting ADC. Within one compartment water may diffuse freely, but if the diffusion time Δ of the experiment is long enough for the water molecules to reach the limits of the compartment, the chance that the water molecules will bounce back to the center of the compartment is greatly increased. As Δ increases, more water molecules will hit "the walls" of the compartment, and the observed $<r^2>$ will be smaller than that expected for free diffusion as illustrated in (▶ Fig. 1.4). Because of this effect it is advisable to keep a constant Δ value unless the intention is to determine the size of tissue compartments.[2]

Influence of the b Factor on the ADC

As described in Equation (1.3) the b factor depends on the characteristics of the applied pulsed field gradients and on the diffusion time Δ. For the reasons already explained it is recommended to maintain Δ as a fixed value and to increase the b

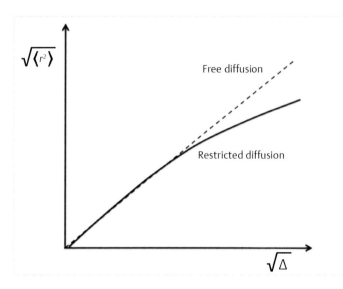

Fig. 1.4 Mean square displacement as a function of diffusion time showing the effect of restriction.

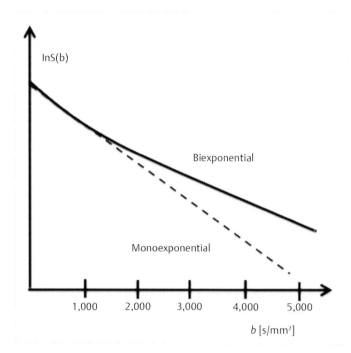

Fig. 1.5 Nonlinearity of diffusion in white matter at high b values.

value only by increasing the diffusion gradient field strength (G). The stronger the applied pulsed field gradients, the higher the capacity of the gradients to cause dephasing, and signal attenuation will be measured even in the presence of very slow diffusion. This means that the higher the b value, the higher the contribution of the slow diffusing compartments will be in the final DWI. As the b value increases (> 1,000 s/mm²) the resulting ADC becomes smaller.[3] This is because the obtained ADC in brain tissues is the average of the diffusion of several tissue compartments in the voxel, and as the b value increases and diffusion rate decreases, the contribution of slow diffusion compartments becomes higher. If signal intensity is plotted on a logarithmic scale as a function of b, the signal intensity decreases almost linearly until a value of 1,000 s/mm² is reached, but above 1,000 s/mm², the slope of the signal attenuation begins to change (▶ Fig. 1.5). For this reason, when using high b values (> 1,000 s/mm²) the signal attenuation is better described with a biexponential model.[3] This biexponential behavior will be encountered only for voxels where compartments with different diffusions coexist, as in the white matter, whereas in the CSF within the ventricles signal attenuation will be monoexponential. By measuring the DWI signal as a function of different b values up to 4,000 to 6,000 s/mm²

Clark and Le Bihan[3] estimated the fast diffusing fraction in brain tissue to be ~ 0.7, too large to be reflecting only the diffusion in the extracellular space, as discussed in their study.

Choice of the b Value

The question now arises as to how high the chosen b value should be. The slower the diffusion in the tissue, the higher the b value needs to be; on the other hand, if the b value is too high, the resulting DWI is very noisy. A b value of ~ 1/ADC of the tissue of interest is suggested to be optimal, but given that the TE needs to be increased with higher b values (due to the use of stronger gradients), and that a longer TE leads to a lower SNR, the optimal b becomes ~ 0.9/ADC.[4,5] For brain studies a b value of 1,000 s/mm² is commonly used and results in an effective compromise between diffusion sensitivity and SNR. Nevertheless, for lesions with a stronger restriction to diffusion than that in normal white matter (i.e., in tumors), it is interesting to use higher b values (i.e. b = 2,000 s/mm²) to increase the sensitivity of the method.[6,7,8] Hence the ability to obtain a valuable DWI will be strongly related to the strength of the gradient coils and the maximum b values that can be achieved.

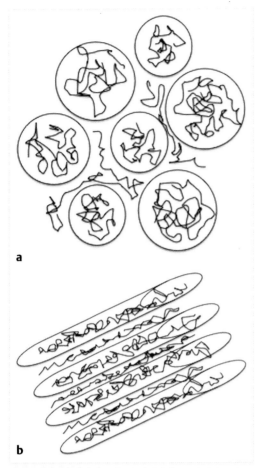

a

b

Fig. 1.6 (a) Isotropic and (b) anisotropic display of the barriers to diffusion.

1.2.5 Anisotropy of Water Diffusion in the Brain

Isotropic and Anisotropic Diffusion

Sometimes the barriers that restrict water diffusion in brain tissues are isotropically distributed (▶ Fig. 1.6a), which means that diffusion will be restricted equally in all directions. At other times these barriers will be distributed anisotropically, resulting in stronger diffusion restrictions perpendicular to the barriers (▶ Fig. 1.6b). In white matter water, diffusion is facilitated parallel to axonal projections and myelin fibers, and it is restricted perpendicular to them. Thus the measured ADC depends on the direction of the applied pulsed field gradient. This is clearly illustrated in ▶ Fig. 1.7a–c, where one can observe the DWI with the diffusion gradients applied in the three

orthogonal directions. When these images are compared important differences are visible, in particular in the region of the splenium of the corpus callosum, where there is high signal intensity for the image acquired with diffusion gradients applied in the z direction, indicating restriction to diffusion in the inferior–superior orientation, and very low signal intensity when the diffusion gradient is applied in the x direction, indicating unhindered diffusion in the right-to-left orientation, parallel to the corpus callosum fibers. This region in the brain is known to have the highest values of diffusion anisotropy. The term *anisotropy* indicates that water diffusion in brain tissue depends on orientation. To obtain DWI results that are independent on orientation, one needs to calculate the average of the three DWIs obtained with the pulsed diffusion gradients applied in the three orthogonal directions (▶ Fig. 1.7a–c). This average image is known as the isotropic DWI and is used to calculate the ADC (▶ Fig. 1.7d).

The Tensor Model

The tensor model was proposed to describe and quantify diffusion anisotropy.[9] In the tensor model, ADC is measured in the three perpendicular directions x, y, and z, and in all combinations of these directions, and instead of referring to a single ADC, we refer to the diffusion tensor[1]:

$$\overline{ADC} = \begin{bmatrix} ADC_{xx} & ADC_{xy} & ADC_{xz} \\ ADC_{yx} & ADC_{yy} & ADC_{yz} \\ ADC_{zx} & ADC_{zy} & ADC_{zz} \end{bmatrix} \qquad (1.6)$$

Because the tensor is symmetric (i.e., $ADC_{xy} = ADC_{yx}$, $ADC_{xz} = ADC_{zx}$, and $ADC_{yz} = ADC_{zy}$) diffusion needs to be measured only in six different gradient directions to fill the nine diffusion elements in the matrix. Such a matrix is determined for each voxel of the image. Afterward the matrix is diagonalized, a mathematical process by which all off-diagonal elements become zero, and the diagonal elements are transformed to coincide with the principal axis of diffusion in the voxel. The new diagonal elements correspond to the three eigenvectors (ε_1, ε_2, and ε_3) with their eigenvalues (λ_1, λ_2, and λ_3), representing the main directions of diffusion and their associated diffusivities, respectively. The eigenvalues are arranged according to their magnitudes so that $\lambda_1 \geq \lambda_2 \geq \lambda_3$.

A graphical representation of this tensor can be obtained with the ellipsoid model (▶ Fig. 1.8a), where the axes of the ellipsoid correspond to the

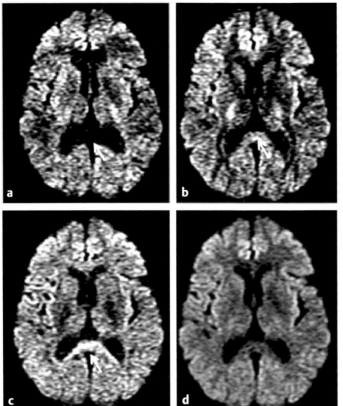

Fig. 1.7 Diffusion weighted images (DWIs) (b = 1,000 s/mm^2) acquired with diffusion gradients applied in the three orthogonal directions: (**a**) right–left, (**b**) anterior–posterior, and (**c**) inferior–superior. Note the marked differences in signal intensity at the splenium of the corpus callosum (arrows) due to the strong orientation of the fibers in this region. (**d**) Isotropic DWI or trace image.

eigenvectors, with the longest axis in the direction of the ε_1. The more stretched the ellipsoid is, the higher the anisotropy in the voxel. On the other hand, in cases of isotropic diffusion, all eigenvectors have the same size, resulting in a sphere (▶ Fig. 1.8b).

The first eigenvalue λ_1 is also known as the axial diffusion because it represents the diffusion parallel to the fiber bundle. ▶ Fig. 1.9a shows the map of axial diffusion and ▶ Fig. 1.9b is its color-coded map indicating the orientation of ε_1. The two other eigenvalues represent the magnitude of diffusion perpendicular to ε_1, and the term *radial diffusion* is introduced to refer to the diffusion perpendicular to the fiber, calculated as $(\lambda_2 + \lambda_3)/2$. Experimental studies suggest that axial diffusion can be used to evaluate axon integrity and that radial diffusion is more sensitive to myelin integrity.[10,11] However, care should be taken because this interpretation is not always straightforward. When comparing different individuals, pathology, and partial volume effects, noise or crossing fibers may change the direction of the calculated ε_1 in a particular voxel with respect to the underlying structure. As a consequence, the direction and size of λ_2 and λ_3

change as well, and the obtained differences in radial diffusivity do not necessarily reflect changes in myelin integrity.[12] Ideally, when comparing axial and radial diffusivities between subjects, the direction of the ε_1 should be taken into account, and voxels with very different directions of ε_1 for both groups should be excluded from the analysis.[12]

Other parameters that aim to quantify the anisotropy in brain tissue are fractional anisotropy (FA), relative anisotropy (RA), and volume ratio (VR) (▶ Fig. 1.10a–c), described by the following:

$$FA = \frac{\sqrt{3\left[(\lambda_1 - \langle\lambda\rangle)^2 + (\lambda_2 - \langle\lambda\rangle)^2 + (\lambda_3 - \langle\lambda\rangle)^2\right]}}{\sqrt{2(\lambda_1^2 + \lambda_2^2 + \lambda_3^2)}}$$

(1.7)

where

$$\langle\lambda\rangle = \frac{Tr(ADC)}{3} = \frac{\lambda_1 + \lambda_2 + \lambda_3}{3}$$

(1.8)

$$RA = \frac{\sqrt{(\lambda_1 - \langle\lambda\rangle)^2 + (\lambda_2 - \langle\lambda\rangle)^2 + (\lambda_3 - \langle\lambda\rangle)^2}}{\sqrt{3}\langle\lambda\rangle}$$

(1.9)

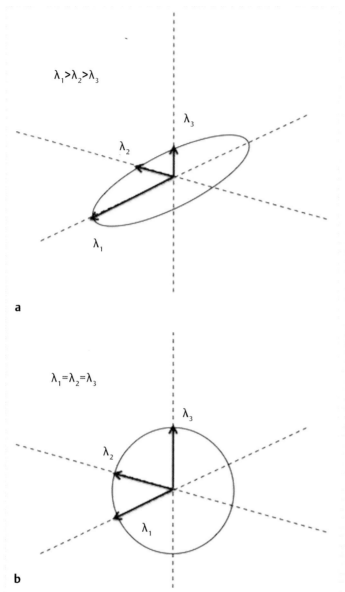

$\lambda_1 > \lambda_2 > \lambda_3$

λ_3

λ_2

λ_1

a

$\lambda_1 = \lambda_2 = \lambda_3$

λ_3

λ_2

λ_1

b

Fig. 1.8 (a) Anisotropic diffusion represented by an ellipsoid and (b) isotropic diffusion represented by a sphere.

$$VR = \frac{\lambda_1 \lambda_2 \lambda_3}{\langle \lambda \rangle^3} \qquad (1.10)$$

Tr(ADC) is the trace of the tensor (the sum of the three eigenvalues), and $\langle \lambda \rangle$ represents the mean diffusivity in the voxel (the average of the three eigenvalues). *VR* represents the ratio of the volume of the ellipsoid describing the anisotropy in the voxel to the volume of a sphere whose radius is the mean diffusivity.[13] Because the volume of the ellipsoid decreases as anisotropy increases, *VR* = 0 indicates a maximum of anisotropy, and *VR* = 1 indicates that diffusion is completely isotropic. *RA* represents the normalized standard deviation of the eigenvalues from $\langle \lambda \rangle$. In case of isotropic diffusion (no deviation) *RA* = 0, and the higher the *RA* the higher the anisotropy. *FA* measures the fraction of the mean diffusion that can be ascribed to anisotropic diffusion, so that *FA* can range from 0 (fully isotropic diffusion) to 1 (fully anisotropic diffusion).[1] *RA* and *FA* present similar parametric

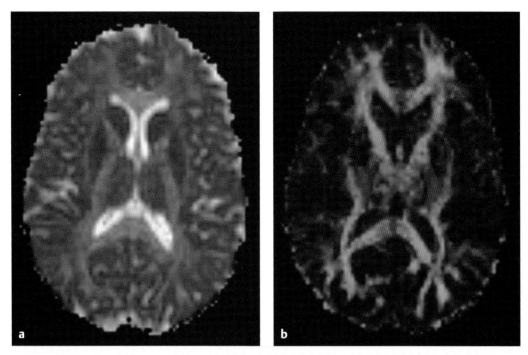

Fig. 1.9 (a) Map of axial diffusion and (b) standard color-coded principal direction map. Red indicates left–right, green indicates anterior–posterior, and blue indicates superior–inferior orientations.

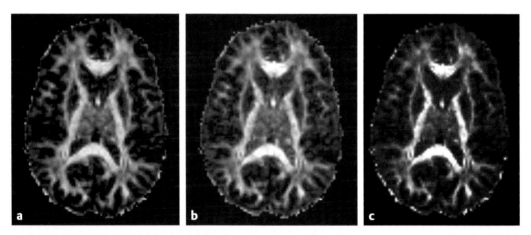

Fig. 1.10 (a) Map of fractional anisotropy, (b) relative anisotropy, and (c) volume ratio.

maps, but it has been shown that *FA* is less affected by noise than *RA*, and that *FA* provides a better contrast-to-noise ratio between grey and white matter.[14] In the healthy brain *FA* is low in cortical gray matter (≈ 0.2), variable in the deep gray matter (0.2–0.4), and higher in the white matter (> 0.1). Regions of very high *FA* are the corpus callosum (≈ 0.8).

1.2.6 Tractography

Tractography is a method for identifying white matter pathways in the brain. It is based on the assumption that the first eigenvector ε_1 derived from the DTI analysis will be parallel to the fiber bundle in the voxel, and different types of algorithms can be applied to reconstruct three-dimensionally these fiber pathways based on the information on each voxel. A basic distinction in the algorithm to be applied is whether it is based on deterministic or probabilistic tractography.[15] The deterministic tractography, most commonly used in clinical applications, is based on the streamline principle, so that, starting from a given region of interest (seed location), adjacent voxels will be integrated to the same streamline as long as their principal eigenvectors are parallel to each other or at least do not deviate too much from the given direction. The limit for this deviation is established by the curvature threshold (commonly 30–60 degrees), so that, if the next voxel has an angle greater than this threshold, it will not be included to the streamline and the tract will stop at that point. Another limit imposed on the growth of this streamline is the value of the fractional anisotropy in the voxel because in voxels with low FA the determination of the eigenvector is associated with large errors. If the next voxel is below an established FA threshold (commonly 0.2–0.3) the tract will stop. Deterministic tractography is often combined with some prior anatomical knowledge that the user can select more than one region of interest through which a white matter tract should pass, and streamlines that do not pass through these selected regions of interests will be excluded from the graphical representation of the white matter tracts. ▶ Fig. 1.11 shows an example of how the white matter tracts of the corpus callosum can be reconstructed based on the anisotropy information of individual voxels.

An important limitation of tractography is that its resolution (~ 2 mm) is too low to identify the orientation of individual white matter fibers (with a diameter on the order of 1 μm). Even if these white matter tracts are largely coherently organized in fiber bundles containing hundreds of thousands of axons, in many of the DTI voxels fiber bundles will cross, split, or merge. The effect of these "crossing fibers" is that the obtained ε_1 will not represent the correct fiber orientation in the voxel because it contains more than one fiber orientation. The coexistence of more than one fiber orientation results in low FA for the voxel, below the established threshold for streamline tractography, which causes interruption of the fiber tracking. As opposed to deterministic tractography, probabilistic tractography is better able to handle the problem of crossing fibers given that, instead of stopping the fiber tracking, the uncertainty for a given fiber orientation is calculated for every voxel, so that afterward the most likely white matter pathways that connect two different regions can be reconstructed. Many new acquisition methods and processing algorithms have been proposed to deal more effectively with crossing fibers, such as, q-space imaging (QSI), diffusion spectrum imaging (DSI), q-ball imaging (QBI), composite hindered and restricted model of diffusion (CHARMED), and

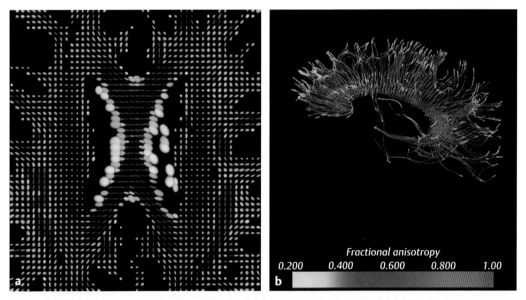

Fig. 1.11 (a) Graphical representation of the diffusion ellipsoids for each voxel and (b) the resulting tractography in the corpus callosum.

high angular resolution diffusion imaging (HARDI). More detailed descriptions of these methods can be found elsewhere.[15]

1.3 Diffusion Imaging Techniques

1.3.1 DWI with Spin-Echo-Echo-Planar Imaging

Up until now we have spoken about the diffusion technique as just the modified SE version of Stejskal and Tanner, a technique used in vitro to measure the self-diffusion coefficient of liquids. The first attempts by Le Bihan to adapt this technique to *in vivo* MRI measurements of diffusion were discouraging and suffered from gradient strength limitations and motion artifacts,[16] but in 1986 he managed to publish the first application of MRI diffusion in the brain.[17] Clinical applications of DWI became feasible after overcoming motion artifacts by combining DWI with echo-planar imaging (EPI), a strategy of rapidly filling the k-space.[18] In the single-shot SE-EPI acquisition all echoes required to build the image derive from the same excitation pulse, and just by switching the polarity of the frequency-encoding gradients a train of gradient-echoes is rapidly formed, capable of filling the whole k-space of a single image (▶ Fig. 1.12a) in about 50 to 100 ms.

1.3.2 DWI with Periodically Rotated Overlapping Parallel Lines with Enhanced Reconstruction (PROPELLER)

A great disadvantage of the SE-EPI acquisition is that this type of sequence is prone to strong susceptibility artifacts. The next section discusses how EPI parameters need to be chosen to minimize this type of artifact, but even after parameter optimization, the regions close to the temporal bones, ears, and sinuses will suffer from distortions, precluding the diagnostic evaluation of these regions. This problem was overcome by combining the periodically rotated overlapping parallel lines with enhanced reconstruction (PROPELLER) technique,[19] insensitive to motion artifacts, with DWI. In the PROPELLER technique (called also Blade or MultiVane) the k-space is filled in blades as shown in ▶ Fig. 1.12b so that the center of the k-space is

sampled with every echo, which turns the acquisition-insensitive to in-plane motion artifacts. Because motion artifacts are not a problem with the PROPELLER technique, this strategy can be combined with pulse sequences, such as fast SE (FSE) or multishot EPI techniques, which require longer acquisition times resulting in less susceptibility artifacts.[20,21] ▶ Fig. 1.13 shows improvement of the image in areas of low field homogeneity by using the DWI-FSE PROPELLER technique.

1.3.3 DWI with Fluid-Attenuated Inversion Recovery

Cerebrospinal fluid (CSF) has a much higher ADC than brain parenchyma, so any contamination with CSF might influence drastically the measured ADC. CSF signal can be suppressed from the DWI by adding an inversion pulse at the beginning of the pulse sequence and applying the 90-degree excitation pulse at exactly the moment when CSF longitudinal magnetization is passing through the null point, a technique known as fluid attenuated inversion recovery (FLAIR). The result is a DWI with CSF signal suppression (▶ Fig. 1.14), which can be of utility when analyzing regions close to the ventricles or sulci. The disadvantage of this technique is that, due to the long inversion time required to suppress CSF, the acquisition time also becomes long.

1.3.4 DWI Parameters

In addition to the *b* value, which has already been discussed other parameters also affect DWI quality. Susceptibility effects lead to errors in phase encoding and consequently image distortion in the phase-encoding direction of EPI. For this reason the phase-encoding direction should always lie along the axis of less susceptibility gradients, which, on an axial slice in the brain, is the anterior–posterior axis. ▶ Fig. 1.15 shows the effect of the phase-encoding direction on the EPI. Reducing the slice thickness also helps to minimize the effect of field inhomogeneity.

Phase-encoding errors are propagated in time from echo to echo in the EPI echo train. Hence it is possible to minimize these artifacts by reducing the echo train length, either by reducing the number of echoes or by speeding up the acquisition (i.e., reducing echo spacing). Reducing the

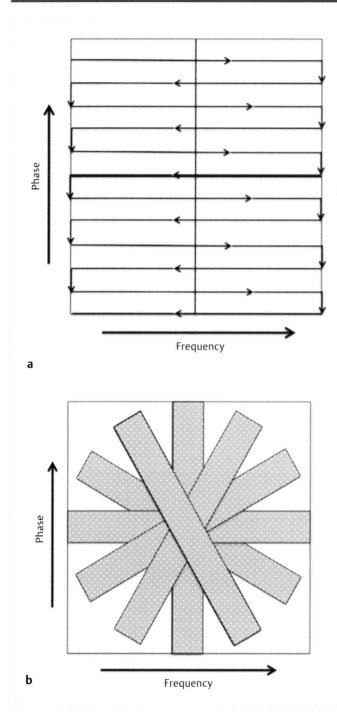

Phase

Frequency

a

Phase

Frequency

b

Fig. 1.12 (**a**) The k-space filling of all lines in a single shot using an echo-planar imaging (EPI) sequence and (**b**) k-space filling of blades using a PROPELLER sequence.

acquisition matrix (spatial resolution) in the phase-encoding direction and using a parallel imaging technique will reduce the number of echoes in the train. Increasing the receiver bandwidth and reducing the matrix (spatial resolution) in the frequency-encoding direction will reduce echo spacing. The optimum acceleration factor R in parallel acquisition will depend on the coil configuration (g-factor of the coil), and usually an acceleration factor of 2 to 3 will provide a good compromise between susceptibility artifact reduction and SNR. To maximize SNR and to reduce

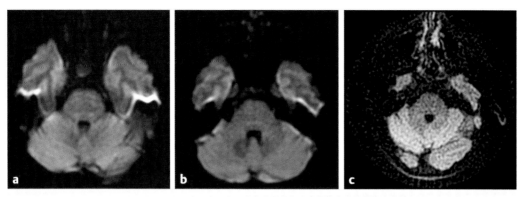

Fig. 1.13 (a) Echo-planar image showing distortion in the regions of low field homogeneity. (b) A small improvement is gained by using parallel acquisition (R = 2). (c) There is no susceptibility artifact with the PROPELLER diffusion weighted imaging sequence.

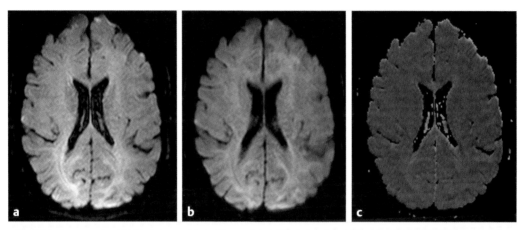

Fig. 1.14 An example of fluid-attenuated inversion recovery diffusion weighted imaging (FLAIR-DWI). (a) Non-DWI ($b = 0$ s/mm^2) with suppression of cerebrospinal fluid, (b) DWI ($b = 1,000$ s/mm^2). (c) Corresponding apparent diffusion coefficient map.

susceptibility artifacts the TE should also be as short as possible, although a limitation to short TE is the b value: the higher the b value the longer the TE becomes. In summary, for optimizing image quality in the DWI-EPI acquisition a smaller matrix (i.e., 128 × 128), maximum gradient strength and speed, maximum receiver bandwidth, minimum TE, and parallel imaging should be used. The choice of these parameters differs according to the application of the diffusion study, whether we are interested in obtaining only DWI or DTI, or if we are interested in tractography. For the latter application, it is very important to have high and isotropic spatial resolution (1 2 mm^2) and to apply a large number of different gradient directions, ideally about at least 30 unique orientations.[15]

1.4 Diffusion Pitfalls

1.4.1 Perfusion Effects

DWI is also sensitive to the motion of water spins in the vascular space caused by blood perfusion. It is even possible to quantify this perfusion contribution by the intravoxel incoherent motion (IVIM) method, where DWI is acquired as a function of several different b values, increasing it in small steps from 0 to about 1,000 s/mm^2 (i.e., 0, 10, 20, 40, 80, 110, 140, 170, 200, 300, 400, 500, 600, 700, 800, and 900 s/mm^2), so it is possible to observe that the signal decays biexponentially, with a rapid decay at the beginning (up to a b value of 200 s/mm^2) and a

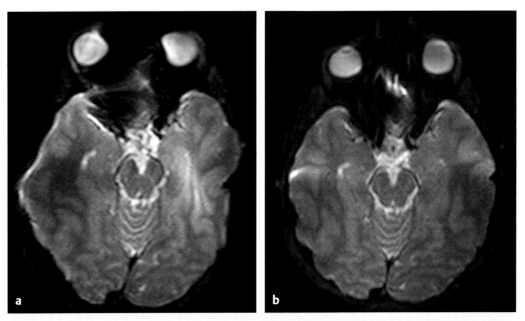

Fig. 1.15 (a) Echo-planar imaging acquired with phase encoding in the x (right–left) direction. (b) Reduction of image distortion by swapping the phase encoding to the y (anterior–posterior) direction.

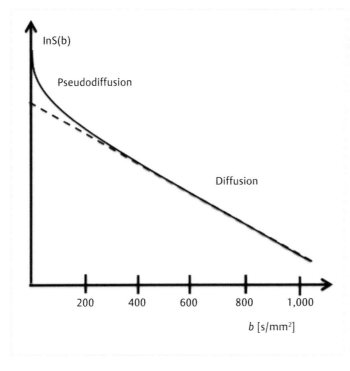

Fig. 1.16 Biexponential behavior of signal attenuation when the effect of perfusion is considered. Perfusion contribution is accounted for by introducing a pseudo diffusion coefficient.

slower decay for higher *b* values (▶ Fig. 1.16). In the IVIM method this biexponential behavior is ascribed to a two-compartment diffusion model, with a microvascular (*f*) and a nonvascular compartment (*1 − f*), characterized, respectively, by a pseudo diffusion coefficient D^* (faster decay) and an apparent diffusion coefficient D (slower decay)[22]:

$$\frac{S(b)}{S_0} = f \times e^{-bD^*} + (1 - f) \times e^{-bD} \qquad (1.11)$$

In an IVIM study of brain gliomas it was found that the perfusion fraction f was significantly higher in high-grade gliomas when compared to low-grade gliomas.[22]

From ► Fig. 1.16 it can be concluded that the contribution of blood perfusion to the ADC measurement can be suppressed by using a b value > 200 s/mm² as the low b value, instead of the standard b = 0 s/mm²,[23] resulting in "flow compensated" ADC. Because the vascular fraction in healthy brain is low (5–8%), this perfusion effect is usually negligible. However, when ADC is used to monitor brain tumor growth any changes in tumor perfusion can represent an important confounding factor and the use of flow compensated ADC is preferable.[23]

1.4.2 Motion Artifacts

Head motion should be minimized as much as possible by placing pads around it within the coil. Residual head motion can be corrected for by including in the postprocessing a registration step of DWI to the non-DWI (b = 0), allowing correction of rotation and translation in three directions (a total of six degrees of freedom). Most DTI software packages include this postprocessing step; however, not all of them correct for the effect of head motion on the direction of the applied diffusion gradients. The list of applied gradient directions used to calculate the diffusion tensor is valid only if there is no head motion during the entire acquisition. If head motion occurs, the gradient directions for each acquired image should be corrected for the motion occurring in the image.

1.4.3 Cerebrospinal Fluid Pulsation Effects

The motion effect of CSF cannot be corrected for and is most prominent during the systolic phase of the cardiac cycle. It has been shown that CSF pulsation affects measured diffusion in brain regions contaminated by CSF, with the effect being stronger in the periventricular regions. This effect can be minimized by obtaining FLAIR-DWI acquisitions, by choosing a minimum b value > b = 0 s/mm² to minimize the contribution of the fast-diffusing water of CSF in the measurement, or by timing the DWI acquisition with the cardiac cycle.

This last option can lead to longer acquisition times depending on the heart rate.[15]

1.4.4 Nyquist Ghosts

EPI acquisitions are characterized by a unique way of filling the k-space, whereby one line is frequency encoded with a positive gradient (from left to right), and the next one is encoded with a negative gradient in the opposite direction (from right to left) (see ► Fig. 1.12a). Timing errors between sampling and gradient application, eddy currents, and frequency offsets can cause asymmetries between odd and even echoes that result in a ghost image after Fourier transformation. This ghost image, known as a Nyquist ghost, is displaced by half the field of view (FOV) in the phase-encoding direction, as illustrated in ► Fig. 1.17. If the Nyquist ghost overlaps with actual regions of interest it may be difficult to make a correct estimation of the ADC and other DTI parameters.[24] Visual inspection of the non-DWI (b = 0), the image of a higher SNR, will allow one to see if the Nyquist ghost is obscuring the real signal or region of interest. In that case it is advisable to repeat the acquisition with a larger FOV so that the Nyquist ghost does not overlap with the region of interest.

1.4.5 Eddy Current Artifacts

The gradients applied in DWI are very high in amplitude and need to be switched on and off

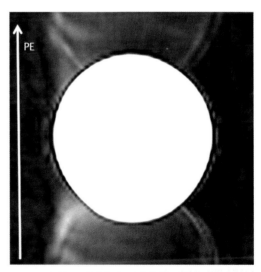

Fig. 1.17 Characteristic Nyquist ghost in echo-planar imaging. The artifactual image is displaced by half the field of view in the phase encoding (PE) direction.

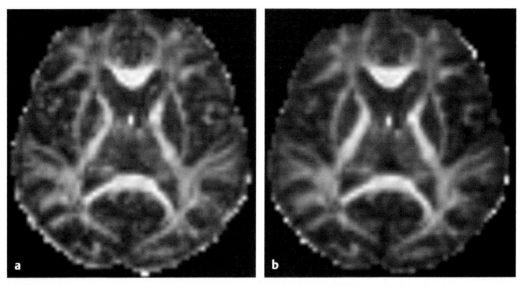

Fig. 1.18 (a) Effect of eddy currents in the diffusion weighted imaging. (b) Same image after correction of eddy currents.

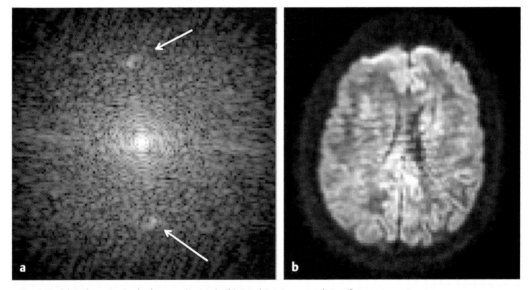

Fig. 1.19 (a) Spike noise in the k-space (arrows). (b) Resulting image spike artifact.

rapidly, which causes eddy currents that introduce errors in the spatial encoding process. The result is that the obtained image can be shifted, compressed, stretched, or sheared depending on the diffusion encoding direction. If this problem is not corrected a false high-anisotropy rim can be seen at the edge of the images (▶ Fig. 1.18a). This effect can be corrected by coregistering the DWI to the non-DWI ($b = 0$) (▶ Fig. 1.18b).

1.4.6 Spike Artifacts

As mentioned previously, DWI leads to high demands on gradient performance, which can lead to spike noise artifacts. Spike noise represents a sporadic and erroneous signal intensity change during data collection that is registered as a spot in k-space (▶ Fig. 1.19a), and after Fourier transformation it causes a ripple artifact over the entire

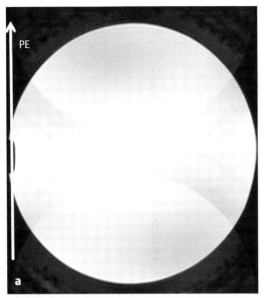

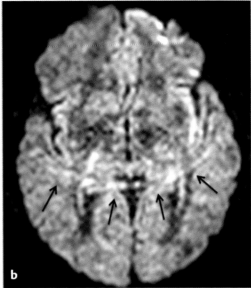

Fig. 1.20 SENSE artifact in the phase encoding (PE) direction resulting from parallel acquisition (**a**) in a phantom and (**b**) in a patient.

image (▶ Fig. 1.19b). Images with such spike noise artifacts should be excluded from the DWI or DTI analysis or the erroneous data points in k-space should be corrected before Fourier transformation. Chavez et al proposed outlier detection-based de-spiking (ODD), an automatic correction method that detects, localizes, and corrects diffusion weighted data sets corrupted by spike noise.[25] If this artifact occurs often, it is advisable to contact the scanner service engineers to elucidate the source of the spike noise.

1.4.7 Sense Artifact

As previously discussed, parallel acquisition schemes (i.e., SENSE= SENSitivity Encoding; iPA-T=integrated Parallel Acquisition Techniques; ASSET=Array coil Spatial Sensitivity Encoding) considerably reduce geometric distortions observed in EPI. When using multichannel head coils parallel acquisition improves image quality in DWI; however, one must be aware that the special reconstruction algorithms used with this technique lead to a very unique and nonhomogeneous noise distribution in the image, which may result in artifacts known as SENSE artifacts (▶ Fig. 1.20). These artifacts can be minimized by reducing the acceleration factor R of the parallel acquisition or by improving the SNR of the image.

1.5 Summary

DWI is a powerful technique to detect and quantify pathological changes in brain tissues. ADC reflects the amount of water diffusion in the brain and by measuring the diffusion tensor it is possible to quantify diffusion anisotropy and identify the principal fiber orientation in voxels. Care must be taken with the details of the pulse sequence used to measure diffusion because it can change the obtained quantitative values and result in artifacts.

References

[1] Le Bihan D, Mangin JF, Poupon C, et al. Diffusion tensor imaging: concepts and applications. J Magn Reson Imaging 2001; 13(4): 534–546

[2] Moonen CTW, van Zijl PCM, Le Bihan D, DesPres D. In vivo NMR diffusion spectroscopy: 31 P application to phosphorus metabolites in muscle. Magn Reson Med 1990; 13(3): 467–477

[3] Clark CA, Le Bihan D. Water diffusion compartmentation and anisotropy at high b values in the human brain. Magn Reson Med 2000; 44(6): 852–859

[4] Jones DK. Fundamentals of diffusion MR imaging. In: Gillard JH, Waldman AD, Barker PB, eds. Clinical MR Neuroimaging. Cambridge: Cambridge University Press; 2005:54–85

[5] Wheeler-Kingshott CAM, Barker GJ, Steens SCA, van Buchem MA. D: the diffusion of water. In: Tofts P, ed. Quantitative MRI of the Brain: Measuring Changes Caused by Disease. West Sussex: John Wiley & Sons; 2003:203–256

[6] Bano S, Waraich MM, Khan MA, Buzdar SA, Manzur S. Diagnostic value of apparent diffusion coefficient for the accurate assessment and differentiation of intracranial meningiomas. Acta Radiol Short Rep 2013; 2(7): 2047981613512484

[7] Hui ES, Cheung MM, Chan KC, Wu EX. B-value dependence of DTI quantitation and sensitivity in detecting neural tissue changes. Neuroimage 2010; 49(3): 2366–2374

[8] Ronen I, Ugurbil K, Kim DS. How does DWI correlate with white matter structures? Magn Reson Med 2005; 54(2): 317–323

[9] Basser PJ, Mattiello J, LeBihan D. MR diffusion tensor spectroscopy and imaging. Biophys J 1994; 66(1): 259–267

[10] Song SK, Sun SW, Ramsbottom MJ, Chang C, Russell J, Cross AH. Dysmyelination revealed through MRI as increased radial (but unchanged axial) diffusion of water. Neuroimage 2002; 17(3): 1429–1436

[11] Song SK, Sun SW, Ju WK, Lin SJ, Cross AH, Neufeld AH. Diffusion tensor imaging detects and differentiates axon and myelin degeneration in mouse optic nerve after retinal ischemia. Neuroimage 2003; 20(3): 1714–1722

[12] Wheeler-Kingshott CAM, Cercignani M. About "axial" and "radial" diffusivities. Magn Reson Med 2009; 61(5): 1255–1260

[13] Pierpaoli C, Basser PJ. Toward a quantitative assessment of diffusion anisotropy. Magn Reson Med 1996; 36(6): 893–906

[14] Hasan KM, Alexander AL, Narayana PA. Does fractional anisotropy have better noise immunity characteristics than relative anisotropy in diffusion tensor MRI? An analytical approach. Magn Reson Med 2004; 51(2): 413–417

[15] Johansen-Berg H, Behrens TEJ, eds. Diffusion MRI: From Quantitative Measurement to In Vivo Neuroanatomy. London: Academic Press (Elsevier); 2009

[16] Le Bihan D. Diffusion MRI: what water tells us about the brain. EMBO Mol Med 2014; 6(5): 569–573

[17] Le Bihan D, Breton E, Lallemand D, Grenier P, Cabanis E, Laval-Jeantet M. MR imaging of intravoxel incoherent motions: application to diffusion and perfusion in neurologic disorders. Radiology 1986; 161(2): 401–407

[18] Turner R, Le Bihan D, Maier J, Vavrek R, Hedges LK, Pekar J. Echo-planar imaging of intravoxel incoherent motion. Radiology 1990; 177(2): 407–414

[19] Pipe JG. Motion correction with PROPELLER MRI: application to head motion and free-breathing cardiac imaging. Magn Reson Med 1999; 42(5): 963–969

[20] Pipe JG, Farthing VG, Forbes KP. Multishot diffusion weighted FSE using PROPELLER MRI. Magn Reson Med 2002; 47(1): 42–52

[21] Wang FN, Huang TY, Lin FH, et al. PROPELLER EPI: an MRI technique suitable for diffusion tensor imaging at high field strength with reduced geometric distortions. Magn Reson Med 2005; 54(5): 1232–1240

[22] Federau C, Meuli R, O'Brien K, Maeder P, Hagmann P. Perfusion measurement in brain gliomas with intravoxel incoherent motion MRI. AJNR Am J Neuroradiol 2014; 35(2): 256–262

[23] Cohen AD, LaViolette PS, Prah M, et al. Effects of perfusion on diffusion changes in human brain tumors. J Magn Reson Imaging 2013; 38(4): 868–875

[24] Porter DA, Calamante F, Gadian DG, Connelly A. The effect of residual Nyquist ghost in quantitative echo-planar diffusion imaging. Magn Reson Med 1999; 42(2): 385–392

[25] Chavez S, Storey P, Graham SJ. Robust correction of spike noise: application to diffusion tensor imaging. Magn Reson Med 2009; 62(2): 510–519

2 Brain Edema: Pathophysiology

Falgun H. Chokshi and Amit M. Saindane

Key Points

- Vasogenic edema results from leakage of fluid through a disrupted blood–brain barrier (BBB).
- Excitotoxic brain injury (EBI) includes temporary or permanent dysfunction of excitatory amino acid homeostasis.
- Aquaporin-4 (AQP-4) channels are found in the brain and allow massive free water transport across the astroglial endfeet membranes.
- Vasogenic edema is bright on apparent diffusion coefficient (ADC) maps, whereas cytotoxic edema is dark.
- An understanding of the pathophysiology of water diffusion in vasogenic and cytotoxic edema is fundamental in understanding diffusion weighted imaging/diffusion tensor imaging (DWI/DTI) characteristics.

2.1 Introduction

Several forms of edema have been identified under the larger rubric of "brain edema." These generally fall into the cellular or extracellular forms. *Cellular edema* denotes cytotoxic edema (CE). *Extracellular edema* refers to vasogenic edema (VE) and "special" forms of osmotic edema and hyperemic edema.[1,2] The pathophysiology of these forms of brain edema were characterized and defined more than 50 years ago.[1]

This chapter defines the two most common forms of brain edema (VE and CE), discusses their imaging characteristics, and presents representative disease processes that can be readily investigated using diffusion weighted imaging (DWI) and diffusion tensor imaging (DTI). The text incorporates causes of excitotoxic brain injury (EBI), which

ultimately leads to cytotoxic edema. VE and CE can present separately or in combination. This chapter demonstrates a wide variety of representative and commonly seen adult-specific conditions that have DWI and DTI findings, spanning multiple categories of diseases, including vascular, infectious, inflammatory, neoplastic, and demyelinating diseases. Subsequent chapters provide in-depth discussions of additional diseases and their DWI and DTI findings.

2.2 Pathophysiology

2.2.1 Vasogenic Edema

VE results from leakage of fluid through a disrupted blood–brain barrier (BBB). Although extracellular protein breakdown has been shown to attenuate fluid clearance, no evidence to date suggests that the protein breakdown products result in fluid exiting the vascular space.[3] Through a combination of bulk flow and diffusion of water, fluid accumulates preferentially in the usually tightly bundled white matter. If the BBB is reconstituted early in the process, the VE can be reversed.[4]

2.2.2 Cytotoxic Edema and Excitotoxic Brain Injury

Excitotoxic Brain Injury

EBI includes temporary or permanent dysfunction of excitatory amino acid homeostasis. Among the excitatory amino acids glutamate, aspartate, and glycine, glutamate is the most important. It is involved in numerous functions, such as cognition, memory, movement, and sensation.[5] Abnormal levels of glutamate can cause neuronal injury and demise related to activation of the *N*-methyl-d-aspartate (NMDA) receptor subtype of the glutamate receptor.[6]

In the acute phase, three mechanisms are known to cause excessive extracellular glutamate: (1) glutamate leakage from disrupted axonal membranes, (2) abnormal neuronal membrane depolarization causing further glutamate release, and (3) dysfunctional reuptake of extracellular glutamate. These mechanisms can self-propagate in a transaxonal or transsynaptic manner along white matter tracts.[5,6,7]

Cytotoxic Edema

Abnormal increases in intracellular water content cause CE. On the molecular level, the sodium–potassium (Na+-K+) adenosine triphosphatase (ATPase) and calcium ion pumps become dysfunctional, resulting in net diffusion of water into the cell. The BBB remains intact initially, yielding stable extracellular water content. Continuous insults cause BBB breakdown and subsequent VE. Apoptotic pathways are activated as well.[7]

The discovery of various subtypes of aquaporin (AQP) channel proteins has shed light on another mechanism of CE.[8] Specifically, AQP-4 channels are found in the brain and allow massive free water transport across the astroglial endfeet membranes.[9] These findings are supported by numerous mouse model studies[10,11]; however, the relationship between these water channels and cerebral edema in humans remains to be demonstrated.

2.3 Diseases Associated With Cerebral Edema

2.3.1 Vasogenic Edema

On magnetic resonance imaging (MRI), VE is T1 hypointense and T2 hyperintense, predominantly within the white matter. VE is bright on both DWI and ADC maps. Decreased fractional anisotropy (FA) is seen on DTI sequences.[4]

Neoplasm-Related Vasogenic Edema

Both benign and malignant neoplasms can cause VE due to tumor angiogenesis and BBB breakdown and show increased diffusivity on DWI and ADC maps. Type-1 peritumoral VE is associated with low-grade (▶ Fig. 2.1) and nonglial tumors, such as metastases and meningiomas. Parenchymal compression causes ischemia and necrosis, which can persist after the tumor is removed.

Type-2 peritumoral edema is associated with high-grade glial neoplasms, which show highly infiltrative behavior and significant destruction of the BBB. VE extension beyond the vicinity of enhancing tumor is characteristic and represents tumor microinvasion (▶ Fig. 2.2). Partial to complete resolution of VE can occur after removal of the tumor. Relative to type-1 VE, type-2 edema shows more increased ADC signal and further diminishment of FA on DTI, likely related to greater tissue destruction by malignant neoplasms.

2.3.2 Cytotoxic Edema/Excitotoxic Brain Injury

Computed tomography shows a loss of gray–white matter differentiation early in CE/EBI. In subacute phases, BBB breakdown can show white matter hypoattenuation of VE, presenting a mixed edema picture. MRI reveals swelling of the gray matter and loss of gray–white matter differentiation. ADC dark and DWI bright areas are present in CE/EBI; FA is decreased on DTI.[4]

Arterial Infarction

Hypoxia caused by acute arterial infarction leads to rapid depletion of adenosine triphosphate (ATP) and resultant CE.[4] Excitotoxicity causes sodium–potassium pump failure and rapid influx of water into the cell. Intracellular calcium increases causing release of lipase and protease, ultimately leading to cell death.[5] Experimental studies on NMDA-type glutamate receptor antagonists (MK-801)

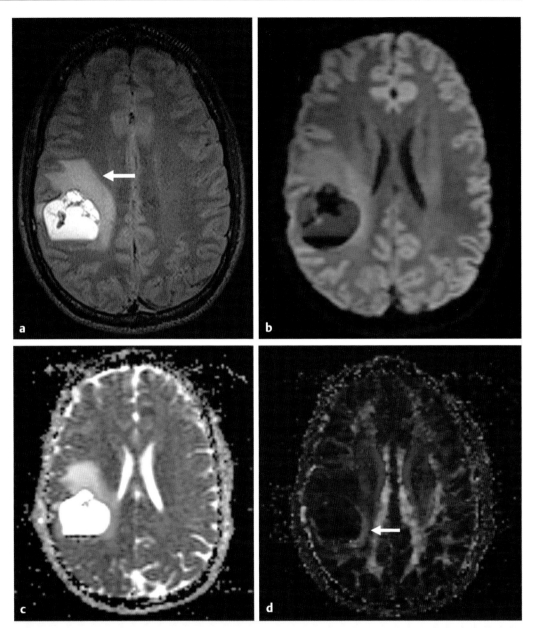

Fig. 2.1 A 42-year-old man with a supratentorial pilocytic astrocytoma with surrounding edema displacing adjacent white matter tracts. (a) T2-fluid=attenuated inversion recovery image showing a well-defined tumor in the right parietal lobe with internal cystic components and layering debris, along with surrounding vasogenic edema (arrow). (b) Diffusion weighted imaging shows slight hyperintensity in the surrounding edema. (c) Apparent diffusion coefficient map confirms that this surrounding area is T2 shine-through. (d) Color fractional anisotropy map shows displacement of deep white matter tracts (arrow) without evidence of disruption or destruction.

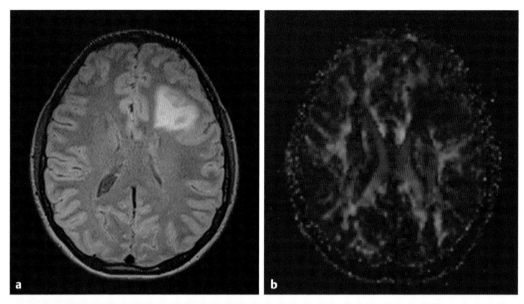

Fig. 2.2 A 27-year-old woman with left frontal anaplastic astrocytoma with infiltration of regional fiber tracts. **(a)** T2-fluid-attenuated inversion recovery image showing a relatively well defined left frontal T2 hyperintense mass extending to the anterior body of the corpus callosum. **(b)** Axial diffusion tensor imaging color fractional anisotropy map shows destruction of fiber tracts in the region of the mass and infiltration of fiber tracts at the medial margin as shown by loss of the normal white matter tracts (compare to right hemisphere for reference).

have shown a reduced volume of ischemic injury after occlusion of the middle cerebral artery (MCA).[12] Accordingly, excitotoxic injury related to glutamate is associated with the pathophysiological findings of ischemic penumbra.[5,12]

Within 30 minutes CE develops, often peaking between 24 and 72 hours, and can persist for up to 24 hours after reperfusion. Detection of hyperacute infarction (< 30 min from onset of neurological deficit) is most sensitive on DWI[4] (▶ Fig. 2.3a–c). As the infarction evolves, the CE (DWI bright, ADC dark) will be surrounded by VE (DWI bright, ADC bright) and associated mass effect. ADC can show pseudonormalization between 10 and 15 days, with persistent DWI hyperintensity due to T2 shine-through of VE[13] (▶ Fig. 2.3d–f). Chronic infarction shows ADC bright signal due to encephalomalacia and gliosis.[14]

Cerebral Venous Infarction

Venous infarction is caused by thrombus in the dural venous sinuses, cortical veins, or deep cerebral veins. The area of infarction does not correspond to an arterial distribution and has a propensity to undergo hemorrhagic transformation. Risk factors include chronic inflammation, infection, thrombophilic states (e.g., dehydration, hypercoagulation disorders, cancer), and cranial surgery.[15] CE surrounded by VE and mass effect is typically seen (▶ Fig. 2.4). CT or magnetic resonance venography can identify thrombus.

Multiple Sclerosis

CE in multiple sclerosis (MS) plaques is rarely captured on MRI. As seen in the early (hyperacute and acute) phases of MS, these lesions are profoundly

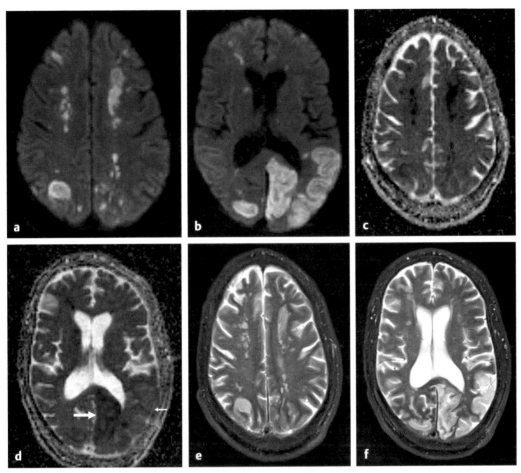

Fig. 2.3 A 45-year-old man with human immunodeficiency virus and staphylococcal bacteremia with endocarditis and multiple septic emboli of various ages. (**a**) Diffusion weighted imaging (DWI) showing multiple watershed distribution infarctions. (**b**) DWI showing additional areas of infarction, including left medial and parietal cortical infarctions. (**c**) Apparent diffusion coefficient (ADC) shows that watershed infarctions are dark and therefore acute. (**d**) ADC shows that medial left parietal infarction is dark and therefore acute (arrow), whereas the lateral parietal infarction is pseudonormalized and therefore subacute (small arrow). (**e**) T2-weighted image with high T2 signal in the areas of watershed infarction. (**f**) T2-weighted image with high signal in both the medial and lateral parietal infarctions, but also showing gyral swelling in the subacute infarction laterally.

hypointense on ADC maps and bright on DWI[5] (▶ Fig. 2.5).

Glutamate excitotoxicity damages oligodendrocytes, myelin sheaths, and axons in these patients,[16] with glutamate and aspartate levels being elevated in cerebrospinal fluid analysis of patients with acute MS.[17] Histologically,

intramyelinic edema is found within the cytotoxic plaques.[5]

Creutzfeldt–Jakob Disease

Clinical manifestations of Creutzfeldt–Jakob Disease (CJD) include rapidly progressive dementia,

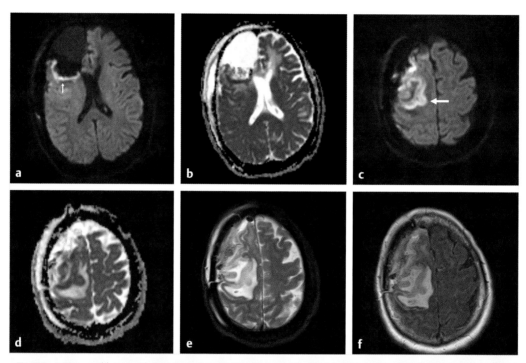

Fig. 2.4 A 58-year-old man with right frontal anaplastic oligoastrocytoma status post–prior resection, radiation therapy, and recent repeat resection. (**a**) Diffusion weighted imaging (DWI) shows high signal along the right frontal surgical cavity indicative of devitalized tissue (arrow). (**b**) Apparent diffusion coefficient (ADC) map confirms reduced diffusion at the margin of the surgical cavity. (**c**) More superiorly and distant from the surgical cavity is a large area of high signal on DWI (arrow). (**d**) On ADC this area is bright, indicating T2 shine-through. (**e**) On T2-weighted images this was a new area of edema and local mass effect due to a cortical venous injury and venous infarction during the surgery. (**f**) T2-fluid-attenuated inversion recovery image also demonstrates the area of postoperative venous infarction in the right frontal lobe

myoclonus, and ataxia. A characteristic pattern of diffusion restriction occurs in CJD explained by the spatially variable, yet functionally profound, abnormalities in glutamate receptors.[18] The cerebral cortex and bilateral basal ganglia show T2-hyperintense lesions (▶ Fig. 2.6). In variant CJD, the pulvinar of both thalami and the periaqueductal gray matter are affected,[19] although sporadic CJD is associated with such lesions as well.[20] These lesions are DWI bright and ADC dark.[21] Decreased ADC is attributed to focal swelling (vacuolization) of both axonal and dendritic processes on electron microscopy.[22]

Hypoxic Ischemic Encephalopathy

Hypoxic ischemic encephalopathy (HIE) results from diminishment of oxygen delivery caused by a host of etiologies, such as hypoxia (e.g., respiratory failure, strangulation, and altitude sickness), hypoxemia (e.g., carbon monoxide poisoning), and ischemia (e.g., shock, cardiac arrest, acute intracranial pressure increases). The resultant depletion of energy is due to mitochondrial dysfunction and impedes glutamate reabsorption. Thus increased extracellular glutamate results in neuronal and glial toxicity.[5]

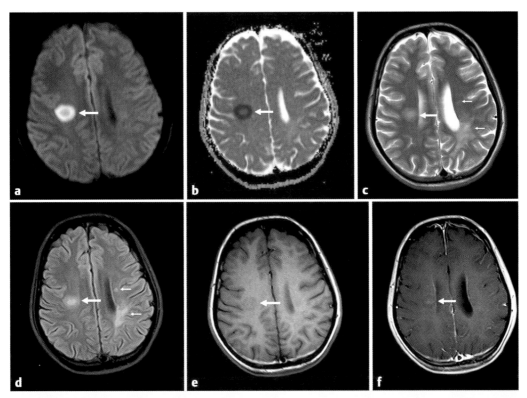

Fig. 2.5 A 26-year-old woman with acute demyelinating lesion from multiple sclerosis (MS). (**a**) Diffusion weighted image shows a peripherally bright ring lesion in the right centrum semiovale (arrow). (**b**) Apparent diffusion coefficient map confirms that periphery of this lesion is dark (arrow) representing reduced diffusion. (**c**) T2-weighted image shows a centrally hyperintense and peripherally gray matter isointense signal to the lesion (arrow). Additional other T2 hyperintense white matter lesions are noted (small arrows). (**d**) T2-fluid-attenuated inversion recovery image shows to better advantage the ringlike lesion (arrow) and additional lesions (small arrows). (**e**) T1-weighted image demonstrates gray matter isointense to slightly hyperintense signal to the periphery of the ring lesion (arrow). (**f**) Postcontrast T1-weighted image shows central enhancement of the lesion (arrow).

In adults, the basal ganglia (especially the globus pallidus), thalamus, hippocampus, corpus callosum, and perirolandic cortex are disproportionally affected due to their high metabolic demand and arterial watershed territories of the basal ganglia.[4,5] DWI shows a pattern of relatively symmetric cytotoxic edema in these regions with bright DWI and dark ADC signal, even though conventional T1- and T2-weighted sequences may appear normal to near normal[4] (▶ Fig. 2.7 and ▶ Fig. 2.8).

Herpes Encephalitis

Excitotoxic injury in herpes encephalitis is attributed to abnormally increased concentrations of glutamate and glycine in the cerebrospinal fluid (CSF).[23] Free radical release during immune system response to the infections causes the excitotoxicity-instigating release of glutamate.[5] In adults, herpes encephalitis is due to *Herpes simplex* type 1 and usually affects the insula, inferior frontal lobes, and medial temporal lobes. On DWI, CE is present

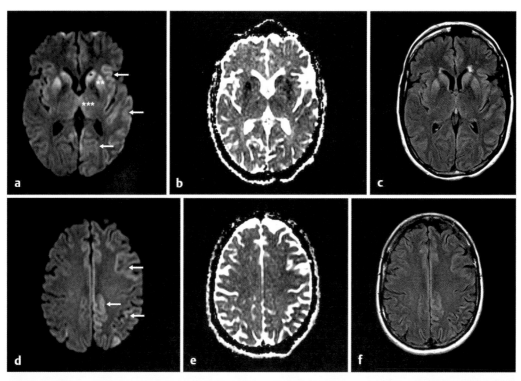

Fig. 2.6 A 56-year-old woman with Creutzfeldt–Jakob disease (CJD). (**a**) Diffusion weighted imaging (DWI) shows high signal in the caudate head (*), putamen (**), medial thalamus (***), and areas of cortex (small arrows). (**b**) Apparent diffusion coefficient (ADC) map confirms that these areas are dark and represent reduced diffusion. (**c**) T2-fluid-attenuated inversion recovery (FLAIR) image shows high signal in these deep gray matter structures and cortex. (**d**) DWI more cranially shows extensive cortical high signal (small arrows). (**e**) ADC map confirms that these areas are dark and represent reduced diffusion. (**f**) T2-FLAIR image shows slight high signal in these areas of cortex.

in these areas, variably associated with hemorrhage and necrosis[5] (► Fig. 2.9).

Limbic Encephalitis

Limbic encephalitis is the most common inflammatory disease that affects the hippocampus. Three subtypes have been identified: paraneoplastic, nonparaneoplastic, and infectious.[24,25] In contradistinction to herpes encephalitis, limbic encephalitis does not show diffusion restriction on DWI unless there is also seizure-associated postictal CE. In general, intermediate to high ADC values are present, with DWI hyperintensity usually representing T2 shine-through as confirmed by hyperintense signal on ADC images[24] (► Fig. 2.10).

Osmotic Myelinolysis

Both central pontine and extrapontine forms of osmotic myelinolysis are caused by destruction of myelin sheaths in the cerebrum and brainstem. Rapid correction of severe hyponatremia causes the release of a host of excitotoxins, including betamine, glutamate, and taurine.[26] Early in the disease, DWI is bright and ADC is dark, signifying CE[5] (► Fig. 2.11).

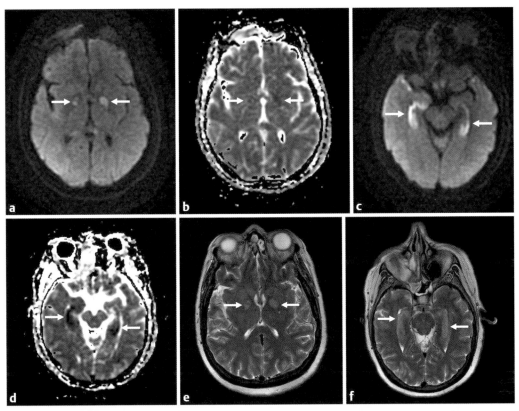

Fig. 2.7 A 66-year-old woman with respiratory failure following sepsis and meningitis. Hypoxic Injury. (a) Diffusion weighted imaging (DWI) showing high signal in both globus pallidi (arrows). (b) Apparent diffusion coefficient (ADC) map confirms that areas are dark and represent reduced diffusion (arrows). (c) DWI showing high signal in both hippocampi (arrows). (d) ADC map confirms that areas are dark and represent reduced diffusion (arrows). (e) T2-weighted image showing high signal in both globus pallidi (arrows). (f) T2-weighted image showing high signal in both hippocampi (arrows).

Status Epilepticus

In status epilepticus, excitotoxic edema results from excessive release of glutamate, which binds to both NMDA and non-NMDA receptors.[27] Both neurons and glial cells are affected. Transient CE from this glutamate release subsides once the astrocytes detoxify the excess extracellular glutamate.[28] The encephalopathy associated with status epilepticus affects NMDA receptor–rich regions, such as the hippocampus, limbic system components, thalamus, and cerebellum.[29] Cerebral hemispheres and insular cortices can also be involved (▶ Fig. 2.12). DWI and ADC images show restricted diffusion in these regions, often decreasing or resolving on subsequent MRI scans.[28]

Focal Lesion in the Splenium of the Corpus Callosum in Epilepsy

In the immediate postictal state, focal, transient CE can be present in the splenium of the corpus callosum. Medications, seizures, or both can cause the lesions.[30] Fibers decussating in the splenium of the corpus callosum serve as a conduit for transhemispheric propagation of the seizure activity.[5] Additionally, abrupt stoppage of antiseizure

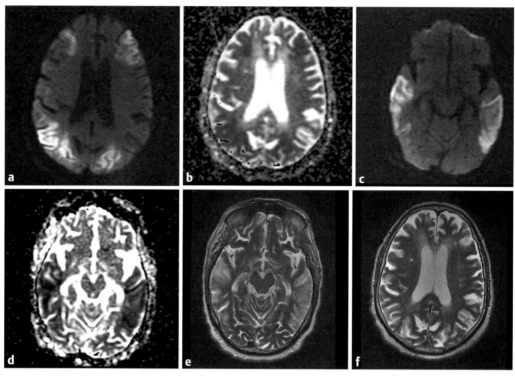

Fig. 2.8 A 75-year-old man with end stage renal disease with hypoxic ischemic injury from a severe hypotensive episode during hemodialysis. (**a**) Diffusion weighted imaging (DWI) showing high signal within the bilateral frontal and parietal lobes at the anterior and middle cerebral artery (ACA-MCA) border zones. (**b**) Apparent diffusion coefficient (ADC) map confirms that these areas are dark and represent reduced diffusion. (**c**) DWI showing high signal within the bilateral posterior temporal lobes. (**d**) ADC map confirms that areas are dark and represent reduced diffusion. (**e**) T2-weighted image showing high signal in the areas of reduced diffusion at the ACA-MCA border zones. (**f**) T2-weighted image showing high signal in the areas of reduced diffusion in the posterior temporal lobes.

medications (e.g. phenytoin, carbamazepine) can result in this lesion due to transient excitotoxicity causing CE via imbalance of both glutamate homeostasis and imbalance of the arginine–vasopressin system. DWI shows a DWI bright, ADC dark lesion in the splenium of the corpus callosum[5] (▶ Fig. 2.13).

Diffuse Axonal Injury

Excitotoxicity involving glutamate and NMDA receptors underlies diffuse axonal injury. Damage to the axon occurs at the node of Ranvier, allowing glutamate leakage into the extracellular space.

Lesions are characteristically located in the brainstem, cerebellar peduncles, corpus callosum, fornix, and gray–white matter junction (▶ Fig. 2.14).

2.4 Summary

DWI has revolutionized neuroimaging, offering a powerful tool in the arsenal of MRI sequences. The pathophysiology of cytotoxic, excitotoxic, and vasogenic edema dictates the DWI characteristics in a plethora of pathological conditions. Recall of these principles can enrich the interpretation by the radiologist.

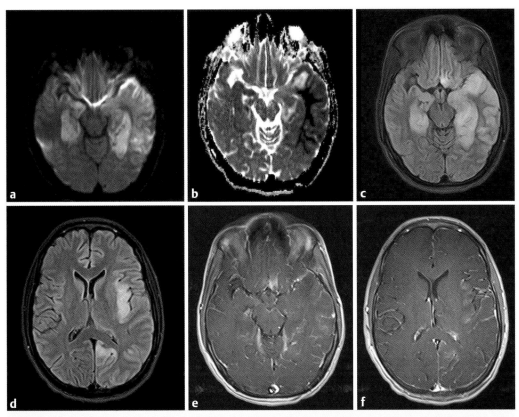

Fig. 2.9 A 27-year-old man with acute onset of abnormal behavior with herpes simplex virus encephalitis. (**a**) Diffusion weighted imaging showing high signal within the bilateral hippocampi and lateral left temporal lobe. (**b**) Apparent diffusion coefficient map confirms that portions of the hippocampi and left lateral temporal lobe are dark and represent reduced diffusion. (**c**) T2-fluid-attenuated inversion recovery (FLAIR) image shows swelling and high signal in these areas as well as the inferior left frontal lobe. (**d**) T2-FLAIR image shows additional swelling and high signal in the left insula and left retrosplenial region. (**e**) Postcontrast T1-weighted image shows faint enhancement in the inferior left frontal and temporal lobe. (**f**) Post-contrast T1-weighted image shows faint enhancement in the left insula and retrosplenial region.

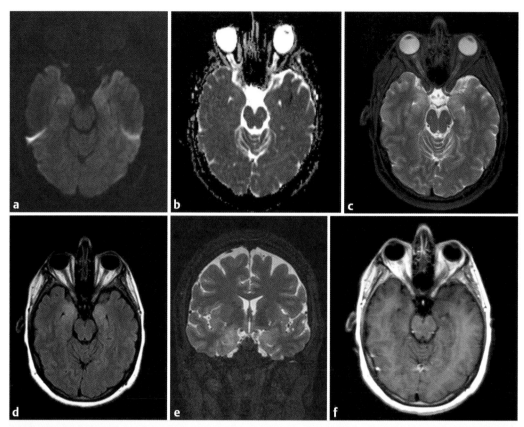

Fig. 2.10 A 36-year-old woman with ovarian cancer and seizures with imaging consistent with paraneoplastic limbic encephalitis. (**a**) Diffusion weighted imaging shows slight high signal in both anteromedial temporal lobes. (**b**) Apparent diffusion coefficient map shows slight high signal indicating T2 shine-through effect. (**c**) T2-weighted image demonstrating high T2 signal in the anteromedial temporal lobes. (**d**) T2-fluid-attenuated inversion recovery image shows better conspicuity of the findings of abnormal increased signal. (**e**) Coronal T2-weighted image again shows high T2 signal in the amygdala and hippocampus. (**f**) Postcontrast T1-weighted image shows no abnormal enhancement.

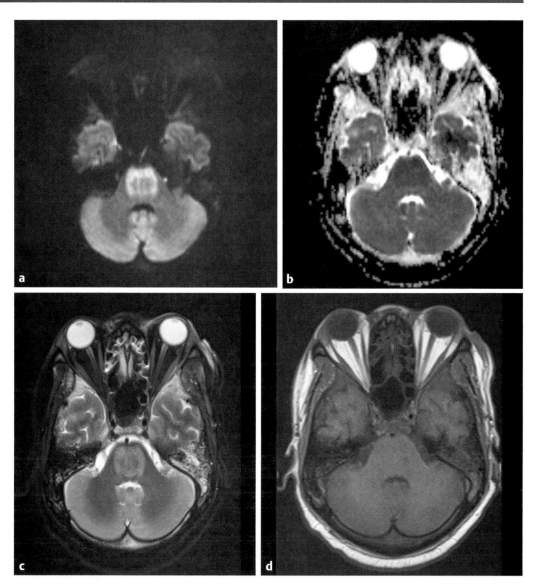

Fig. 2.11 A 47-year-old man with multiple medical problems and acute mental decline secondary to rapid correction of hyponatremia resulting in osmotic demyelination. (**a**) Diffusion weighted imaging shows high signal in the pons with relative sparing of the descending corticospinal tracts. (**b**) Apparent diffusion coefficient map confirms that areas are dark and represent reduced diffusion. (**c**) T2-weighted image shows high signal of the areas of reduced diffusion. (**d**) Corresponding T1-weighted image does not demonstrate any abnormality.

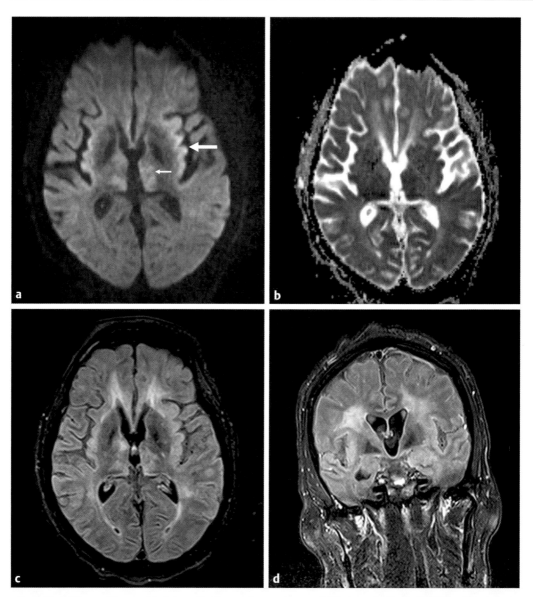

Fig. 2.12 A 55-year-old man with status epilepticus and unusual areas of diffusion reduction in the bilateral insula and thalami. (**a**) Diffusion weighted imaging shows high signal in the bilateral thalami (large arrow) and insula (small arrow) that was new from a prior magnetic resonance imaging scan (not shown). (**b**) Apparent diffusion coefficient map confirms that areas are dark and represent reduced diffusion. (**c**) T2-fluid-attenuated inversion recovery (FLAIR) image shows these areas are T2 bright, as well as extensive additional areas of T2-FLAIR abnormality in the cerebral white matter. (**d**) Coronal T2-FLAIR image also shows these areas are T2 bright, as well as extensive additional areas of T2-FLAIR abnormality in the cerebral white matter.

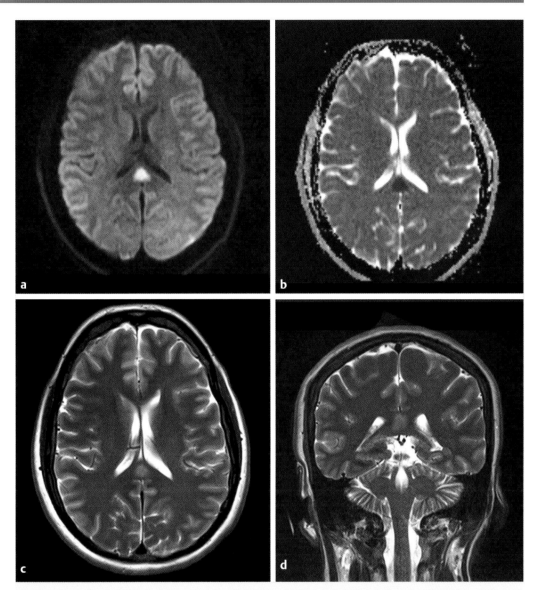

Fig. 2.13 A 42-year-old woman with chronic epilepsy taking multiple antiepileptic medications. This finding was found incidentally on a magnetic resonance imaging scan for evaluation of epilepsy. (**a**) Diffusion weigthed imaging shows a triangular bright lesion in the splenium of corpus callosum. (**b**) Apparent diffusion coefficient map confirms this area is dark and represents reduced diffusion. (**c**) T2-weighted image shows high signal in this triangular lesion. (**d**) Coronal T2-weighted image also shows high signal in this lesion.

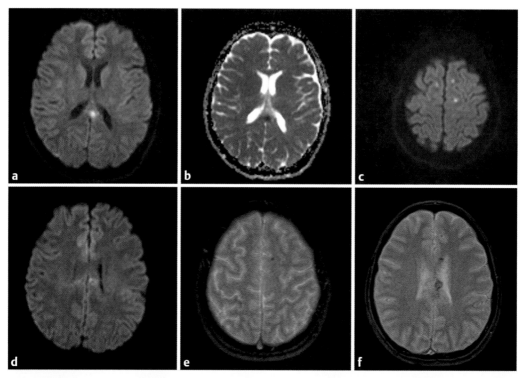

Fig. 2.14 A 20-year-old woman found unresponsive with external signs of trauma and magnetic resonance imaging findings of diffuse axonal injury. (**a**) Diffusion weighed imaging (DWI) shows high signal in the splenium of the corpus callosum. (**b**) Apparent diffusion coefficient (ADC) map confirms that this area is dark and represents reduced diffusion. (**c**) DWI shows additional areas of reduced diffusion in the subcortical frontal lobes (areas were dark on corresponding ADC map). (**d**) DWI shows small additional areas of reduced diffusion in the body of the corpus callosum (areas were dark on corresponding ADC map). (**e**) T2*-weighted image shows area of susceptibility artifact associated with one of the left frontal subcortical lesions indicative of hemorrhage. (**f**) T2*-weighted image shows additional areas of susceptibility artifact associated with the corpus callosum lesions indicative of hemorrhage.

References

[1] Klatzo I. Presidental address. Neuropathological aspects of brain edema. J Neuropathol Exp Neurol 1967; 26(1): 1–14

[2] Vajda Z, Nielsen S, Sulyok E, Dóczi T. Aquaporins in cerebral volume regulation and edema formation [in Hungarian]. Orv Hetil 2001; 142(5): 223–225

[3] Gröger U, Marmarou A. Importance of protein content in the edema fluid for the resolution of brain edema. Adv Neurol 1990; 52: 215–218

[4] Ho ML, Rojas R, Eisenberg RL. Cerebral edema. AJR Am J Roentgenol 2012; 199(3): W258–73

[5] Moritani T, Smoker WR, Sato Y, Numaguchi Y, Westesson PL. Diffusion weighted imaging of acute excitotoxic brain injury. AJNR Am J Neuroradiol 2005; 26(2): 216–228

[6] Lipton SA, Rosenberg PA. Excitatory amino acids as a final common pathway for neurologic disorders. N Engl J Med 1994; 330(9): 613–622

[7] Nag S, Manias JL, Stewart DJ. Pathology and new players in the pathogenesis of brain edema. Acta Neuropathol 2009; 118(2): 197–217

[8] Venero JL, Vizuete ML, Machado A, Cano J. Aquaporins in the central nervous system. Prog Neurobiol 2001; 63(3): 321–336

[9] Nielsen S, Nagelhus EA, Amiry-Moghaddam M, Bourque C, Agre P, Ottersen OP. Specialized membrane domains for water transport in glial cells: high-resolution immunogold cytochemistry of aquaporin-4 in rat brain. J Neurosci 1997; 17(1): 171–180

[10] Vespa PM. Slow rewarming: a cool model of posttraumatic hypothermia. Crit Care Med 2001; 29(11): 2224–2225

[11] Manley GT, Fujimura M, Ma T, et al. Aquaporin-4 deletion in mice reduces brain edema after acute water intoxication and ischemic stroke. Nat Med 2000; 6(2): 159–163

[12] Buchan AM, Slivka A, Xue D. The effect of the NMDA receptor antagonist MK-801 on cerebral blood flow and infarct volume in experimental focal stroke. Brain Res 1992; 574 (1–2): 171–177

[13] Copen WA, Schwamm LH, González RG, et al. Ischemic stroke: effects of etiology and patient age on the time course of the core apparent diffusion coefficient. Radiology 2001; 221(1): 27–34

[14] Allen LM, Hasso AN, Handwerker J, Farid H. Sequence-specific MR imaging findings that are useful in dating ischemic stroke. Radiographics 2012; 32(5): 1285–1297, discussion 1297–1299

[15] Star M, Flaster M. Advances and controversies in the management of cerebral venous thrombosis. Neurol Clin 2013; 31(3): 765–783

[16] Matute C, Alberdi E, Domercq M, Pérez-Cerdá F, Pérez-Samartín A, Sánchez-Gómez MV. The link between excitotoxic oligodendroglial death and demyelinating diseases. Trends Neurosci 2001; 24(4): 224–230

[17] Stover JF, Pleines UE, Morganti-Kossmann MC, Kossmann T, Lowitzsch K, Kempski OS. Neurotransmitters in cerebrospinal fluid reflect pathological activity. Eur J Clin Invest 1997; 27(12): 1038–1043

[18] Ferrer I, Puig B. GluR2/3, NMDAepsilon1 and GABAA receptors in Creutzfeldt-Jakob disease. Acta Neuropathol 2003; 106(4): 311–318

[19] Molloy S, O'Laoide R, Brett F, Farrell M. The "Pulvinar" sign in variant Creutzfeldt-Jakob disease. AJR Am J Roentgenol 2000; 175(2): 555–556

[20] Haïk S, Brandel JP, Oppenheim C, et al. Sporadic CJD clinically mimicking variant CJD with bilateral increased signal in the pulvinar. Neurology 2002; 58(1): 148–149

[21] Murata T, Shiga Y, Higano S, Takahashi S, Mugikura S. Conspicuity and evolution of lesions in Creutzfeldt-Jakob disease at diffusion weighted imaging. AJNR Am J Neuroradiol 2002; 23(7): 1164–1172

[22] Matoba M, Tonami H, Miyaji H, Yokota H, Yamamoto I. Creutzfeldt-Jakob disease: serial changes on diffusion weighted MRI. J Comput Assist Tomogr 2001; 25(2): 274–277

[23] Launes J, Sirén J, Viinikka L, Hokkanen L, Lindsberg PJ. Does glutamate mediate brain damage in acute encephalitis? Neuroreport 1998; 9(4): 577–581

[24] Förster A, Griebe M, Gass A, Kern R, Hennerici MG, Szabo K. Diffusion weighted imaging for the differential diagnosis of disorders affecting the hippocampus. Cerebrovasc Dis 2012; 33(2): 104–115

[25] Sureka J, Jakkani RK. Clinico-radiological spectrum of bilateral temporal lobe hyperintensity: a retrospective review. Br J Radiol 2012; 85(1017): e782–e792

[26] Lien YH. Role of organic osmolytes in myelinolysis. A topographic study in rats after rapid correction of hyponatremia. J Clin Invest 1995; 95(4): 1579–1586

[27] Fountain NB. Status epilepticus: risk factors and complications. Epilepsia 2000; 41 Suppl 2: S23–S30

[28] Kim JA, Chung JI, Yoon PH, et al. Transient MR signal changes in patients with generalized tonicoclonic seizure or status epilepticus: periictal diffusion weighted imaging. AJNR Am J Neuroradiol 2001; 22(6): 1149–1160

[29] Mark LP, Prost RW, Ulmer JL, et al. Pictorial review of glutamate excitotoxicity: fundamental concepts for neuroimaging. AJNR Am J Neuroradiol 2001; 22(10): 1813–1824

[30] Kim SS, Chang KH, Kim ST, et al. Focal lesion in the splenium of the corpus callosum in epileptic patients: antiepileptic drug toxicity? AJNR Am J Neuroradiol 1999; 20(1): 125–129

3 Supratentorial White Matter Tracts and Their Organization

Christopher P. Hess and Jason M. Johnson

Key Points

- Eloquent brain function emerges from the coordinated activity of multiple cortical and subcortical brain regions; the white matter defines a supporting network for the efficient transfer of information of these regions within and between cerebral hemispheres.
- Although the organization of white matter is complex, diffusion magnetic resonance imaging (MRI) consistently visualizes a relatively small group of association (intrahemispheric), commissural (interhemispheric), and projection (afferents or efferents from the periphery to the brain) pathways.
- Precise delineation of white matter tracts requires diffusion data of high technical quality, reconstruction algorithms capable of representing complex white matter architecture, and familiarity with normal connectional anatomy.
- Color fractional anisotropy (FA) images and fiber tractography can be used to understand the location of normal white matter tracts, infiltration and distortion of tracts, and the relationship between lesions and surrounding pathways.

3.1 Introduction

Beneath the convolutions of the gray matter of the cerebral hemispheres lies the white matter, a woven mass of brain tissue composed of myelinated axons and supporting glial cells. The uniform signal intensity of the white matter on conventional anatomical imaging belies a highly complex network of pathways interconnecting different brain regions and exchanging information with the peripheral nervous system through the spinal cord and cranial nerves. This intricate architecture serves as the scaffolding for higher brain function and as the target of many neurological disorders. An understanding of basic connectional neuroanatomy is essential for the radiologist to relate symptoms to lesion location, to guide neurosurgical interventions in the brain, and to recognize tumors and other diseases that spread along white matter tracts.

This chapter is written for the reader interested in developing a practical understanding of white matter anatomy. The chapter begins by briefly outlining technical aspects of diffusion imaging relevant to the accurate depiction of fiber tracts. The location and function of the supratentorial white matter pathways that are most consistently visualized with modern 3 tesla clinical diffusion protocols are then summarized. Given space constraints, the discussion necessarily omits cerebellar and brainstem tracts. The reader specifically interested in brainstem tractography is referred to a number of excellent papers on the subject.[1,2,3]

3.2 Technical Considerations

As discussed elsewhere in this text, the addition of a diffusion gradient to a magnetic resonance imaging (MRI) pulse sequence renders acquired images sensitive to the random motion of water molecules along directions parallel to the orientation of the diffusion gradient.[4,5] Early experiments revealed that brain images vary significantly with changes in the direction of the applied diffusion gradient; *diffusion is highly anisotropic in white matter*. In addition to this orientational variability, varying the strength of the gradient (the diffusion weighting, or *b* value) sensitizes the image to water diffusing over different distances; stronger gradients encode motion over smaller distances (tens or hundreds of micrometers), and weaker gradients are sensitive only to bulk shifts in water occurring over larger distances (millimeters). By systematically varying the magnitude and direction of the applied diffusion gradients, it is possible to characterize the probability of water movement over various spatial scales along each direction in space.

Restricted by microscopic cellular barriers, especially neuronal and myelin membranes, diffusion preferentially occurs along directions parallel to axons. Within each voxel, the relationship between the diffusion sensitized image data and the three-dimensional white matter architecture depends on the technique that is used to represent the underlying diffusion probability. Diffusion tensor imaging (DTI), high angular resolution diffusion imaging (HARDI), and diffusion spectrum imaging (DSI) are three different classes of diffusion acquisition and reconstruction strategies.[6] From a data acquisition standpoint, DTI can be performed with a relatively small number of measured directions and low b values, making the technique fast and easy to achieve using lower-specification gradient coils than are used with HARDI and DSI. These advantages come with the important shortcoming that DTI is unable to represent more than one fiber population within each voxel, a significant drawback in light of the fact that 90% or more of the white matter contains more than a single fiber population.[7]

By acquiring a larger number of diffusion directions with stronger diffusion weighting, HARDI can overcome this limitation and reveals multiple crossing fibers (at the expense of longer imaging times and a requirement for high-performance gradient coils). DSI, which probes diffusion over multiple b values and diffusion directions, permits an even more complete characterization of intra-voxel diffusion. However, long imaging times and low signal-to-noise ratios preclude DSI in patients on clinical scanners at the present time. At the time of this writing, white matter mapping at our institution is accomplished in clinical patients within a 7 minute scan time at isotropic 2.2 mm spatial resolution (55 diffusion directions with $b = 2,000$ or $3,000$ s/mm^2) using a 3 tesla MRI scanner equipped with an eight-channel coil. With continued improvements in technology, such as multiband and multichannel parallel imaging acquisition, it is likely that DSI too will soon find its way into clinical practice.

Diffusion data are used to generate an estimate of water diffusion probability in three dimensions within each voxel in space (a six-dimensional function!). This complex function is conveniently visualized in DTI using color-encoded maps of fractional anisotropy (FA). With these images, the intensity of each voxel represents the directional coherence of diffusion, and the color encodes the dominant direction of diffusion. The standard color scheme is to use *red* for left–right diffusion orientation, *green* for posterior–anterior, and *blue* for inferior–superior (note that diffusion is not able to distinguish polarity, however, and that right–left diffusion appears the same as left–right diffusion, etc.). ▶ Fig. 3.1 and ▶ Fig. 3.2 show how color FA maps can be useful to localize lesions within specific white matter tracts.

Fiber-tracking algorithms further exploit the estimated diffusion probabilities to follow axonal bundles through space from voxel to voxel and thereby identify specific tracts. These algorithms can be divided into deterministic and probabilistic techniques; the former following "streamlines" from individually placed "seed regions" and the latter exploiting uncertainty in the measurements in order to define a probability of connectivity of each voxel with adjacent voxels.[8,9] Probabilistic techniques are more robust in that they more accurately estimate tract extent, but they are less specific because they are more likely to result in spurious estimates of connectivity. Most clinical diffusion applications to date use deterministic tractography methods such as fiber assignment by continuous tracking (FACT), a technique initially introduced more than a decade ago.[10]

Most current tractography algorithms perform "whole brain" tractography, in which connectivity throughout the brain is precomputed. This results in a set of "streamlines" throughout the brain, each corresponding to a single putative connection between two specific brain regions. Using anatomical landmarks and familiarity with connectional anatomy, regions of interest (ROIs) are then placed by the operator to cull specific tracts in a process that has been referred to as virtual dissection. The resulting pathways can then be assessed visually for distortion from locally destructive lesions, infiltrative disease, or other abnormalities. In many centers, they can also be incorporated directly into neurosurgical navigation systems to display white matter tracts of interest in relation to lesions undergoing open surgical intervention.

Streamlines, whittled by the expert into recognizable tracts, do not represent true neuronal fibers. But together the streamlines provide an estimate as to the spatial extent of a tract of interest in the individual patient. Tractography is powerful but biased in this regard, however, and it is important to remember several caveats when interpreting streamlines and the results of tractography.[11] First, tracts represent the final product of a multistep reconstruction process and are thus prone to accumulation of errors. The radiologist should always review the original data for acquisition artifacts and patient motion. ROIs used to delineate tracts must be carefully defined. Second, tractography is highly dependent on the spatial resolution and signal to noise quality of the acquired diffusion data. The extent of tracts may be under- or overestimated with low spatial resolution, and spurious tracts should be anticipated

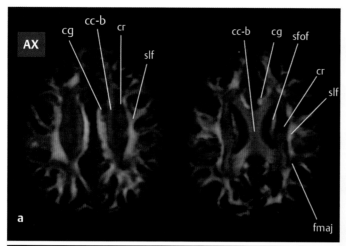

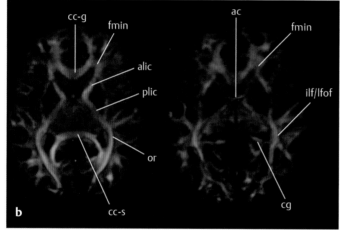

Fig. 3.1 Axial color fractional anisotropy maps at four levels through a normal brain, (a) from the level of the corona radiata through (b) the anterior commissure with white matter structures labeled. ac, anterior commissure; alic, anterior limb internal capsule; c-g, genu of the corpus callosum; cc-b, body of the corpus callosum; cc-s, splenium of the corpus callosum; cg, cingulum bundle; cr, corona radiata; fmaj, forceps major; fmin, forceps minor; fx, fornix; ifof, inferior fronto-occipital fasciculus; ilf, inferior longitudinal fasciculus; or, optic radiation; plic, posterior limb internal capsule; sfof, superior fronto-occipital fasciculus; slf, superior longitudinal fasciculus; and uf, uncinate fasciculus.

with noisy data. Third, the results of tractography vary with multiple other technical factors, including the *b* value and the number of acquired diffusion directions. It is thus recommended that radiologists performing tractography settle on a single acquisition and reconstruction protocol and become familiar with the appearance of tracts that are achieved with this technique. Finally, it is important to emphasize that streamlines in tractography are mathematical entities, not actual fibers, and as such their distribution does not directly correlate with the properties of the underlying axons. For example, the density of the streamlines visualized within a pathway is not directly proportional to the packing density of the neurons within that tract. Subject to these provisos, tractography is a powerful tool for radiologists to use to understand white matter organization in the individual patient.

3.3 White Matter Tract Categorization

Current knowledge of white matter organization derives from both invasive tract tracing and tract dissection studies in specimens and primate models, and from diffusion fiber tractography in normal volunteers.[12,13,14] Based on the nature of the information that they carry, supratentorial fiber tracts can be assigned into one of three categories:

1. **Association pathways** are *intrahemispheric* tracts that interconnect different cortical areas within the same hemisphere. Short "subcortical U" fibers that link adjacent gyri are short association tracts; bundles in the deep white matter have a much greater physical length. Because longer association tracts are frequently oriented from anterior to posterior, association fibers often appear green on color FA images.

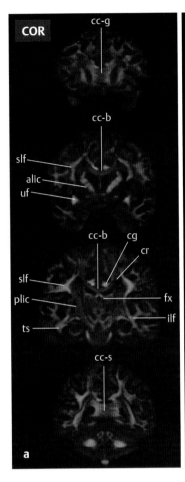

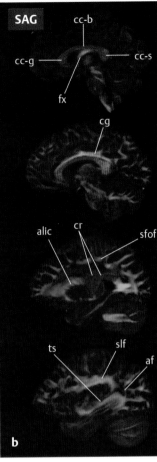

Fig. 3.2 (a) Coronal and (b) sagittal color fractional anisotropy maps at four levels through a normal brain. From the top row down, coronal images are from anterior to posterior and sagittal images are from the midline to the lateral aspect of the brain. ac, anterior commissure; alic, anterior limb internal capsule; c-g, genu of the corpus callosum; cc-b, body of the corpus callosum; cc-s, splenium of the corpus callosum; cg, cingulum bundle; cr, corona radiata; fmaj, forceps major; fmin, forceps minor; fx, fornix; ifof, inferior fronto-occipital fasciculus; ilf, inferior longitudinal fasciculus; or, optic radiation; plic, posterior limb internal capsule; sfof, superior fronto-occipital fasciculus; slf, superior longitudinal fasciculus; and uf, uncinate fasciculus.

2. **Commissural pathways** are *interhemispheric* tracts that link cortical or subcortical areas across hemispheres. These are described as either *homotopic*, connected to homologous regions in either hemisphere, or *heterotopic*, spanning different areas within each hemisphere. Commissural tracts are often red (right–left oriented) on color FA maps.

3. **Projection tracts** originate (motor) or terminate (sensory) in the cortex and connect the cortex to subcortical structures such as the basal ganglia, cerebellum, or spinal cord. Many of these tracts are blue (craniocaudally oriented) on color FA images. Afferent and efferent nerve bundles conveying information through cranial nerves, such as the optic radiations, are also considered to be projection fibers. In what follows, the most commonly described white matter tracts are organized into three categories: association tracts, commissural pathways, and projection tracts.

3.3.1 Association Tracts

The association tracts include the cingulum bundle, superior longitudinal fasciculus, arcuate fasciculus, inferior longitudinal fasciculus, uncinate fasciculus, and fronto-occipital fasciculi.

Cingulum Bundle

The cingulum (Latin for "band" or "belt") bundle (CB) is a belt-shaped tract with an inferior segment that lies within the temporal lobe and a superior frontoparietal portion that encircles the corpus callosum (▶ Fig. 3.3). Part of the limbic circuit of Papez, the CB is a bidirectional conduit for information transfer between different elements of the limbic system and between the limbic system and the hemispheres. Fibers within this tract travel within the cingulate gyrus superiorly and within the parahippocampal gyrus of the temporal lobe inferiorly, making these bundles easy to

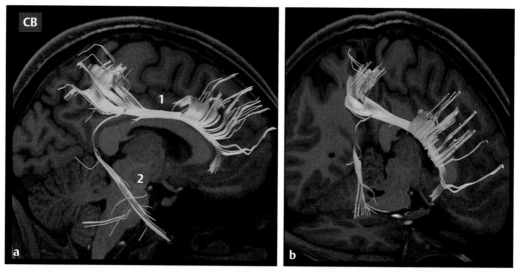

Fig. 3.3 (a) Sagittal and (b) oblique images showing tractography of the cingulum bundle (CB), depicting the anterior arm (1) of the tract extending posteriorly around the corpus callosum (the retrosplenial cingulum) to enter the ipsilateral temporal lobe (2) as the parahippocampal cingulum. Note the dense contributions to this tract from the anterior frontal and parietal white matter.

visualize as paired green structures surrounding the corpus callosum on color FA maps (▸ Fig. 3.1 and ▸ Fig. 3.2). The CB contains both short- and long-association fibers; the proportion of long fibers connecting the frontal and temporal lobes is small compared to the number of short fibers joining and leaving the bundle along its length. The anterior component of the CB has been tied closely to emotion and behavior, whereas the more posterior ("retrosplenial cingulum") and inferior ("parahippocampal cingulum") portions are important for cognitive functions, including attention, spatial orientation, and memory.[15] Abnormalities within the CB have been linked to a variety of disorders, including traumatic brain injury, depression, and schizophrenia. Declining FA within the parahippocampal cingulum may be useful for discrimination of mild cognitive impairment from normal aging in the setting of hippocampal atrophy.[16] The CB also serves as a major pathway for seizure propagation.

Superior Longitudinal Fasciculus

The largest associative bundle in the brain, the superior longitudinal fasciculus (SLF) is a major bidirectional pathway for the widespread distribution of information between the frontal, parietal, occipital, and temporal lobes within each hemisphere. The tract lies above the insula and lateral to the centrum semiovale (▸ Fig. 3.4). The SLF can be divided into three distinct components based on their anatomical location: SLF I superomedially, SLF III inferolaterally, and a larger central SLF II portion between SLF I and SLF III.[17] The arcuate fasciculus (see below) is also considered by most authors to be part of the SLF. The SLF is important for the initiation and regulation of motor behavior (SLF I), perception of visual space (SLF II), and the transfer of somatosensory information and working memory for language articulation

Arcuate Fasciculus

The arcuate (Latin for "curved") fasciculus (AF) is a c-shaped pathway that connects the temporal and parietal lobes with the ipsilateral frontal cortex (▸ Fig. 3.5). Among the different regions linked together by the AF are the Broca area within the inferior frontal gyrus and the Wernicke area within the superior temporal gyrus, cortical regions critical to language comprehension and production. Lesions within the AF frequently result in conduction aphasia, in which patients exhibit intact auditory comprehension but have difficulty with speech production. The pathway is also at risk of injury during the resection of insular gliomas, especially tumors located in the left hemisphere. Inferiorly within the superior temporal gyrus, the AF curves dorsally around the sylvian

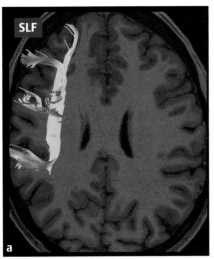
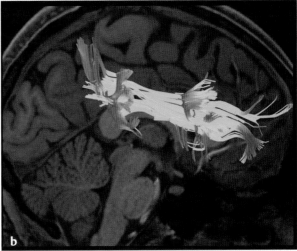

Fig. 3.4 (a) Axial and (b) sagittal depictions of the large superior longitudinal fasciculus (SLF), which connects the anterior hemisphere to the posterior hemisphere through the centrum semiovale and frontal operculum.

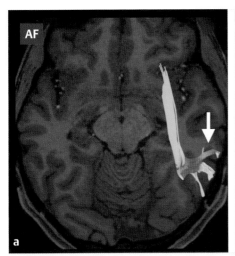
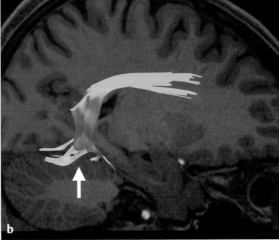

Fig. 3.5 (a) Axial and (b) sagittal illustrations of the left arcuate fasciculus (AF), a major pathway for normal language function that connects the superior temporal gyrus (arrows) to the ipsilateral frontal lobe.

fissure and passes below the SLF into the frontal lobe. Portions of the tract ramify along its course into the surrounding perisylvian frontal, parietal, and temporal lobes. The tract is larger on the left in the majority of people. Interestingly, the degree of asymmetry in volume and anisotropy observed between the hemispheres varies throughout the population, with marked left lateralization in 60% of subjects, bilateral representation but predominantly left lateralization in 20%, and bilateral symmetrical representation in 20%.[18]

Inferior Longitudinal Fasciculus

The inferior longitudinal fasciculus (ILF) extends from the anterior temporal lobe to the ipsilateral occipital lobe and is critical to visual memory and object recognition, including face recognition.[19] The ILF lies laterally within the temporal lobe and passes below the optic radiations and lateral to the ventricular atria as it enters the occipital lobes (▶ Fig. 3.6). Patients with lesions to the ILF suffer from visual neglect, prosopagnosia, visual amnesia,

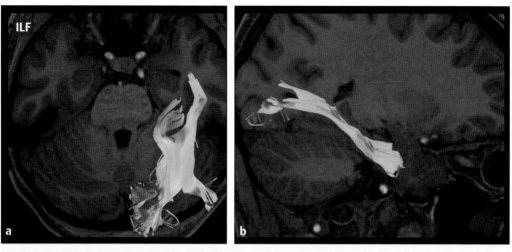

Fig. 3.6 Reconstructions of the inferior longitudinal fasciculus (ILF), projected onto (**a**) axial and (**b**) sagittal T1-weighted images and running laterally and inferiorly to the optic radiations along the temporal horn and atrium of the lateral left ventricle to connect the ipsilateral temporal and occipital lobes.

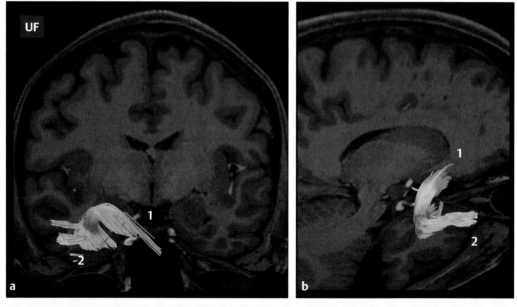

Fig. 3.7 The right uncinate fasciculus (UF), which links the orbitofrontal cortex (1) to structures within the limbic and extralimbic temporal lobe (2), shown as (**a**) coronal and (**b**) oblique sagittal projections.

and, sometimes, visual hallucinations. It has also been suggested that this tract is disrupted in autistic spectrum disorder.

Uncinate Fasciculus

Like the cingulum, the uncinate fasciculus (UF) (▶ Fig. 3.7) is considered part of the limbic system.

This tract contributes to the processing of information related to memory (especially episodic memory), visual learning, and emotion.[20] It can serve as an important pathway for seizure propagation from the temporal into the frontal lobe in patients with temporal lobe epilepsy and is disrupted in patients with Alzheimer disease. The pathway has a curved trajectory that connects the anterior

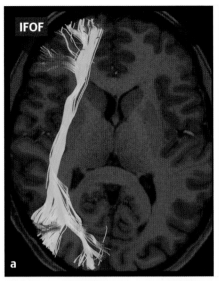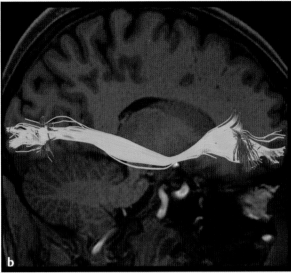

Fig. 3.8 (a) Axial and (b) sagittal images depicting the large right inferior fronto-occipital fasciculus (IFOF), which connects the occipital and frontal lobes. As this bundle runs through the external capsule, it passes above the uncinate fasciculus.

temporal lobe with the ipsilateral medial and lateral orbitofrontal cortices. Originating within the anterior temporal lobe lateral to the amygdala, the UF curves posteriorly and superiorly through the temporal stem and passes behind and above the middle cerebral artery en route to the orbitofrontal cortex.

Fronto-occipital Fasciculus

Whereas the SLF is the largest associative tract, the inferior fronto-occipital fasciculus (IFOF) (▶ Fig. 3.8) is the longest associative tract and probably the only direct connection between occipital and frontal lobes. Its function remains poorly understood but is thought to be related to semantic processing for reading and writing. The tract runs slightly superior and medial to the ILF and lateral to the optic radiation, passing just above and possibly intermingling with fibers from the uncinate fasciculus at the level of the external capsule.[21,22]

The superior fronto-occipital fasciculus (SFOF) is a much smaller pathway that transmits information regarding spatial awareness and visual perception between the frontal lobe and ipsilateral parietal lobe (making the name of the tract misleading). The tract is controversial, but some authors describe it as passing immediately lateral to the superior margin of the caudate and medial

to the fibers of the SLF (▶ Fig. 3.9). This tract is frequently difficult to distinguish from the medial SLF and thalamocortical radiations passing through the anterior limb of the internal capsule.

3.3.2 Commissural Pathways

The commissural pathways include the corpus callosum and anterior commissure.

Corpus Callosum

Above the lateral ventricles, the prominent corpus callosum (CC) is the largest commissural tract in the brain and connects homologous regions of cortex across the midline. This structure is responsible for the coordinated exchange of sensory and other information across the hemispheres. Fibers are transversely oriented in the body of the callosum but arch anteriorly and posteriorly to reach the poles of either convexity. Axons within the CC are topographically arranged, with fibers passing through the genu, body, and splenium of the callosum linking the orbitofrontal lobes and the frontoparietal and occipital cortices, respectively (▶ Fig. 3.10). Posteriorly within the splenium, the anterior posterior arrangement of fibers also corresponds to the peripheral-foveal organization of the medial and lateral visual cortex.

43

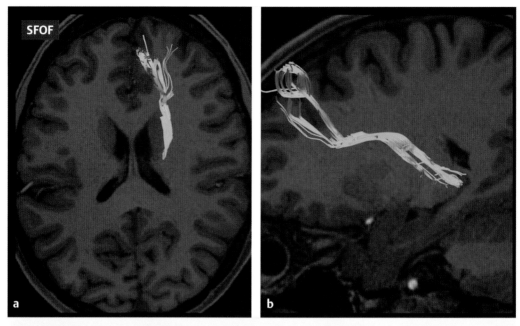

Fig. 3.9 The superior fronto-occipital fasciculus (SFOF) in (**a**) axial and (**b**) sagittal projections, this tract passes lateral to the caudate and medial to the corona radiata.

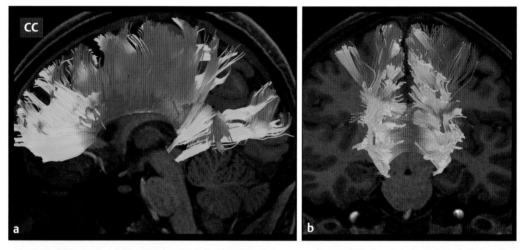

Fig. 3.10 (**a**) Sagittal and (**b**) coronal projections of the massive corpus callosum (CC) show how branches of this bundle follow a topographic arrangement from anterior to posterior, connecting many homologous areas of the cortex across the hemispheres.

Although the tract is very easily identified in the midline on color FA images as a large red bundle, the tract becomes more difficult to resolve laterally, where its fibers intermingle with the corona radiata and large associative pathways, such as the SLF. Anteriorly and posteriorly, densely packed fibers passing through the genu and splenium of the callosum fan out within the adjacent frontal and occipital white matter in regions referred to as forceps minor and major, respectively. Here, fibers fan out peripherally and intercalate with multiple other pathways. Injuries to the CC may be associated with deficits from the failure of coordinated function across the cerebral hemispheres. These

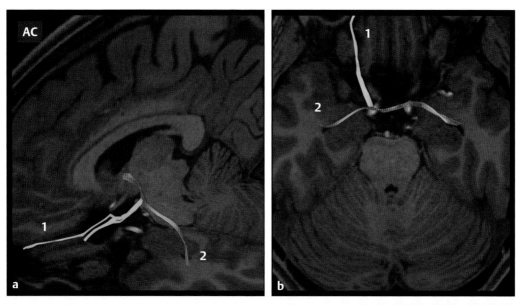

Fig. 3.11 Dominant anterior (1) and posterior (2) branches of the anterior commissure (AC) extending to the olfactory region of the right frontal cortex and temporal lobes and communicating in the midline, as shown on (**a**) oblique sagittal and (**b**) axial images.

disconnection: syndromes also follow a topological arrangement, with anterior callosal disruption resulting in disorders such as "alien hand syndrome" and more posterior interruption resulting in hemispatial neglect, visual, and amnestic disorders[23].

Anterior Commissure

The anterior commissure connects portions of the temporal, occipital, and orbitofrontal cortex are thought to allow interhemispheric transfer of visual, auditory, and olfactory information.[24] This moustache-shaped pathway is seen well in the midline with color-encoded FA maps as a rounded red bundle anterior to the third ventricle and between the anterior and posterior columns of the fornices. The larger posterior limb of these commissural fibers extends laterally, posteriorly, and inferior to the striatum (▶ Fig. 3.11), medial to and paralleling the uncinate fasciculus, then traveling into the temporal stem to branch into the white matter of the inferior temporal and occipital lobes. These more posterior aspects of the branches of the tract are difficult to visualize with conventional diffusion MRI because these fibers mingle with those of the UF and ILF. The smaller anterior limb extends toward the region of the olfactory bulbs, olfactory tracts, and amygdala, but these are frequently not well resolved in clinical diffusion MRI examinations.

3.3.3 Projection Tracts

The third category, projection tracts, includes pyramidal tracts and optic radiation.

Pyramidal Tracts

The corticospinal tract (CST) and corticobulbar tract (CBT) contain the upper motor neurons that together constitute the primary descending motor tracts responsible for voluntary movement of the face, arms, trunk, and legs. About a third of the fibers from these tracts actually arise from the motor cortex of the precentral gyrus, the remainder connecting to the adjacent premotor, supplementary motor, and parietal cortices. As known from lesion studies and tract dissection, both exhibit a somatotopic arrangement of fibers from the cortex, through the corona radiata, posterior internal capsule, cerebral peduncle, and brainstem, where axons in the CBT synapse with motor brainstem nuclei, and the CST fibers continue inferiorly into the spinal cord. Lesions of the CST and CBT result in contralateral upper motor neuron weakness.

Due to its prominent craniocaudal orientation, the CST is easily identified within the subcortical

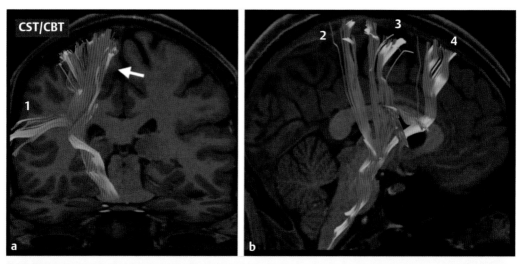

Fig. 3.12 Best seen on **(a)** coronal images, the lateral branches of the pyramidal tract (1) project to the lateral precentral gyrus, and are more difficult to identify than the dominant medial branches (white arrow). These branches are not depicted well with diffusion tensor imaging (DTI) tractography, and require high angular resolution diffusion imaging (HARDI) or diffusion spectrum imaging (DSI) to be visualized. **(b)** Note on sagittal projection that the pyramidal tract extends not only to the precentral gyrus (3), but also to the parietal lobe (2) and the supplementary motor area (4). CST, corticospinal tract; CBT, corticobulbar tract.

white matter of the precentral gyrus, corona radiata, internal capsule, and brainstem as blue voxels in these regions on color FA images (▶ Fig. 3.12). The medial extent of this fiber bundle is consistently depicted well with tractography. However, a well-known limitation of conventional deterministic DTI tractography is its inability to consistently track corticobulbar fibers to the lateral motor cortex. This shortcoming arises from the inability of DTI to distinguish these lateral projections as they intersect with crossing fibers from the corpus callosum and SLF within the centrum semiovale. Because depiction of the entire extent of this pathway is highly desirable in order to preserve eloquent motor function during neurosurgical brain tumor resection, many institutions prefer to use diffusion techniques, such as HARDI, that are capable of characterizing crossing fibers.

Optic Radiation

The optic radiation, also referred to as the geniculolocalcarine tract, carries input from the contralateral visual field via the lateral geniculate nucleus (LGN). Fibers from the LGN pass posteriorly through the retrolenticular internal capsule, along the lateral margin of the posterior lateral ventricle into the occipital lobes (▶ Fig. 3.13). Although classically divided into upper and lower divisions, three distinct bundles within this pathway can be identified using diffusion tractography.[25] The largest *dorsal bundle* carries information regarding the inferior visual field directly to the ipsilateral superior calcarine cortex. A smaller *ventral bundle* supplying the superior visual field projects to the inferior calcarine cortex. Finally, between these two bundles, a very small *central* bundle representing macular vision projects to both sides of the medial calcarine cortex. The ventral bundle is also referred to as the Meyer loop, a bundle of fibers notable for a characteristic "knee" of fibers that pass anteriorly into the temporal lobe prior to coursing posteriorly. From the LGN, the Meyer loop extends anteriorly over the roof of the temporal horn then loops posteriorly to pass along the lateral aspect of the temporal horn and through the temporal stem en route to the occipital cortex.

Superior quadrantanopia is relatively common after anterior temporal lobectomy, occurring in varying degrees of severity in 50 to 90% of patients. This postoperative result occurs due to transection of fibers within the Meyer loop, the anterior extent of which varies by 1.5 to 1.7 cm among different subjects. Although there is no

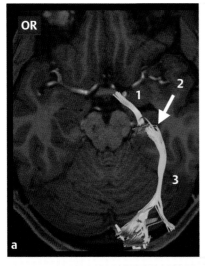
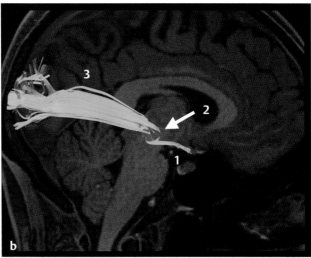

Fig. 3.13 (a) Axial and (b) sagittal images of the left optic tract (1) and optic radiation (OR) (3), carrying topographically organized information from the right visual field to the occipital cortex. From the lateral geniculate nucleus, anterior fibers from this pathway extend a variable length into the ipsilateral temporal lobe (2) before sweeping back into the occipital lobe within the sagittal striatum. Disruption of this segment, the Meyer loop of the optic radiations, gives rise to superior quadrantanopia.

direct relationship between the size of the resection and the severity of the visual field deficit, the magnitude of the resulting quadrantanopia can be more accurately predicted by the extent of resection within the Meyer loop characterized using diffusion tensor tractography.[26]

3.4 Clinical Application: Neurosurgical Planning

Armed with an understanding of the foregoing white matter tracts, the radiologist is equipped to describe the location and significance of lesions within the white matter in patients undergoing biopsy or resection. Because preservation of eloquent function remains a major goal of neurosurgery, tractography of the corticospinal, visual, and language pathways is now routinely performed at many centers. Consider the example in ▶ Fig. 3.14, which shows images from a surgical planning MRI in a patient presenting with mild right hemiparesis. Color FA images illustrate how the ipsilesional CST is compressed but maintained within the corona radiata, whereas the normally green portions of the SLF are not visualized and are likely infiltrated with tumor. The degree of mass effect on the CST is appreciated using fiber tractography. With modern neurosurgical navigation systems in

the operating room, this information from tractography can decrease operative time because it provides the surgeon with an initial map of where resection might result in postoperative hemiparesis.

3.5 Summary

DTI of high technical quality allows consistent visualization of a relatively small group of association, commissural, and projection pathways. Color FA images and fiber tractography can display the location of normal white matter tracts, infiltration and distortion of tracts by lesions, and the relationship between them and the surrounding pathways.

3.5.1 Acknowledgment

Data used for ▶ Fig. 3.1 through ▶ Fig. 3.13 were provided by the Human Connectome Project, WU-Minn Consortium (Principal Investigators: David Van Essen and Kamil Ugurbil; 1U54MH091657) funded by the 16 NIH Institutes and Centers that support the NIH Blueprint for Neuroscience Research; and by the McDonnell Center for Systems Neuroscience at Washington University.

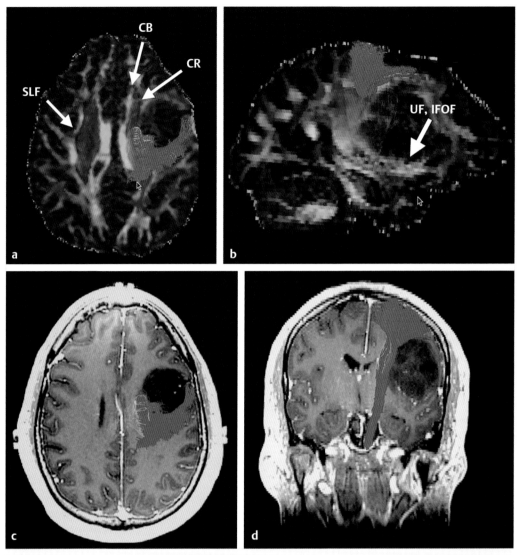

Fig. 3.14 (a) Axial and (b) sagittal color fractional anisotropy (FA) maps, and (c) axial and (d) coronal projections of the left corticospinal tract (CST) in a patient with a left frontal opercular grade 2 anaplastic astrocytoma. The posterior margin of the tumor closely approximates the anterior aspect of the CST, which appears splayed posteriorly around the mass. Color FA images show that the corona radiata (CR) (blue) is largely preserved, the cingulum bundle (CB) is displaced medially by mass effect, and the uncinate fasciculus (UF) and inferior fronto-occipital fasciculus (IFOF) are displaced inferiorly within the external capsule. In contrast to the normal right superior longitudinal fasciculus (SLF), the left SLF is not well seen and is likely involved.

References

[1] Nagae-Poetscher LM, Jiang H, Wakana S, Golay X, van Zijl PC, Mori S. High-resolution diffusion tensor imaging of the brain stem at 3T. AJNR Am J Neuroradiol 2004; 25(8): 1325–1330

[2] Habas C, Cabanis EA. Anatomical parcellation of the brainstem and cerebellar white matter: a preliminary probabilistic tractography study at 3T. Neuroradiology 2007; 49(10): 849–863

[3] Ford AA, Colon-Perez L, Triplett WT, Gullett JM, Mareci TH, Fitzgerald DB. Imaging white matter in human brainstem. Front Hum Neurosci 2013; 7: 400

[4] Basser PJ, Jones DK. Diffusion tensor MRI: theory, experimental design and data analysis - a technical review. NMR Biomed 2002; 15(7–8): 456–467

[5] Mukherjee P, Berman JI, Chung SW, Hess CP, Henry RG. Diffusion tensor MR imaging and fiber tractography: theoretic underpinnings. AJNR Am J Neuroradiol 2008; 29(4): 632–641

[6] Hagmann P, Jonasson L, Maeder P, Thiran JP, Wedeen VJ, Meuli R. Understanding diffusion MR imaging techniques: from scalar diffusion weighted imaging to diffusion tensor imaging and beyond. Radiographics 2006; 26 Suppl 1: S205–S223

[7] Jeurissen B, Leemans A, Tournier JD, Jones DK, Sijbers J. Investigating the prevalence of complex fiber configurations in white matter tissue with diffusion magnetic resonance imaging. Hum Brain Mapp 2013; 34(11): 2747–2766

[8] Mori S, van Zijl PC. Fiber tracking: principles and strategies - a technical review. NMR Biomed 2002; 15(7–8): 468–480

[9] Mukherjee P, Chung SW, Berman JI, Hess CP, Henry RG. Diffusion tensor MR imaging and fiber tractography: technical considerations. AJNR Am J Neuroradiol 2008; 29(5): 843–852

[10] Mori S, Crain BJ, Chacko VP, van Zijl PCM. Three-dimensional tracking of axonal projections in the brain by magnetic resonance imaging. Ann Neurol 1999; 45(2): 265–269

[11] Jones DK, Cercignani M. Twenty-five pitfalls in the analysis of diffusion MRI data. NMR Biomed 2010; 23(7): 803–820

[12] Wakana S, Jiang H, Nagae-Poetscher LM, van Zijl PC, Mori S. Fiber tract-based atlas of human white matter anatomy. Radiology 2004; 230(1): 77–87

[13] Catani M, Thiebaut de Schotten M. A diffusion tensor imaging tractography atlas for virtual in vivo dissections. Cortex 2008; 44(8): 1105–1132

[14] Hess CP, Mukherjee P. Visualizing white matter pathways in the living human brain: diffusion tensor imaging and beyond. Neuroimaging Clin N Am 2007; 17(4): 407–426, vii

[15] Jones DK, Christiansen KF, Chapman RJ, Aggleton JP. Distinct subdivisions of the cingulum bundle revealed by diffusion MRI fibre tracking: implications for neuropsychological investigations. Neuropsychologia 2013; 51(1): 67–78

[16] Jhoo JH, Lee DY, Choo IH, et al. Discrimination of normal aging, MCI and AD with multimodal imaging measures on the medial temporal lobe. Psychiatry Res 2010; 183(3): 237–243

[17] Makris N, Kennedy DN, McInerney S, et al. Segmentation of subcomponents within the superior longitudinal fascicle in humans: a quantitative, in vivo, DT-MRI study. Cereb Cortex 2005; 15(6): 854–869

[18] Catani M, Allin MPG, Husain M, et al. Symmetries in human brain language pathways correlate with verbal recall. Proc Natl Acad Sci U S A 2007; 104(43): 17163–17168

[19] Catani M, Jones DK, Donato R, Ffytche DH. Occipito-temporal connections in the human brain. Brain 2003; 126(Pt 9): 2093–2107

[20] Von Der Heide RJ, Skipper LM, Klobusicky E, Olson IR. Dissecting the uncinate fasciculus: disorders, controversies and a hypothesis. Brain 2013; 136(Pt 6): 1692–1707

[21] Forkel SJ, Thiebaut de Schotten M, Kawadler JM, Dell'Acqua F, Danek A, Catani M. The anatomy of fronto-occipital connections from early blunt dissections to contemporary tractography. Cortex 2014; 56: 73–84

[22] Caverzasi E, Papinutto N, Amirbekian B, Berger MS, Henry RG. Q-ball of inferior fronto-occipital fasciculus and beyond. PLoS ONE 2014; 9(6): e100274

[23] DORON K, GAZZANIGA M (2008). Neuroimaging techniques offer new perspectives on callosal transfer and interhemispheric communication. Cortex, 44(8), 1023-1029. http://doi.org/10.1016/j.cortex.2008.03.007

[24] Peltier J, Verclytte S, Delmaire C, Pruvo JP, Havet E, Le Gars D. Microsurgical anatomy of the anterior commissure: correlations with diffusion tensor imaging fiber tracking and clinical relevance. Neurosurgery 2011; 69(2) Suppl Operative: ons241–ons246, discussion ons246–ons247

[25] Hofer S, Karaus A, Frahm J. Reconstruction and dissection of the entire human visual pathway using diffusion tensor MRI. Front Neuroanat 2010; 4: 15

[26] Yogarajah M, Focke NK, Bonelli S, et al. Defining Meyer's loop-temporal lobe resections, visual field deficits and diffusion tensor tractography. Brain 2009; 132(Pt 6): 1656–1668

4 Diffusion Weighted Imaging and Diffusion Tensor Imaging of the Brain during Early Brain Development: The First Two Years of Life

Wei Gao, John H Gilmore, and Weili Lin

Key Points

- Temporal maturation of the major white matter tracts follows a nonlinear pattern, with the most significant growth during the first year of life, followed by a slower pace in the second year of life.
- Spatial maturation of the major white matter tracts follows a central-to-peripheral, caudal-to-rostral trend during early brain development.
- Significant genetic effects on the development of both global and local white matter diffusion properties are present, whereas common environmental effects are restricted to specific tracts during the first 2 years of life.
- Lateralization of white matter is observed in the fiber bundles associated with language and sensorimotor functions, whereas gender effects are subtle during infancy.
- Significant diffusion cognition correlations have been observed in infancy, and abnormal development of white matter has been associated with different brain diseases/disorders.

4.1 Introduction

An understanding of early brain development is of great clinical importance because many neurological and neurobehavioral disorders have their developmental origins during this period.[1,2] Conventional T1-/T2-weighted magnetic resonance imaging (MRI) has been routinely used for the clinical assessment of brain maturation processes, including gray/white matter growth, water content changes, and myelination.[3,4] Although anatomical/morphological developments are readily apparent in conventional MRI, insights into the development of white matter (WM), particularly the myelination status of WM with age, have been more challenging to obtain until the introduction of diffusion tensor imaging (DTI).[5,6] The underlying physical mechanism of DTI is that the relative angle between the directions of the applied diffusion gradients and water diffusion determines the extent to which magnetic resonance signal intensity is altered in the presence of diffusion gradients; the maximum signal-intensity reduction occurs at a 0-degree angle (i.e., parallel), whereas, theoretically, no signal-intensity change is anticipated at 90 degrees (i.e., perpendicular). Therefore, applying diffusion gradients along noncollinear directions, a tensor matrix can be employed to characterize the directions of water diffusion. Subsequently, the three eigenvalues/eigenvectors obtained through matrix diagonalization of the tensor matrix can be used not only to measure rotation-invariant water diffusion properties, such as mean diffusivity and fractional anisotropy (FA), but also to provide the preferred direction of water diffusion in a given voxel.

Major WM growth occurs prenatally. After the completion of neuronal migration during the last trimester of gestation, interneuron connections are built at two ends: neurons develop dendritic trees to make synaptic connections with other neurons within the gray matter and extend long axons running through the WM to establish long-distance connections. Although almost all prominent WM tracts can be identified using DTI after term birth despite low anisotropy values,[7] continued growth of WM tracts occur postnatally, including increases of axon diameter, improvements of tract organization, developments of miscellaneous axonal cell organs, and, most importantly, development of myelin sheaths for insulating major fiber bundles.[8] Life span examinations of the WM growth consistently show nonlinear developmental patterns featuring the most dramatic development of all major diffusion properties during the first 2 years of life,[9,10] a critical period for WM development. This chapter reviews the recent literature on the use of DTI to study WM development during the first 2 years of life. The chapter discusses the temporal/spatial pattern of WM maturation and the issues related to lateralization and gender effects. Recent evidence is reviewed on the genetic control of early brain WM maturation and its behavioral correlations. Finally, the chapter summarizes recent progress on the clinical findings of DTI in early brain development.

4.2 Temporal Growth Pattern of Major White Matter Tracts

Measurements of intracranial gray matter, and WM volumes have consistently shown nonlinear brain growth, featuring dramatic growth during the first year, followed by more refined and slow growth during the second year of life.[3] Total brain volume increases 105% during the first but only 15% during the second year of life.[3] These temporal brain volume increases have been attributed to reflect different structural events, including synaptogenesis,[11,12] dendrite elaboration,[13] myelination,[14,15] and continued subplate developmental changes,[16] which have all been documented to undergo the fastest development during the first year. With these microstructural developments, it is highly plausible that water diffusion will be modified owing to the alteration of the biological microenvironment (barriers) such that a similar temporal pattern could be observed with DTI. Indeed, regardless of different diffusion parameters, results reported in the literature have generally converged on a nonlinear developmental trend.[9,17] Specifically, using a region of interest (ROI)-based approach, Gao et al[18] examined the spatial temporal development of eight ROIs located at the genu/splenium/body of the corpus callosum (CC), the internal capsule, the cortical spinal tract, the optic radiation, and the frontal/posterior peripheral white matter regions. All eight ROIs exhibit highly significant increases of FA in neonates to 1-year-olds, followed by a modest increase during the second year of life (▸ Fig. 4.1). Although FA represents a highly informative metric capable of characterizing the degree of anisotropy of the underlying water diffusion within a given voxel, it does not separately evaluate water diffusion parallel or perpendicular to the long axis of axonal bundles. In contrast, axial diffusivity

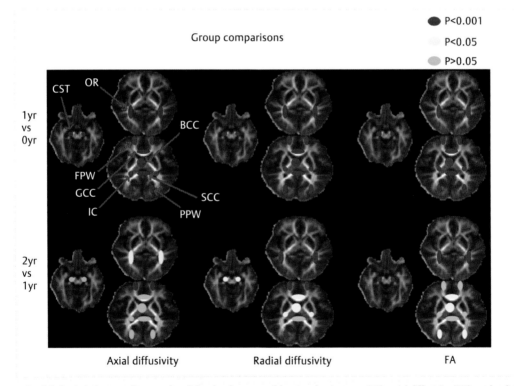

Fig. 4.1 Statistical comparison results of the development of fractional anisotropy (FA), axial diffusivity (AD), and radial diffusivity (RD) across the first 2 years of life. Red/yellow/green regions of interest are shown for illustration of the relative significance in age-dependent development (red: $p < 0.001$; yellow: $p < 0.05$; green: $p > 0.05$). GCC, genu of the corpus callosum; SCC, splenium of the corpus callosum; BCC, body of the corpus callosum; IC, internal capsule; CST, cortical spinal tract; OR, optic radiation; FPW, frontal peripheral white matter; PPW, posterior peripheral white matter. (Reproduced from Gao et al, with permission,[15] original Fig. 3.)

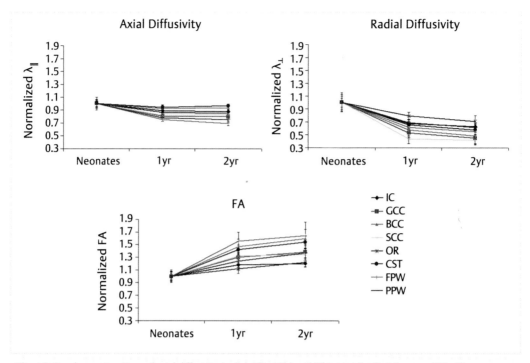

Fig. 4.2 Development pattern of axial diffusivity, radial diffusivity, and FA across the first 2 years of life. The experimentally measured Life values of the 1- and 2-year-old groups are normalized to those of the neonates. GCC, genu of the corpus callosum; SCC, splenium of the corpus callosum; BCC, body of the corpus callosum; IC, internal capsule; CST, cortical spinal tract; OR, optic radiation; FPW, frontal peripheral white matter; PPW, posterior peripheral white matter. (Reproduced from Gao et al, with permission,[15] original Fig. 4.)

(AD) and radial diffusivity (RD) separately quantify water diffusivity parallel and perpendicular to the main axis of water diffusion, respectively, potentially offering additional insights into the microarchitecture of axonal bundles. Using these two metrics, Gao et al further demonstrated that, although a temporal developmental pattern similar to that seen with FA was observed for axial and radial diffusivities during the first 2 years of life (see ▶ Fig. 4.1), a more rapid reduction of radial diffusivity to 44% to 69% of that at birth is observed during the second year of life, whereas the axial diffusivity decreases to only ~ 75 to 95% of the neonatal value (▶ Fig. 4.2). These findings suggest a more rapid development of radial constraints (e. g., myelination) than the growth of axonal structures during the first year of life. Consistent with these DTI findings, Haynes et al[8] conducted a histological study with growth-associated phosphoprotein (GAP-43) staining, a marker of axonal growth and elongation. They showed a high level of GAP43 staining from 24 to 64 postconceptional (PC) weeks, implying rapid axonal development

spanned from pre- to postnatal periods. Subsequently, a slower, adult-like level of axonal development was observed beyond 17 postnatal months (1.5 postnatal year). In contrast, myelination begins from 54 PC weeks (2.5 postnatal months) and develops at a high speed until 72 to 92 PC weeks (6.5 postnatal months to 11.5 postnatal months), spanning approximately the entire first year after birth. Together, these results suggest that the onset of axonal growth is earlier (prenatal) and fastest during the first 5 postnatal months, whereas myelin maturation begins about 2.5 months postnatally and continues at a fast growth pace throughout the first year of life. Therefore, these histological results by Haynes et al[8] suggest the potential physiological underpinnings of the observed relatively faster decrease of radial diffusivity than axial diffusivity by Gao et al[15] because the maturation of myelin is likely the dominant process during this period of life.

More information could be revealed by considering the relationship between axial/radial diffusivity and FA changes. For example, when examining FA alone, three of the eight ROIs evaluated by Gao et al showed no changes in FA (i.e., splenium of the corpus callosum, internal capsule, and frontal peripheral WM) implying nonsignificant growth during the second year of life. However, further inspection of the radial and axial diffusivity revealed completely different pictures (see ▶ Fig. 4.1). Specifically, consistent with the finding of FA, the splenium of the corpus callosum exhibited no changes in both axial and radial diffusivities. In contrast, significant changes of both axial and radial diffusivities were observed in frontal WM, indicating continuing myelination and axonal growth. However, the extent to which axial and radial diffusivities were altered appeared to cancel their contributions in the formulation of FA calculation, leading to a stable FA. Finally, a significant reduction of radial diffusivity in the internal capsule was observed, suggesting continuing myelination. Furthermore, although a significant elevation of FA was observed in the genu/splenium/ body of the corpus callosum, the cortical spinal tract, and peripheral WM between 1 and 2 years of age, these regions exhibited significant changes only in radial and not in axial diffusivity, suggesting that their growth is dominated by continued myelination rather than axonal growth. Together, these results underscore the importance of combined examination of both FA and axial/radial diffusivity measures for a better depiction of the complex underlying microstructural changes during the first 2 years of life.

In contrast, to examine regional maturation patterns of WM, Geng et al[19] exploited a tract-based approach where several major WM tracts were evaluated. The findings observed were similar to those reported using ROI-based approaches regarding the temporal developmental trend of WM fiber tracts during the first 2 years of life. Specifically, they examined the growth of FA, axial diffusivity (AD), and radial diffusivity (RD) for 10 major WM fiber tracts: commissural bundles of the genu, body, and splenium of the corpus callosum; projection fiber tracts of the bilateral anterior/posterior limb of the internal capsule, motor, and sensory tracts; and association tracts of the bilateral uncinate fasciculus tracts, inferior longitudinal fasciculus, and arcuate fasciculus tracts. All fiber tracts showed increasing FA (16.1–55%) and decreasing RD (24.4– 46.4%) and AD (13.3–28.2%) in the first 2 years of life (▶ Fig. 4.3), featuring faster development in the first year than the second year. Consistently, RD showed larger changes than AD, in line with the ROI-based findings.

4.3 Spatial Growth Pattern of Major White Matter Tracts

As previously described, extensive myelination processes of major WM tracts occur during the first year of life are likely the dominant factor attributes to the observed changes of WM diffusivities during infancy. Spatial maturation of WM tracts has been documented following a central-to-peripheral and caudal-to-rostral pattern. Specifically, myelination increases from the splenium of the corpus callosum and optic radiation (at 3–4 months), the occipital and parietal lobes (at 4–6 months), and, finally, to the genu of the corpus callosum and frontal and temporal lobes (at 6–8 months).[20] Consistent with histological studies, DTI findings also show a similar pattern. Zhai et al[17] demonstrated that the central WM areas consistently exhibit higher FA and lower mean diffusivity (MD) values when compared to the peripheral WM regions in neonates. Gao et al[15] further showed that the general maturation pattern begins centrally (genu/splenium/body of the corpus collosum), followed by the cortical spinal tract, internal capsule, optic radiation, and peripheral WM. Moreover, the occipital matures earlier than the frontal peripheral WM regions (▶ Fig. 4.4). Additionally, Chen et al[21] inspected linear (Cl) and planar (Cp) anisotropy. The linear anisotropy is defined as the trace normalized difference between the primary and second eigenvalues, quantifying percentages of the shape of a diffusion tensor matrix attributable to a cylindrical object. In contrast, planar anisotropy quantifies percentages of the shape of a diffusion tensor matrix attributable to a planar object. Their results showed that the central WM had a significantly higher Cl and lower Cp when compared to the peripheral WM during infancy, suggesting that highly organized fiber bundles have already formed at birth in the central major WM regions. In addition, the observed rapid growth velocity of Cl during the first 2 years further enhances the cylindrical shapes of diffusion tensors in these major WM regions, likely driven by the rapid myelination process. Similar findings were observed using tract-based analysis[19]; callosal bundles show larger FA changing rates in central than in peripheral regions. Motor and sensory tracts show a higher rate of changes of FA and RD in anatomical locations close to the cortical regions when compared to those close to the cerebral peduncle. The splenium of the CC is one of the tracts that has the

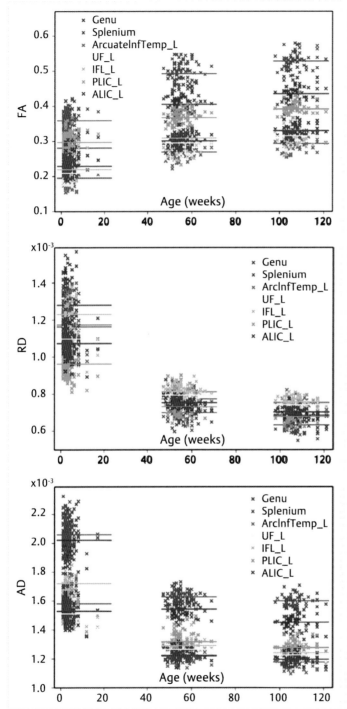

Fig. 4.3 Scatter plots of average fractional anisotropy (FA), axial diffusivity (AD), and radial diffusivity (RD) along seven representative tracts versus postnatal age. Horizontal lines represent the overall mean of the average values in one age group. Different tracts are visualized in different colors. UF, uncinate fasciculus; ILF, inferior longitudinal fasciculus; ALIC, anterior limb of internal capsule; PLIC, posterior limb of internal capsule. (Reproduced from Geng et al., with permission[19])

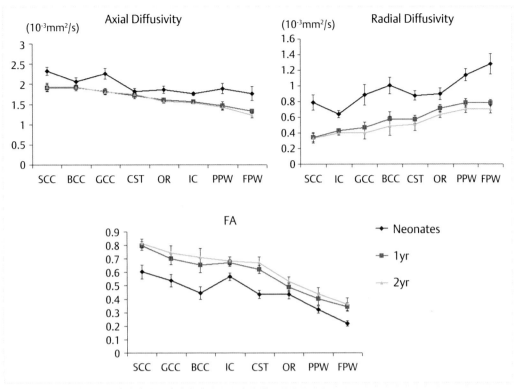

Fig. 4.4 Spatial development pattern of axial diffusivity (upper left), radial diffusivity (upper right), and fractional anisotropy (bottom) across regions of interest during the first 2 years of life. GCC, genu of the corpus callosum; SCC, splenium of the corpus callosum; BCC, body of the corpus callosum; IC, internal capsule; CST, cortical spinal tract; OR, optic radiation; FPW, frontal peripheral white matter; PPW, posterior peripheral white matter. (Reproduced from Gao et al, [15] with permission, original Fig. 5.)

largest FA and smallest RD in the first year, and maintains this high level of maturation in the second year. The genu of the CC has a relatively small RD until the second year of life. Overall, DTI measures reveal a central-to-peripheral and caudal-to-rostral pattern. These findings have profound functional implications and are consistent with the notion that brain functional development starts from basic brain functions, such as motor, sensory, and visual functions and proceeds to higher-order brain function.[22] Maturation of the primary sensory functions requires either rapid up-down information relaying through center projection fibers (e.g., the cortical spinal tract) or interhemispheric communication through midbrain callosal fibers, consistent with the early maturation of central WM. In contrast, higher-order brain functions likely require the maturation of peripheral and anterior WM tracts,[22] which undergo continuing maturation through adolescence and young adult life.

4.4 Genetic Control and Environmental Effects

Genes play a significant role in the variability of global and local brain gray/white matter volumes, cortical thickness, and surface area.[23,24,25,26] Brain functions and functional brain networks are also genetically modulated.[27,28] Therefore, quantitative measures of diffusion properties of the major WM tracts during early brain development should also reflect the modulation of genetic factors. Geng et al[29] studied the genetic and environmental effects on the spatiotemporal growth of different major WM fiber tracts using a model of additive genetic and common and specific environmental variance components. Genetic and environmental contributions to both global and local diffusion parameters were estimated, including FA, RD, and AD. Their results indicate that the individual differences in the global WM microstructure characterized by all three metrics (i.e., FA, RD, and AD) are heritable

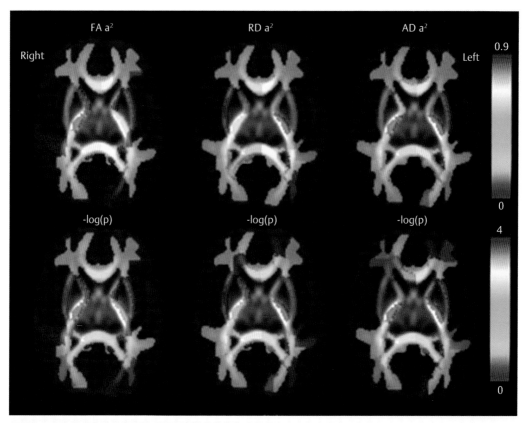

Fig. 4.5 Heritability of white matter diffusivity in the neonatal brain. Heritability values of fractional anisotropy (FA), radial diffusivity (RD) and axial diffusivity (AD) over each region of interest (top row) and their corresponding p-values (bottom row, normalized using $-\log(p)$, $-\log(0.05) = 1.3$, and $-\log(0.0001) = 4$). (Reproduced from Geng et al., with permission[29])

($\blacktriangleright$ Fig. 4.5). Specifically, global FA had the highest heritability of 60%, followed by AD (57%), and RD (53%). There was significant heritability in both hemispheres of FA and RD, but AD heritability appeared to be lateralized to the right hemisphere only. There is a significant positive correlation between RD heritability and mean RD, and similarly between AD heritability and mean AD. Combined with the decreasing trend of both RD and AD during development, these findings seem to suggest that the more mature the region is, the less genetic variation it shows. This conclusion is also consistent with the lower heritability estimates reported in adults than in pediatric subjects.

For the environmental effects, the bilateral anterior/posterior limb of internal capsule, external capsule, uncinate fasciculus, and left middle cerebellar peduncle show high shared environmental effects in RD (57–82%). Similarly, the bilateral external capsule, middle cerebellar peduncle, and inferior frontal occipital fasciculus also have a large proportion of shared environmental effects in AD (47–71%). Particularly, shared environmental effects are substantial for the RD of the bilateral external capsule (left/right: 73%/82%). Together with the anterior–posterior limb of the internal capsule, the external capsule may have started myelination earlier prenatally than other association fibers[30] and demonstrated a lower RD. The authors postulated that prenatal neurohormonal and uterine environment may affect the maturation process of the external capsule, which might lead to the observed shared environmental variation. In general, the authors observed substantial heritability of diffusion properties during infancy, which is higher than that reported in adults. However, genetic effects are heterogeneous over different WM regions (see ▸ Fig. 4.5). The significant positive correlation between heritability and diffusion measures suggests that regional genetic effects may be modulated by maturation status—the more mature the region, the less heritable its variation. Common environmental effects are present in fewer regions that tend to be characterized by a low RD.

4.5 Cognitive Correlations

There are numerous reports on the correlations of DTI measures between different WM fiber tracts and cognitive performance in adults.[31,32,33] However, such investigations are extremely scarce during early brain development, likely due to the lack of robust cognitive assessment strategies for such young ages. Krishnan et al[34] hypothesized that higher WM apparent diffusion coefficient values at term-equivalent age in preterm infants without overt lesions are associated with poorer developmental performance in later childhood. Mean apparent diffusion coefficient values at the level of the centrum semiovale were determined at term-equivalent age. The children were assessed using the Griffiths Mental Development Scales to obtain a developmental quotient (DQ) at 2 years' corrected age. Significant negative correlations between apparent diffusion coefficient values at term-equivalent age and Griffiths Mental Development Scales at 2 years' corrected age were observed, indicating that WM abnormality may represent cerebral damage that gives rise to lower DQ scores, which might be mediated through the associated cortical and deep gray matter deficits. Short et al[35] measured FA, AD, and RD in WM fiber bundles and hypothesized a relation between WM maturation and the development of working memory in 12-month-old infants ($n = 73$). They

showed robust associations between infants' visuospatial working memory performance and microstructural characteristics of widespread WM that connect brain regions known to support working memory in older children and adults (genu, anterior and superior thalamic radiations, anterior cingulum, arcuate fasciculus, temporal–parietal segment) (▸ Fig. 4.6). These studies underscore the potential utility of DTI measures in understanding cognitive development in early infancy.

4.6 Lateralization and Gender Effects

In the adult brain, language and handedness are among the most well recognized brain functional lateralization. Consistently, functional and anatomical lateralization in the speech perception–production network and in the sensorimotor system has been reported.[36] However, only studies in early life can inform how such functional lateralization arises in relation to lateralization. Aiming to address this question, Dubios et al[37] examined the whole brain diffusion properties in infants from 1 to 4 months of age. DTI measures reveal asymmetry in the arcuate fasciculus and cortical spinal tract, thought to be related to language and sensorimotor functions, respectively, providing convincing evidence on the lateralization of diffusion property early in life that might be critical to the later lateralization of corresponding functions. Specifically, they reported that the temporal lobe part of the arcuate fasciculus is larger on the left; the left parietal part of the arcuate fasciculus has a higher FA than the right; and the cortical spinal tract between the cerebral peduncles and the posterior limb of the internal capsule has a higher FA in the left hemisphere than in the right. More recently, the finding of arcuate fasciculus asymmetry was replicated by Geng et al,[19] showing that the left arcuate-superior tract possesses > 20% larger FA values than the right in the first year.

Sexual dimorphism in brain volumetric measures is present at birth, with males having larger total brain cortical gray and white matter volumes than females.[4] However, only subtle gender

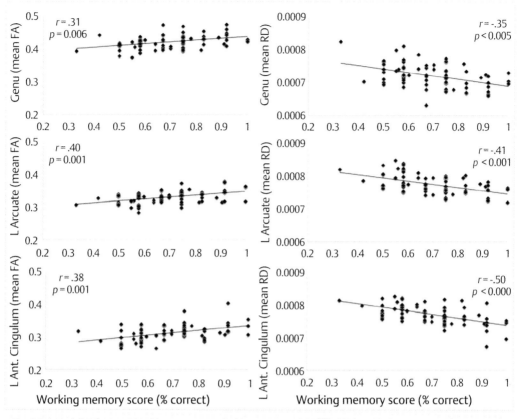

Fig. 4.6 Association between working memory and white matter tracts diffusivity properties at 1 year of age. Scatter plots highlight examples of significant associations between infants' working memory and key white matter tracts: genu, arcuate, and anterior cingulum. Plots show the positive association of working memory with fractional anisotropy (FA) and the negative association with radial diffusivity (RD). Only the left (L) arcuate and left cingulum are shown above; however, scatter plots for these tracts in the right hemisphere are very similar. (Reproduced from Short et al., with permission[35])

differences in the brain diffusion measures were reported during infancy. Geng et al[19] found minor differences in several localized fiber tracts in the right brain: males show a smaller FA in the right sensory tract, a larger AD in the right arcuate superior and motor tracts, and a smaller AD in the right uncinate fasciculus. Several studies focusing on the development of WM from late childhood to adolescence[38,39,40] also failed to detect significant sex effects. Therefore, more studies are needed to delineate the potential mechanisms of the observed sex differences in diffusion in adults.[41]

4.7 Clinical Applications

The use of DTI to characterize brain developmental disorders has also been extensively reported. Yuan

et al[42] retrospectively analyzed DTI in children with hydrocephalus during early infancy to quantify abnormal WM regions. Their results revealed significantly lower FA, higher MD, and higher RD values within the corpus callosum in infants with hydrocephalus. Moreover, the age-dependent increase of FA of the corpus callosum that is typically observed in normal developing infants was absent in their study cohort. In the case of a more devastating genetic disease, Krabbe disease, unrelated umbilical cord transplantation, the only available treatment for this fatal neurodegenerative condition, is only effective if administered before clinical symptoms appear. Escolar et al[43] evaluated the use of DTI in identifying early changes of the major motor tracts of asymptomatic neonates with infantile Krabbe disease.

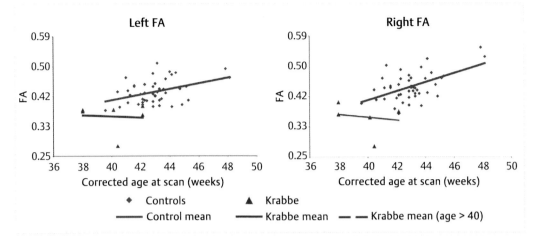

Fig. 4.7 Raw mean fractional anisotropy (FA) values for patients with infantile Krabbe disease and controls. Each point represents a child's mean FA across the central portion of the corticospinal tract. The red triangles represent the six patients with Krabbe disease, whereas the blue diamonds show the typical controls. The red and blue lines represent the linear trend related to the corrected age at the time of the magnetic resonance imaging. (Reproduced from Escolar et al. with permission[43])

Their results showed that patients with Krabbe disease had significantly lower FA values than the controls after adjusting for gestational age, gestational age at birth, birth weight, sex, and race (▶ Fig. 4.7). Quantitative tractography results also showed significant differences in the corticospinal tracts of asymptomatic neonates who had the early-onset form of Krabbe disease. Therefore, DTI could potentially serve as an important biomarker of disease progression in neonates diagnosed with Krabbe through statewide neonate screening programs. DTI could also play a critical role in autism spectrum disorders (ASDs). Specifically, Wolff et al[44] showed that the FA trajectories of 12 of 15 major WM fiber tracts differed significantly between the infants who developed ASDs and those who did not, which is characterized by higher FA values at 6 months followed by a slower change over time relative to infants without ASDs (▶ Fig. 4.8). Overall, studies based on DTI measurements of the early brain's wiring structures have great potential to derive quantitative biomarkers for disease-onset prediction, monitoring, and treatment, and more studies using the longitudinal design are desired to push this field forward.

4.8 Summary

Numerous studies have demonstrated dramatic development of the brain diffusion properties in WM during the first 2 years of life. Temporally, different diffusion properties follow nonlinear growth featuring the most significant changes during the first year of life. Spatially, the WM maturation generally follows a central-to-peripheral, caudal-to-rostral trend. During this time period, significant genetic effects on the development of both global and local WM diffusion properties were observed, whereas common environmental effects were restricted to specific tracts. Lateralized development of WM diffusion was mostly concentrated on the fiber bundles linked to language and sensorimotor functions. Sex effects on WM development during infancy were subtle and local. There are significant diffusion cognition correlations observed in infancy, and abnormal development of WM has been associated with different brain diseases/disorders, supporting the great potential of this noninvasive neuroimaging technique in clinical use.

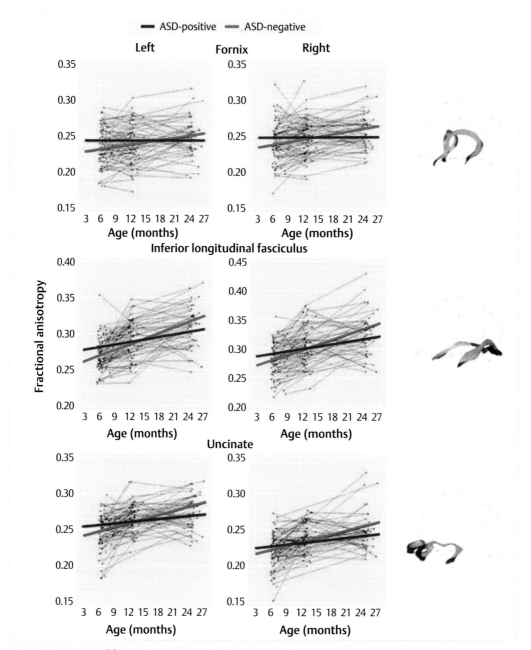

Fig. 4.8 Trajectories of fractional anisotropy in limbic and association white matter fiber tracts in 92 high-risk Infants with (red curves) and without (blue curves) evidence of autism spectrum disorders (ASDs) at 24 months of age. (Reproduced from Wolff et al. with permission[44])

References

[1] Owen MJ, O'Donovan MC, Thapar A, Craddock N. Neurodevelopmental hypothesis of schizophrenia. Br J Psychiatry 2011; 198(3): 173–175

[2] Paloyelis Y, Mehta MA, Kuntsi J, Asherson P. Functional MRI in ADHD: a systematic literature review. Expert Rev Neurother 2007; 7(10): 1337–1356

[3] Knickmeyer RC, Gouttard S, Kang C, et al. A structural MRI study of human brain development from birth to 2 years. J Neurosci 2008; 28(47): 12176–12182

[4] Gilmore JH, Lin W, Prastawa MW, et al. Regional gray matter growth, sexual dimorphism, and cerebral asymmetry in the neonatal brain. J Neurosci 2007; 27(6): 1255–1260

[5] Basser PJ, Mattiello J, LeBihan D. Estimation of the effective self-diffusion tensor from the NMR spin echo. J Magn Reson B 1994; 103(3): 247–254

[6] Basser PJ, Pierpaoli C. Microstructural and physiological features of tissues elucidated by quantitative-diffusion tensor MRI. J Magn Reson B 1996; 111(3): 209–219

[7] Huang H, Zhang J, Wakana S, et al. White and gray matter development in human fetal, newborn and pediatric brains. Neuroimage 2006; 33(1): 27–38

[8] Haynes RL, Borenstein NS, Desilva TM, et al. Axonal development in the cerebral white matter of the human fetus and infant. J Comp Neurol 2005; 484(2): 156–167

[9] Hüppi PS, Warfield S, Kikinis R, et al. Quantitative magnetic resonance imaging of brain development in premature and mature newborns. Ann Neurol 1998; 43(2): 224–235

[10] Mukherjee P, Miller JH, Shimony JS, et al. Diffusion tensor MR imaging of gray and white matter development during normal human brain maturation. AJNR Am J Neuroradiol 2002; 23(9): 1445–1456

[11] Elston GN, Oga T, Fujita I. Spinogenesis and pruning scales across functional hierarchies. J Neurosci 2009; 29(10): 3271–3275

[12] Rakic P, Bourgeois JP, Eckenhoff MF, Zecevic N, Goldman-Rakic PS. Concurrent overproduction of synapses in diverse regions of the primate cerebral cortex. Science 1986; 232 (4747): 232–235

[13] Petanjek Z, Judas M, Kostović I, Uylings HB. Lifespan alterations of basal dendritic trees of pyramidal neurons in the human prefrontal cortex: a layer-specific pattern. Cereb Cortex 2008; 18(4): 915–929

[14] Flechsig P. Developmental (myelogenetic) localisation of the cerebral cortex in the human. Lancet 1901; 158 (4077): 1027–1030

[15] Gao W, Lin W, Chen Y, et al. Temporal and spatial development of axonal maturation and myelination of white matter in the developing brain. AJNR Am J Neuroradiol 2009; 30(2): 290–296

[16] Kostović I, Jovanov-Milošević N, Radoš M, et al. Perinatal and early postnatal reorganization of the subplate and related cellular compartments in the human cerebral wall as revealed by histological and MRI approaches. Brain Struct Funct 2014; 219(1): 231–253

[17] Zhai G, Lin W, Wilber KP, Gerig G, Gilmore JH. Comparisons of regional white matter diffusion in healthy neonates and adults performed with a 3.0-T head-only MR imaging unit. Radiology 2003; 229(3): 673–681

[18] Gao W, Gilmore JH, Giovanello KS, et al. Temporal and spatial evolution of brain network topology during the first two years of life. PLoS ONE 2011; 6(9): e25278

[19] Geng X, Gouttard S, Sharma A, et al. Quantitative tract-based white matter development from birth to age 2years. Neuroimage 2012; 61(3): 542–557

[20] Deoni SC, Mercure E, Blasi A, et al. Mapping infant brain myelination with magnetic resonance imaging. J Neurosci 2011; 31(2): 784–791

[21] Chen Y, An H, Zhu H, et al. Longitudinal regression analysis of spatial-temporal growth patterns of geometrical diffusion measures in early postnatal brain development with diffusion tensor imaging. Neuroimage 2011; 58(4): 993–1005

[22] Tau GZ, Peterson BS. Normal development of brain circuits. Neuropsychopharmacology 2010; 35(1): 147–168

[23] Peper JS, Brouwer RM, Boomsma DI, Kahn RS, Hulshoff Pol HE. Genetic influences on human brain structure: a review of brain imaging studies in twins. Hum Brain Mapp 2007; 28(6): 464–473

[24] Posthuma D, De Geus EJ, Baaré WF, Hulshoff Pol HE, Kahn RS, Boomsma DI. The association between brain volume and intelligence is of genetic origin. Nat Neurosci 2002; 5(2): 83–84

[25] Thompson PM, Cannon TD, Narr KL, et al. Genetic influences on brain structure. Nat Neurosci 2001; 4(12): 1253–1258

[26] Panizzon MS, Fennema-Notestine C, Eyler LT, et al. Distinct genetic influences on cortical surface area and cortical thickness. Cereb Cortex 2009; 19(11): 2728–2735

[27] Glahn DC, Winkler AM, Kochunov P, et al. Genetic control over the resting brain. Proc Natl Acad Sci U S A 2010; 107 (3): 1223–1228

[28] Gao W, Elton A, Zhu H, et al. Intersubject variability of and genetic effects on the brain's functional connectivity during infancy. J Neurosci 2014; 34(34): 11288–11296

[29] Geng X, Prom-Wormley EC, Perez J, et al. White matter heritability using diffusion tensor imaging in neonatal brains. Twin Res Hum Genet 2012; 15(3): 336–350

[30] Kinney HC, Brody BA, Kloman AS, Gilles FH. Sequence of central nervous system myelination in human infancy. II. Patterns of myelination in autopsied infants. J Neuropathol Exp Neurol 1988; 47(3): 217–234

[31] Madden DJ, Bennett IJ, Burzynska A, Potter GG, Chen NK, Song AW. Diffusion tensor imaging of cerebral white matter integrity in cognitive aging. Biochim Biophys Acta 2012; 1822(3): 386–400

[32] Charlton RA, Barrick TR, McIntyre DJ, et al. White matter damage on diffusion tensor imaging correlates with age-related cognitive decline. Neurology 2006; 66(2): 217–222

[33] Tsujimoto M, Senda J, Ishihara T, et al. Behavioral changes in early ALS correlate with voxel-based morphometry and diffusion tensor imaging. J Neurol Sci 2011; 307(1–2): 34–40

[34] Krishnan ML, Dyet LE, Boardman JP, et al. Relationship between white matter apparent diffusion coefficients in preterm infants at term-equivalent age and developmental outcome at 2 years. Pediatrics 2007; 120(3): e604–e609

[35] Short SJ, Elison JT, Goldman BD, et al. Associations between white matter microstructure and infants' working memory. Neuroimage 2013; 64: 156–166

[36] Toga AW, Thompson PM. Mapping brain asymmetry. Nat Rev Neurosci 2003; 4(1): 37–48

[37] Dubois J, Hertz-Pannier L, Cachia A, Mangin JF, Le Bihan D, Dehaene-Lambertz G. Structural asymmetries in the infant language and sensori-motor networks. Cereb Cortex 2009; 19(2): 414–423

[38] Bava S, Thayer R, Jacobus J, Ward M, Jernigan TL, Tapert SF. Longitudinal characterization of white matter maturation during adolescence. Brain Res 2010; 1327: 38–46

[39] Lebel C, Beaulieu C. Longitudinal development of human brain wiring continues from childhood into adulthood. J Neurosci 2011; 31(30): 10937–10947

[40] Giorgio A, Watkins KE, Douaud G, et al. Changes in white matter microstructure during adolescence. Neuroimage 2008; 39(1): 52–61

[41] Inano S, Takao H, Hayashi N, Abe O, Ohtomo K. Effects of age and gender on white matter integrity. AJNR Am J Neuroradiol 2011; 32(11): 2103–2109

[42] Yuan W, Mangano FT, Air EL, et al. Anisotropic diffusion properties in infants with hydrocephalus: a diffusion tensor imaging study. AJNR Am J Neuroradiol 2009; 30(9): 1792–1798

[43] Escolar ML, Poe MD, Smith JK, et al. Diffusion tensor imaging detects abnormalities in the corticospinal tracts of neonates with infantile Krabbe disease. AJNR Am J Neuroradiol 2009; 30(5): 1017–1021

[44] Wolff JJ, Gu H, Gerig G, et al. IBIS Network. Differences in white matter fiber tract development present from 6 to 24 months in infants with autism. Am J Psychiatry 2012; 169 (6): 589–600

5 Diffusion Weighted and Diffusion Tensor Imaging in Aging

Andrew Joseph Degnan and Lucien M. Levy

Key Points

- The aging population presents an increasingly substantial challenge worldwide, with greater numbers of individuals living to older age and vulnerable to cognitive decline and dementia, thus requiring higher levels of personal care.
- Diffusion based imaging strategies is sensitive to more subtle age-related changes in white matter integrity, and these methods may enable the differentiation of normal adult aging from mild cognitive impairment and Alzheimer dementia.
- White matter indices are more sensitive to subtle changes than anatomical volumetric analyses examining atrophy in a variety of dementias.
- Cognitive performance in specific domains, such as memory and executive function, corresponds with many diffusion tensor imaging (DTI)-based indicators within specific functionalized regions of the brain during aging.
- Specific patterns of white matter degeneration may be discerned on DTI to distinguish between dementias.

5.1 Physics and Techniques

Both diffusion weighted imaging (DWI) and its related diffusion tensor imaging (DTI) rely on the premise of water diffusion changes as an indirect indicator of underlying brain parenchyma. Understanding the basis of diffusion methods and their limitations as assessments of surrogate measures of white matter tract and axonal integrity is critical for applying diffusion imaging methods clinically to the aging brain. These techniques are summarized in (▶ Table 5.1).

5.1.1 Diffusion Weighted Imaging

DWI uses a magnetic resonance sequence using two *b* values (based on magnetic gradient strength and pulse timing) to observe the motion of water molecules. If water molecules migrate during the interval between these gradients, then signal loss will occur. Such signal loss represents uninhibited random diffusion of water molecules representing *isotropic diffusion*. Diffusion restriction represents constriction of water molecules preventing random motion between gradient pulses and presenting as hyperintense signal on DWI. The apparent diffusion coefficient (ADC) is the quantitative index that separates the T2 shine-through effect from diffusion weighted images.

5.1.2 Diffusion Tensor Imaging

Because molecular water mobility may not be the same in all directions, DTI employs gradients in multiple noncollinear directions in order to quantify diffusion measurements in creating a three-dimensional ellipsoid representing the diffusion vector within a given voxel. In white matter tracts, water is observed to preferentially (nonrandomly) migrate in the direction of axonal fibers in an *anisotropic* manner. The extent to which white matter tracts are maintained *indirectly* influences water diffusion and therefore the measurement of ADC along various axes. DTI selectively highlights densely packed fibers with a highly ordered orientation parallel to each other.

Table 5.1 Fundamental principles of diffusion tensor imaging

Imaging modality	Properties
Diffusion weighted imaging (DWI)	Examines the ability of water to diffuse freely within tissues Diffusion restriction may indicate gross pathology within tissue
Diffusion tensor imaging (DTI)	Examines the orientation of water diffusion by measuring diffusion in multiple directions, forming a vector sensitive to changes in brain microstructure Surrogate marker of white matter integrity Fiber tractography methods can reconstruct white matter tracts

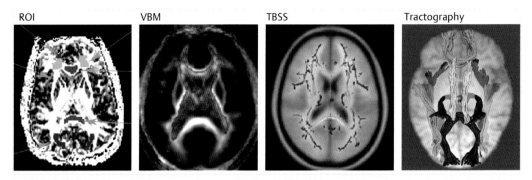

Fig. 5.1 Representations of diffusion tensor imaging data. Multiple methods are available for examining the multidirectional data acquired by diffusion tensor imaging. A region of interest (ROI) analysis method examines individual selected regions. Voxel-based morphometry (VBM) uses group-normalized data to quantitatively analyze white matter properties across the brain. Tract-based spatial statistics (TBSS) employs DTI information to generate putative representations of white matter tracts. Fiber tractography elucidates white matter pathways. (Reproduced with permission from Madden et al, [12] copyright Elsevier 2009.)

The methods used to analyze DTI data are shown in (▶ Fig. 5.1) and are explored in greater technical detail in Chapter 1. Approaches range from region-of-interest methods that examine specific areas of the brain independently to whole brain voxel-based analyses. Tract-based spatial statistics (TBSS) is one means of delineating individual white matter tracts. Deterministic tractography methods are common techniques that examine the most likely white matter structure originating from a selected seed point, whereas probabilistic tractography estimates white matter trajectories for each voxel. These and other newer analytic techniques are being applied to the study of the aging brain. One newer approach, fiber density mapping (FDM), mitigates a key limitation of the aforementioned diffusion analyses, which only examine anisotropy measures for each voxel on an individual basis without the context of surrounding fiber patterns. FDM enhances analysis by examining the surrounding white matter fibers within the axonal bundle passing through a selected voxel.[1]

DTI-Based Measurements

No single characteristic of white matter integrity is directly measured by an individual DTI measure; therefore, multiple DTI-based variables offer insight into multifactorial aspects of white matter physiology. These quantitative calculations provide orientation-independent information on brain architecture and white matter integrity on the basis of a diffusion tensor mathematical matrix construct. The following values (summarized in ▶ Table 5.2)

arise from calculations of the three eigenvectors that constitute the ellipsoid diffusion tensor.

- *Radial diffusivity* (RD) or *perpendicular diffusivity* ($\lambda_\perp$) calculated from the diffusivity perpendicular to the first eigenvector is thought to represent a proxy for myelin integrity because water diffusion across axons would be easier with breakdown of normal myelin structures. RD is generally thought to represent a greater contributor to FA changes.
- *Fractional anisotropy* (FA) is an index measuring intravoxel coherence (essentially, the normalized standard deviation of the three diffusivities) where the value ranges from isotropic (0), a spherical vector, to anisotropic (1), an ellipsoid vector. The FA reflects microstructure integrity.
- *Mean diffusivity* (MD) provides information of the overall diffusion as the average of all three axes of the tensor (eigenvalues) within a selected volume.
- *Axial diffusivity* (AD) or *parallel diffusivity* ($\lambda_{//}$) measured from the diffusivity parallel to the first eigenvector, on the other hand, is inferred to indicate axonal integrity as a measure of fiber diameter and organization.

Of note, ADC can be viewed as an average of these two diffusivity values, RD and AD.

5.2 Clinical Applications

DTI provides detailed anatomical information about the status and directionality of white matter tracts. Because integrated coordination of neural

Table 5.2 Commonly used diffusion tensor imaging metrics and their correlates

Diffusion tensor imaging measure	Quantification	Details
Fractional anisotropy (FA)	$\sqrt{\frac{1}{2}}\dfrac{\sqrt{(\lambda_1-\lambda_2)^2+(\lambda_2-\lambda_3)^2+(\lambda_3-\lambda_1)^2}}{\sqrt{\lambda_1^2+\lambda_2^2+\lambda_3^2}}$	- Calculation involving the diffusivity differences - Values of 0 represent a spherical tensor and 1, an ellipsoid tensor - Provides information on microstructure integrity - Regarded as most robust DTI statistic
Mean diffusivity (MD)	$(\lambda_1+\lambda_2+\lambda_3)\,/\,3$	- Average of eigenvector diffusivities - Provides information on microstructure integrity
Radial diffusivity (RD) - Perpendicular diffusivity	$\dfrac{(\lambda_2+\lambda_3)}{2}$	- Diffusivity perpendicular to the primary eigenvector - Primary contributor to FA - Reflects myelin integrity
Axial diffusivity (AD) - Parallel diffusivity - Longitudinal diffusivity	λ_1	- Diffusion parallel to the primary eigenvector - Influenced by axonal diameter and number

Table 5.3 Spectrum of aging, cognitive impairment and dementia

	Clinical manifestation
Cognitively normal aging	Optimal aging without manifestations of memory loss or cognitive impairment on neuropsychological testing
Normal aging	Generally thought to include self-perceived memory loss without cognitive deficits relative to peers, but may include poorer performance relative to younger cohorts
Mild cognitive impairment (MCI)	An ambiguous definition that includes individuals thought to perform between normal aging and dementia; generally regarded as a transitional period prior to dementia
Amnestic mild cognitive impairment (aMCI)	Subclassification of MCI where individuals demonstrate prominent memory impairment symptoms; these individuals are at greatest risk of Alzheimer disease out of the general MCI population
Dementia	Generic classification for cognitive impairment that interferes with daily functioning; includes cognitive impairments in addition to memory deficits
Alzheimer disease	Most common form of dementia with hallmark neurodegenerative changes definitively diagnosed on autopsy, although frequently diagnosed clinically; targeted amyloid positron emission tomographic imaging is presently available for presumptive diagnosis

Source: Adapted from Small GW, Bookheimer SY, Thompson PM, et al. Current and future uses of neuroimaging for cognitively impaired patients. Lancet neurology. 2008;7(2):161-172. doi:10.1016/S1474-4422(08)70019-X.

activity across distant brain regions is essential to cognition, ascertaining axonal integrity could provide insight into the mechanisms by which cognitive functions are disrupted. Elucidating the basis of cognitive decline is an important problem in the clinical assessment of elderly individuals, which is becoming of pressing concern in most developed countries where aging demographics are generating large burdens on health care and the economy. Determining whether worsening reaction time or memory is related to mild cognitive impairment or "old age" versus a more debilitating dementia, such as Alzheimer disease, provides important information for patients and their families and can guide appropriate treatment strategies. Presently, the clinical definitions of cognitive aging and impairment are varied (▶ Fig. 5.3) and may not correspond well with objective measures. DTI may better assess the degree of neurodegeneration as a surrogate measure of white matter architectural integrity that correlates with pathology. Although not a functional imaging modality, the white matter pathways described by DTI serve as the conduits by which activity in brain networks occurs and may provide some information on functional pathways.[2] Therefore, changes in DTI mirror alterations in functional networks that may be responsible for cognitive decline in aging and dementia.

The application of DTI clinically to the aging patient with cognitive decline or symptoms of dementia remains difficult. Nevertheless, there have been significant advances in the past decade that facilitate the use of DTI to answer clinical questions of differentiating between types of dementia. Most of the earlier studies that provide the fundamental basis for what is known about DTI changes in specific dementia types are based on the comparison of multiple individuals with dementia versus controls using groupwise analysis methods. More recent studies offer evidence to support the use of single-subject DTI studies to diagnose individual patients with neurodegenerative dementias.[3]

5.2.1 Normal Aging

Because white matter volume does not appear to decrease as much as gray matter volumes with aging, volumetric magnetic resonance imaging (MRI) analyses of white matter loss are inadequate to assess the aging brain.[4] Likewise, white matter hyperintense lesion burden does not appear to consistently account for cognitive decline. DTI addresses this limitation by ascertaining the finer detail of subtle changes within axonal structures. As discussed in Chapter 4, normal white matter development leads to MD reduction and FA increase over normal development to middle age, which corresponds to axonal development and myelination with greater time spent maturing frontal–temporal connections.[5] In later age, these developmental changes reverse, with decreasing anisotropy and increasing diffusivity values globally. Both abnormal and normal adult aging may lead to significant decline in white matter organization.[6] While aging changes appear global and symmetric, some have shown the greatest FA decline within the corpus callosum, frontal, limbic, and temporal lobes, although these same regions have the highest anisotropy initially.[1,6] More

specifically, most literature supports an anterior-predominant gradient of FA decline and diffusivity increase (MD, AD, and RD) with age.[7] ▶ Fig. 5.2 demonstrates the normal patterns of aging-related FA and MD changes across several brain regions. Furthermore, application of Fiber density mapping (FDM) to the aging brain reinforces these findings, which were observed to occur globally within white matter to a greater extent within anterior versus posterior regions.[1] Thus it appears that frontal regions are both the latest to develop in maturation and likewise the most susceptible to functional decline in the later years of life, which also concurs with clinical findings of executive (frontal) dysfunction.[8]

Pathophysiology of DTI Changes in Aging

With aging, myelin layers continue to be added with redundant myelin, and this myelin may be formed by oligodendrocytes in a manner making it vulnerable to healthy myelin formed by oligodendrocytes earlier in life. Myelin loss with both declining number and length of myelinated axonal fibers and demyelination are implicated in FA loss and increased diffusivity with increased extracellular space (▶ Fig. 5.3). Another mechanism by which increased diffusion may occur with aging is via splitting of myelin and cavitation within myelin sheaths, thereby also producing increased extracellular space encouraging free diffusion.[8]

5.2.2 Mild Cognitive Impairment

Over the last decade, many studies have demonstrated white matter integrity correlates for neurocognitive deficits seen with aging as described in the preceding section. Defining the distinction between mild cognitive impairment (MCI) and normal aging and discerning at what point MCI progresses into Alzheimer disease are challenging tasks that are not amenable to clear, objective stages. This heterogeneity therefore poses a serious obstacle to integration of DTI studies of MCI because individual studies include participants at varying stages on the aging–cognitive decline–dementia spectrum (the definitions of which differ among investigators). DTI studies of MCI demonstrate widespread changes in diffusion metrics throughout much of the white matter (▶ Fig. 5.4).[9] Therefore, DTI may not enhance our understanding of MCI if analyzed generally without delving

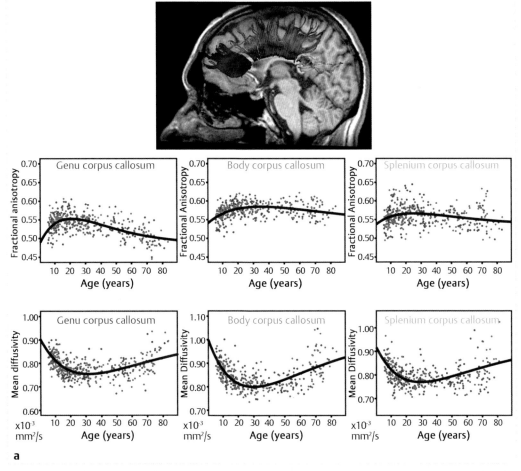

Fig. 5.2 Plots of fractional anisotropy (FA) and mean diffusivity changes with age. (a) The corpus callosum is a vital component of white matter architecture for cognitive function and degeneration is implicated in worsening cognitive measures including reaction time. FA peaks in adulthood and decreases with aging, to a greater extent within the anterior portions. (*continued*)

further into the specific deficits and white matter structures involved.

Association between Specific Cognitive Functions and Diffusion Changes

One of the fundamental clinical concerns regarding aging is the effect of white matter disorganization on cognitive performance. A study of cognitively normal adults observed a statistically significant correlation between increasing reaction time and decreasing FA (particularly, the corpus callosum, superior longitudinal fasciculus, and inferior fronto-occipital fasciculus).[10] These

particular regions correlate with executive function, language tasks, association pathways, and memory. Other variables, including white matter volume or hyperintense lesions, did not explain this relationship.[10] Another study examining typically aging adults using DTI noted that processing speed is more closely associated with cerebral FA than are other cognitive measures, even accounting for age.[11] In this study, global cerebral MD, AD, and RD are associated with cognitive flexibility, and reasoning is associated with prefrontal AD.[11] White matter integrity influences age-related deterioration of cognitive functions by decreasing the speed and efficiency of axonal pathways. In addition, these findings are robust for the specific cognitive domain involved—they are independent

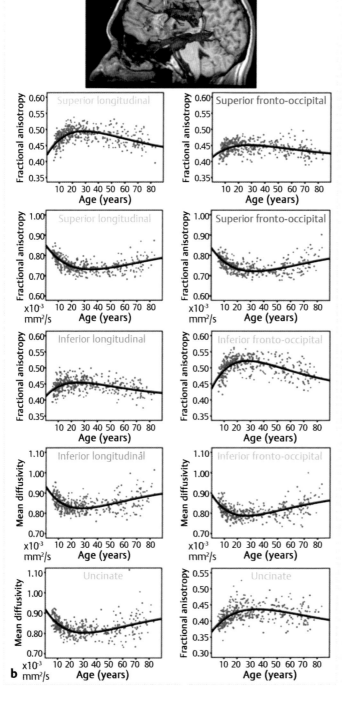

(*continued*) (**b**) Association fibers are integral to the organization of neural activity, and white matter integrity within these fibers preserves higher-order cognition. As in the corpus callosum, FA peaks and mean diffusivity (MD) troughs occur in early adulthood. FA decreases and MD increases with age are slightly greater within the frontal association fibers. (Reproduced with permission from Lebel et al,[5] copyright Elsevier Ltd, 2012.)

Normal axons

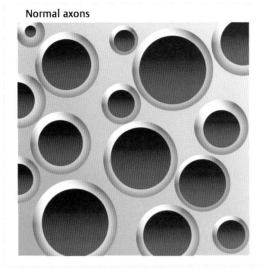

Aging axons

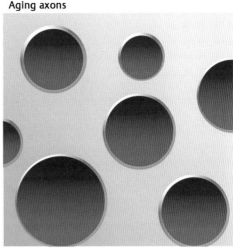

Fig. 5.3 Comparison of normal axons and aging axons. Normal axon integrity exhibits a dense, rich microstructure with normal myelination and little extracellular space. In comparison, the aging brain demonstrates axonal loss and dysmyelination that results in thinning of the myelin sheath and increased extracellular space. The increase in extracellular space and the decreased hindrance of diffusion presented by decreased axonal size and number results in increased diffusivity with age.

of the aging process, arguing for individual clinical significance in the elderly patient with a cognitive deficit.[12]

Across aging, FA corresponds to performance on examinations of balance and gait, suggesting a close relationship between white matter integrity and functional measures that are important indicators of function in the elderly.[13] White matter changes related to aging are diverse and may be affected by many factors. Alcoholic individuals, for example, show FA reductions in key white matter tracts (▶ Fig. 5.5) that inversely correspond to memory dysfunction scores.[14]

Just as these changes may be accelerated by health factors, these alterations are not inexorable, and they may even be ameliorated by health status and cognitive training. One study of elderly master athletes demonstrates increased FA in several regions (right corona radiata and longitudinal fasciculus) compared to sedentary, age-matched counterparts.[15] This and other studies suggest that physical fitness could encourage preservation of regions critical to motor control and visuospatial functions. In a study of memory training, researchers observed alterations in the rate of change of anterior FA with memory improvement compared to controls over an 8 week period, thereby suggesting that neurocognitive training can encourage white matter microstructural conservation.[16]

5.2.3 Alzheimer Disease

As a neurodegenerative disease, Alzheimer disease entails several pathophysiological changes affecting neurons and axons, with the deposition of beta-amyloid and tau representing two major components. Inevitably, axonal loss and injury are the result of these degenerative changes that ultimately culminate with cognitive dysfunction and severe dementia. The ability of imaging indices to detect Alzheimer disease at earlier stages may, in the future, allow for interventions that could alter the trajectory of functional impairment. Even though targeted imaging methods such as florbetapir (^{18}F) are now available to image amyloid effectively, the presence of amyloid alone does not definitively diagnose Alzheimer disease, and the addition of DTI could improve sensitivity of amyloid imaging methods.[17,18] Moreover, neurodegenerative changes and clinical symptoms of dementia may proceed independent of amyloid accumulation.[19]

One difficulty in ascertaining DTI changes in dementias is the concomitant aging-related changes that may be superimposed on pathophysiology. Changes in white matter cytoarchitecture in dementia should not be regarded as simply progression or exaggeration of normal aging phenomena.[12]

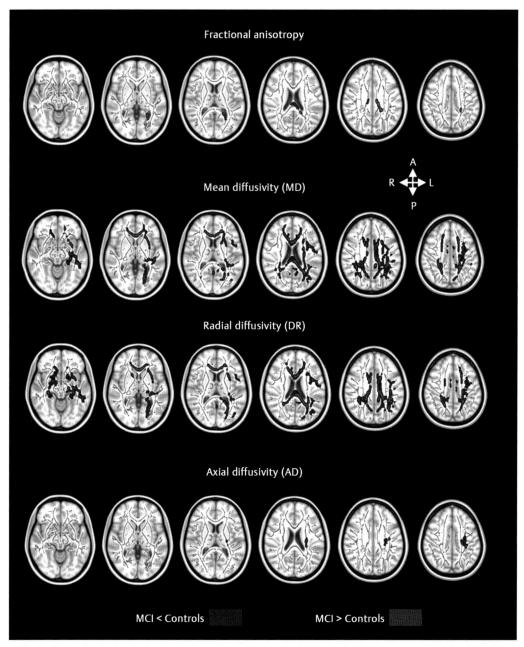

Fig. 5.4 Diffusion imaging metrics in mild cognitive impairment (MCI). Differences in white matter microstructure detected by diffusion tensor imaging in patients with MCI. Different diffusion metrics can be used to differentiate patients with MCI from healthy controls. Effects are often especially strong for mean diffusivity and radial diffusivity. (Reproduced with permission from Amlien and Fjell,[9] copyright Elsevier 2014.)

The white matter deterioration seen in Alzheimer disease and perhaps its prodromal manifestations is thought to reflect axonal fiber loss and Wallerian degeneration mostly, as suggested by greater increases in RD than AD. The theory of Wallerian degeneration assumes the loss of gray matter prior to white matter changes, a finding that is subject to much debate but is supported by a large meta-analysis of DTI studies in Alzheimer disease and MCI.[20] Still others suggest that effects

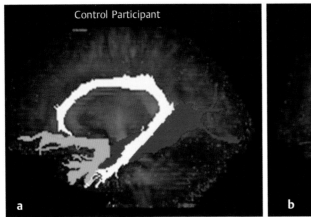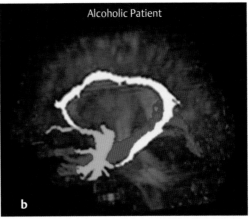

Fig. 5.5 Diffusion tensor imaging abnormalities in alcoholism. Projections of the right inferior longitudinal fasciculus (magenta), cingulum (yellow), and uncinate fasciculus (green) in (**a**) a patient with alcoholism compared with a (**b**) control participant. These regions are decreased in size and fractional anisotropy values, which are associated with memory dysfunction score. (Reproduced with permission from Trivedi et al,[14] copyright Elsevier Ltd, 2013.)

on the white matter microstructure occur early on in Alzheimer disease and that gray matter atrophy with subsequent Wallerian degeneration of white matter does not adequately account for white matter changes seen on DTI.[9]

Even despite the presence of multiple studies confirming significant changes in diffusion properties in Alzheimer disease, the clinical application of these findings to individual patients remains difficult. Changes in Alzheimer disease in a single-subject study were greatest within the posterior cingulate and posterior parietotemporal region, but were relatively minor, pointing to the challenges of detecting subtle changes using DTI on an individual basis.[3] Nevertheless, in many cases the findings of white matter atrophy can be striking, even on an individual patient level ▶ Fig. 5.6. Prominent corpus callosal thinning was seen in a patient with Alzheimer disease when compared with an age-matched healthy individual.[21] However, others have identified significant association of Mini-Mental State Examination scores with precuneal FA changes suggesting that the observed white matter degeneration observed in Alzheimer disease has a direct clinical impact on cognitive function.[22]

Increased diffusivity, specifically MD, within the hippocampus has been proposed as a marker of worsening memory performance and perhaps an indicator of early Alzheimer disease, because tau accumulation occurs first within the hippocampus[23]; MD appears to perform slightly better

than FA in classifying individuals with Alzheimer disease versus normal aging, and adding MD to hippocampal atrophy accurately predicts mild Alzheimer disease versus aging.[11,12] These microstructural white matter changes may also occur in aging within the parahippocampal white matter (▶ Fig. 5.7), which may explain memory deficits in aging, and this overlap slightly complicates solitary application of white matter indices of the hippocampus in diagnosing Alzheimer disease.[24] Nevertheless, others argue white matter deterioration marked by increased diffusivity alone is sufficient and manifests to a greater extent within the hippocampal region in prodromal and mild Alzheimer disease than aging. A study of patients with amnestic MCI suggested that FA reduction or MD increase in the cingulum bundle in particular as an indicator of severe amnestic MCI (aMCI) that will likely progress to Alzheimer disease.[25] Quantitative tractography of apolipoprotein E (ApoE4) carriers at greater risk of developing Alzheimer disease reveals shorter fiber tract lengths in the uncinate fasciculus where other studies previously identified increased MD in the cingulum bundle and corpus callosum in healthy carriers.[26]

Taken together, these studies all suggest that a combination of gray matter atrophy and white matter disruption within parahippocampal and other white matter tracts are implicated in the progression of MCI to Alzheimer disease. These imaging findings could influence the clinical

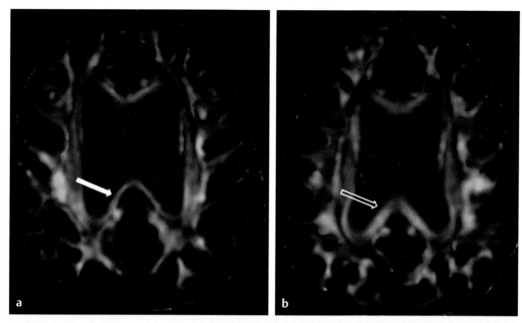

Fig. 5.6 Individual subject comparison of diffusion tensor imaging (DTI) maps in Alzheimer disease (AD). Color-coded map in an 83-year-old with AD (**a**) demonstrates prominent atrophy of the corpus callosum (solid arrow), compared with an 86-year-old normal volunteer (**b**) (open arrow). DTI has allowed greater understanding of the effects of AD in the commissural and association white matter tracts. (Reproduced with permission from Huston and Field,[21] copyright Elsevier 2013.)

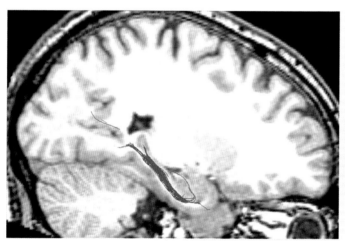

Fig. 5.7 Targeted use of parahippocampal white matter in Alzheimer disease. This figure exemplifies diffusion tensor imaging–based delineation of white matter fiber tracts extending from the parahippocampal white matter. White matter integrity changes may occur as a product of aging, although they can potentially be affected to a greater extent in Alzheimer disease. (Reproduced with permission from Rogalski et al,[24] copyright Elsevier 2012.)

diagnosis of individuals presenting with aMCI or carrying known genetic risk factors for Alzheimer disease. Although no such effective interventions have come to fruition as of yet, imaging with DTI will inevitably also serve a role in assessing treatment response and even perhaps provide information vital to the development of targeted therapeutics for Alzheimer disease.

5.2.4 Other Dementias

Differentiating between specific dementias may influence clinical decision making regarding prognosis and therapy. Although fewer resources have been dedicated to the investigation of less common dementias compared to Alzheimer disease, there have still been significant advances in

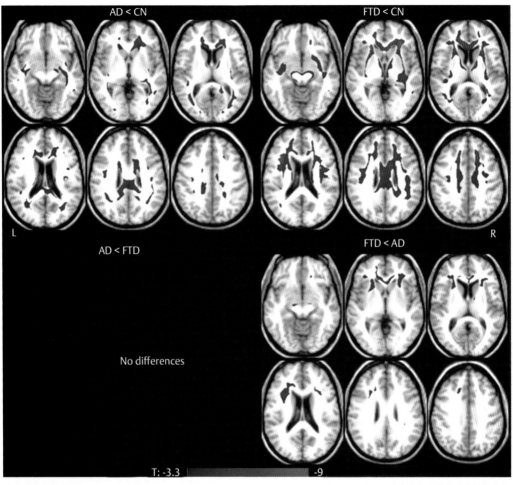

Fig. 5.8 Comparison of frontotemporal dementia (FTD) and Alzheimer disease (AD). Significance maps of systematic brain abnormalities in FTD and AD patients relative to control subjects (CN) (AD < CN and FTD < CN), and direct comparisons between AD and FTD (AD < FTD and FTD < AD). Reduced white matter (WM) fractional anisotropy (FA) (blue color) in AD or FTD overlaid on an axial brain template. FTD patients had widespread FA reductions in frontal and temporal lobes, anterior corpus callosum, and anterior cingulum. Compared to AD, FTD patients had significantly decreased FA values bilaterally in frontal deep WM, anterior corpus callosum, and anterior cingulum. (Reproduced with permission from, open access copyright Zhang et al.[27])

appreciating white matter disruption in a variety of dementia conditions.

Frontotemporal Dementia

Frontotemporal dementia (FTD) is a major constituent of early dementias and may be confused with early-onset Alzheimer disease. A comparison of FTD with Alzheimer disease not surprisingly revealed a greater reduction of FA within frontal regions in FTD (▶ Fig. 5.8)[27]; unlike Alzheimer disease, FTD entails more prominent white matter degeneration. More generally, increased diffusivity

(MD) was seen throughout much of the frontal and temporal lobes in behavioral variant FTD compared to controls.[28] Selective FA reduction has been demonstrated within the superior longitudinal fasciculus in frontal variant FTD, whereas this decrease occurred in the inferior longitudinal fasciculus for temporal variant FTD.[29]

Dementia with Lewy Bodies

Dementia with Lewy bodies (DLB) is another form of neurodegenerative dementia closely related to Alzheimer disease and may overlap clinically with other dementias. DTI is particularly well-suited to DLB because atrophy is not a leading component as in other dementias, and white matter indices may be more helpful than volumetric assessments of atrophy. DTI demonstrates preliminary utility in identifying differences between DLB and Alzheimer disease where DLB selectively involves substantially reduced FA in the precuneus and parieto-occipital tracts involved in visual association in comparison to more diffuse changes observed in Alzheimer disease (▶ Fig. 5.9).[22,30] Diffusivity within the amygdala in DLB also corresponds well with a common measure of parkinsonism motor symptoms.[22] There is a significant decrease in FA within the parahippocampal gyri in Alzheimer disease compared to DLB that aids in distinguishing between these two similar forms of dementia.[30] Although bearing much overlap, early research suggests DTI is capable of differentiating between the neurodegenerative dementias.

Vascular Dementia

Another common cause of cognitive decline is vascular dementia. Because cerebrovascular disease is common in the elderly (including individuals with Alzheimer disease) differentiating vascular dementia from other dementias is an important dilemma. The use of diffusion imaging in vascular disease is an important topic in itself and will be explored in greater detail in the next chapter. Patients with vascular dementia and Alzheimer dementia have regional differences of white matter integrity, with selective reduction of FA in the forceps minor (transcallosal fibers through the genu of the corpus callosum in vascular dementia).[31]

Progressive Supranuclear Palsy

Progressive supranuclear palsy (PSP), although generally manifesting with distinct clinical symptoms, may be confused for Parkinson disease and other conditions, particularly early in the disease process. Therefore, DTI may be helpful in making the diagnosis. In PSP, FA is reduced and MD is increased within the body of the corpus callosum, cingulum, and frontal white matter.[32] In another study of PSP, a selected pattern of decreased FA and increased ADC within the inferior fronto-occipital fasciculus corresponded to severity of frontal cognitive symptoms and personality change in one study.[33] Similarly, a single subject–based DTI study

demonstrated that individuals with either corticobasal degeneration (another Parkinson plus syndrome with prominent motor symptoms) or progressive supranuclear palsy demonstrated widespread FA reductions with an anterior predominance, but did not identify any difference between these two conditions.[3] More recent work showed PSP to have a more symmetric and infratentorial pattern of FA reduction when compared to corticobasal degeneration, despite much overlap (▶ Fig. 5.10).[32] These findings, if validated, could potentially be helpful in distinguishing the two syndromes clinically. One particularly useful conclusion of this study was progression of individuals with nonfluent aphasia to corticobasal degeneration or progressive supranuclear palsy could be predicted by the presence of widespread increased RD and decreased FA on initial DTI examination.[3]

Other Dementias

Although the majority of dementia cases are of Alzheimer etiology, there are a few less common dementia syndromes that may present with unusual symptoms and may be difficult to diagnose. DTI could potentially aid in diagnosing these conditions in order to optimize treatment and prognostication. Posterior cortical atrophy is yet another neurodegenerative disease and is characterized by complex visual functions abnormalities, including acalculia, agnosia, and visual field deficits. This condition appears to occur with atrophy, particularly within the occipital lobe that progresses. DTI has been used to ascertain FA reductions within the occipital lobe and document later involvement of both occipital and parietal lobes within an individual patient—a finding that is distinct from Alzheimer disease, thereby allowing clinical evidence to support a clinical diagnosis of posterior cortical atrophy (▶ Fig. 5.11).[34] Other dementias may be amenable to analysis with DTI, and future research may unveil subtle subtypes within more common neurodegenerative dementias that may have prognostic and pharmacological implications. Much more research is needed to address both the specificity of diffusion imaging findings in dementia types as well as their ramifications for clinical management.

5.3 Summary

- Alterations in the quality of axonal connections in the brain affects neural connectivity and thereby influences cognitive performance.

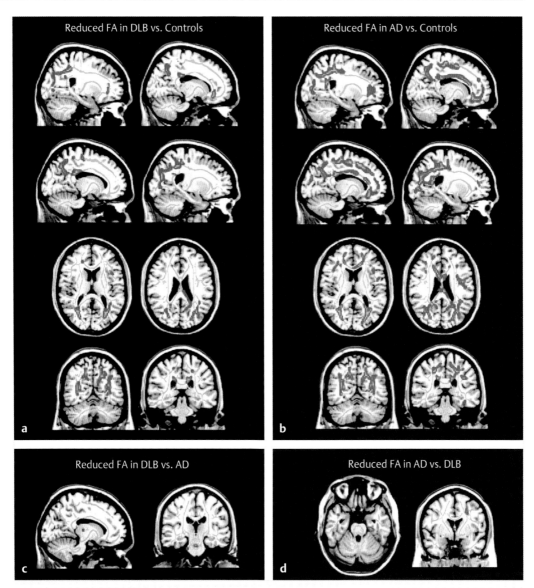

Fig. 5.9 Fractional anisotropy (FA) changes between Alzheimer disease (AD) and dementia with Lewy bodies (DLB). Tract-based spatial statistics maps indicating areas of reduced FA (blue) in DLB and AD (blue), overlaid onto the Montreal Neurological Institute template image and mean FA skeleton (green). (**a**) DLB versus controls: change was identified mainly in the parieto-occipital areas (precuneal and cingulate gyri). Reduced FA in the temporal lobes was in a region of the posterior thalamic radiation that included the optic radiation ($p < 0.05$, corrected). (**b**) AD versus controls: change was more widespread than in DLB and included clusters in the temporal, parieto-occipital, and frontal lobes ($p < 0.05$, corrected). (**c**) DLB versus AD: reduced FA in the pons and left thalamus ($p < 0.05$). (**d**) AD versus DLB: small clusters of reduced FA in the parahippocampal gyri, frontal lobes, and fornix (p < 0.05). (Reproduced with permission from Watson et al,[30] copyright Wolters Kluwer Health, 2012.)

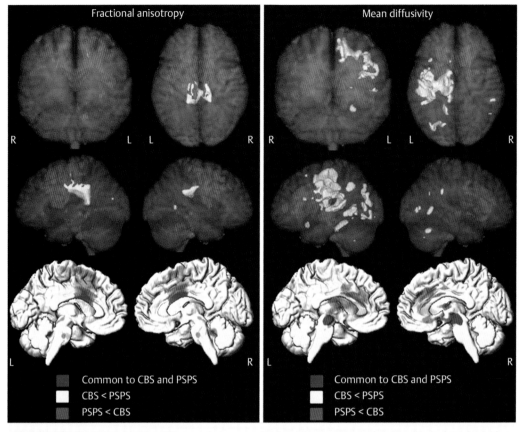

Fig. 5.10 Diffusion tensor imaging differences between corticobasal degeneration and progressive supranuclear palsy. Three-dimensional brain renderings showing regions of overlap and difference between corticobasal degeneration syndrome (CBS) and progressive supranuclear palsy syndrome (PSPS) with much overlap in corpus callosum and frontal white matter changes. Generally, PSPS demonstrated a more infratentorial predominance and was more symmetric than CBS. Results are shown on transparent brain renderings showing front, top, left, and right views, and medial surface renderings (bottom row). Inclusive masking was used to identify regions common to CBS and PSPS (red), and direct comparisons were used to identify regions with greater degeneration in CBS compared to PSPS (yellow), and regions with greater degeneration in PSPS compared to CBS (blue). Results are shown separately for fractional anisotropy and mean diffusivity. L, left/more involved hemisphere; R, right/less involved hemisphere. (Reproduced with permission from Whitwell et al,[32] copyright Elsevier Ltd, 2014.)

- Aging in late adulthood demonstrates deterioration in white matter cytoarchitecture, which is measured noninvasively as declining anisotropy and increasing diffusivity on DTI studies. These changes demonstrate a frontal–posterior gradient in normal aging and may be mitigated by physical and cognitive training.
- DTI can discern differences in white matter integrity in normal aging compared to mild cognitive impairment and Alzheimer disease.
- Alzheimer disease may be suggested by the combination of hippocampal atrophy and disruption of the neighboring parahippocampal white matter tracts.
- Research into DTI-based correlates of white matter integrity in normal aging and dementia may provide improved prognostication and could offer targets for therapeutic intervention in the future.
- The diagnosis of less common and unusual dementia presentations may be aided by the presence of specific sites of involvement on DTI.

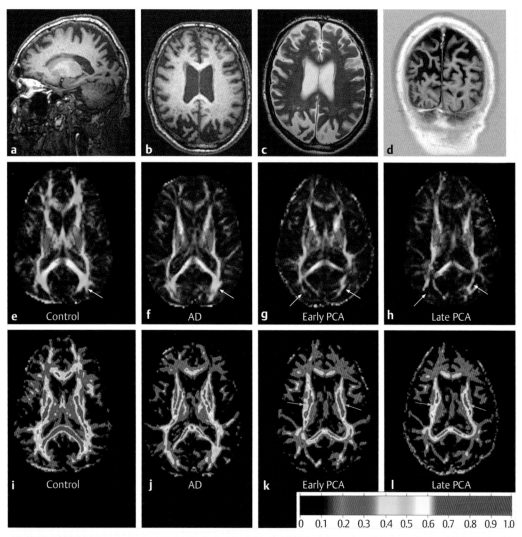

Fig. 5.11 Diffusion tensor imaging in posterior cortical atrophy (PCA) compared to Alzheimer disease (AD). Magnetic resonance images of the patient with posterior cortical atrophy (PCA) showing a global atrophy with occipitoparietal predominance; (a) sagittal and (b) axial T1-weighted three-dimensional two-field echo sequence, (c) axial T2-weighted sequence, and (d) coronal T1-inversion recovery image. (e) fractional anisotropy (FA) maps of a healthy control, (f) a representative patient with AD, (g) and early PCA, and (h) a later PCA, fiber directions (red: left–right, green: anterior–posterior, blue: inferior–superior). (i–l) FA in pseudocolors. Compared with the AD patient and controls, PCA showed a substantial FA reduction in bilateral occipital lobes (white arrows). Whereas the FA reduction in the occipital white matter in the patient with PCA remained stable over a period of 15 months, the overall FA values further decreased, particularly within parietal regions. (Reproduced with permission from Duning et al,[34] copyright BMJ Publishing Group, Inc. 2009.)

References

[1] Stadlbauer A, Ganslandt O, Salomonowitz E, et al. Magnetic resonance fiber density mapping of age-related white matter changes. Eur J Radiol 2012; 81(12); 4005–4012

[2] Greicius MD, Supekar K, Menon V, Dougherty RF. Resting-state functional connectivity reflects structural connectivity in the default mode network. Cereb Cortex 2009; 19(1): 72–78

[3] Sajjadi SA, Acosta-Cabronero J, Patterson K, Diaz-de-Grenu LZ, Williams GB, Nestor PJ. Diffusion tensor magnetic resonance imaging for single subject diagnosis in neurodegenerative diseases. Brain 2013; 136(Pt 7): 2253–2261

[4] Pfefferbaum A, Mathalon DH, Sullivan EV, Rawles JM, Zipursky RB, Lim KO. A quantitative magnetic resonance imaging study of changes in brain morphology from infancy to late adulthood. Arch Neurol 1994; 51(9): 874–887

[5] Lebel C, Gee M, Camicioli R, Wieler M, Martin W, Beaulieu C. Diffusion tensor imaging of white matter tract evolution over the lifespan. Neuroimage 2012; 60(1): 340–352

[6] Moseley M. Diffusion tensor imaging and aging–a review. NMR Biomed 2002; 15(7–8): 553–560

[7] Sullivan EV, Pfefferbaum A. Diffusion tensor imaging and aging. Neurosci Biobehav Rev 2006; 30(6): 749–761

[8] Sullivan EV, Pfefferbaum A. Neuroradiological characterization of normal adult ageing. Br J Radiol 2007; 80(Spec No 2): S99–S108

[9] Amlien IK, Fjell AM. Diffusion tensor imaging of white matter degeneration in Alzheimer's disease and mild cognitive impairment. Neuroscience 2014; 276: 206–215

[10] Kerchner GA, Racine CA, Hale S, et al. Cognitive processing speed in older adults: relationship with white matter integrity. PLoS ONE 2012; 7(11): e50425

[11] Borghesani PR, Madhyastha TM, Aylward EH, et al. The association between higher order abilities, processing speed, and age are variably mediated by white matter integrity during typical aging. Neuropsychologia 2013; 51(8): 1435–1444

[12] Madden DJ, Bennett IJ, Song AW. Cerebral white matter integrity and cognitive aging: contributions from diffusion tensor imaging. Neuropsychol Rev 2009; 19(4): 415–435

[13] Sullivan EV, Adalsteinsson E, Hedehus M, et al. Equivalent disruption of regional white matter microstructure in ageing healthy men and women. Neuroreport 2001; 12(1): 99–104

[14] Trivedi R, Bagga D, Bhattacharya D, et al. White matter damage is associated with memory decline in chronic alcoholics: a quantitative diffusion tensor tractography study. Behav Brain Res 2013; 250: 192–198

[15] Tseng BY, Gundapuneedi T, Khan MA, et al. White matter integrity in physically fit older adults. Neuroimage 2013; 82: 510–516

[16] Engvig A, Fjell AM, Westlye LT, et al. Memory training impacts short-term changes in aging white matter: a longitudinal diffusion tensor imaging study. Hum Brain Mapp 2012; 33(10): 2390–2406

[17] Witte MM, Trzepacz P, Case M, et al. Association between clinical measures and florbetapir F18 PET neuroimaging in mild or moderate Alzheimer's disease dementia. J Neuropsychiatry Clin Neurosci 2014; 26(3): 214–220

[18] Clark CM, Pontecorvo MJ, Beach TG, et al. AV-45-A16 Study Group. Cerebral PET with florbetapir compared with neuropathology at autopsy for detection of neuritic amyloid-β plaques: a prospective cohort study. Lancet Neurol 2012; 11(8): 669–678

[19] Rabinovici GD, Jagust WJ. Amyloid imaging in aging and dementia: testing the amyloid hypothesis in vivo. Behav Neurol 2009; 21(1): 117–128

[20] Sexton CE, Kalu UG, Filippini N, Mackay CE, Ebmeier KP. A meta-analysis of diffusion tensor imaging in mild cognitive impairment and Alzheimer's disease. Neurobiol Aging 2011; 32(12): 2322.e5–2322.e18

[21] Huston JM, Field AS. Clinical applications of diffusion tensor imaging. Magn Reson Imaging Clin N Am 2013; 21(2): 279–298

[22] O'Donovan J, Watson R, Colloby SJ, Blamire AM, O'Brien JT. Assessment of regional MR diffusion changes in dementia with Lewy bodies and Alzheimer's disease. Int Psychogeriatr 2014; 26(4): 627–635

[23] den Heijer T, der Lijn Fv, Vernooij MW, et al. Structural and diffusion MRI measures of the hippocampus and memory performance. Neuroimage 2012; 63(4): 1782–1789

[24] Rogalski E, Stebbins GT, Barnes CA, et al. Age-related changes in parahippocampal white matter integrity: a diffusion tensor imaging study. Neuropsychologia 2012; 50(8): 1759–1765

[25] Liu J, Yin C, Xia S, et al. White matter changes in patients with amnestic mild cognitive impairment detected by diffusion tensor imaging. PLoS ONE 2013; 8(3): e59440

[26] Salminen LE, Schofield PR, Lane EM, et al. Neuronal fiber bundle lengths in healthy adult carriers of the ApoE4 allele: a quantitative tractography DTI study. Brain Imaging Behav 2013; 7(3): 274–281

[27] Zhang Y, Schuff N, Ching C, et al. Joint Assessment of Structural, Perfusion, and Diffusion MRI in Alzheimer's Disease and Frontotemporal Dementia. International Journal of Alzheimer's Disease 2011: Article ID 546871, 11 pages

[28] Whitwell JL, Avula R, Senjem ML, et al. Gray and white matter water diffusion in the syndromic variants of frontotemporal dementia. Neurology 2010; 74(16): 1279–1287

[29] Borroni B, Brambati SM, Agosti C, et al. Evidence of white matter changes on diffusion tensor imaging in frontotemporal dementia. Arch Neurol 2007; 64(2): 246–251

[30] Watson R, Blamire AM, Colloby SJ, et al. Characterizing dementia with Lewy bodies by means of diffusion tensor imaging. Neurology 2012; 79(9): 906–914

[31] Zarei M, Damoiseaux JS, Morgese C, et al. Regional white matter integrity differentiates between vascular dementia and Alzheimer disease. Stroke 2009; 40(3): 773–779

[32] Whitwell JL, Schwarz CG, Reid RI, Kantarci K, Jack CR, Jr, Josephs KA. Diffusion tensor imaging comparison of progressive supranuclear palsy and corticobasal syndromes. Parkinsonism Relat Disord 2014; 20(5): 493–498

[33] Kvickström P, Eriksson B, van Westen D, Lätt J, Elfgren C, Nilsson C. Selective frontal neurodegeneration of the inferior fronto-occipital fasciculus in progressive supranuclear palsy (PSP) demonstrated by diffusion tensor tractography. BMC Neurol 2011; 11: 13

[34] Duning T, Warnecke T, Mohammadi S, et al. Pattern and progression of white-matter changes in a case of posterior cortical atrophy using diffusion tensor imaging. J Neurol Neurosurg Psychiatry 2009; 80(4): 432–436

[35] Small GW, Bookheimer SY, Thompson PM, et al. Current and future uses of neuroimaging for cognitively impaired patients. Lancet neurology 2008; 7(2): 161–172. doi:10.1016/S1474-4422(08)70019-X

6 Diffusion Weighted Imaging in Vascular Pathology

Sangam Kanekar and Chandan Misra

Key Points

- Cytotoxic edema is seen within minutes to hours on diffusion weighted images (DWI) with sensitivity and specificity of 88 to 100% and 86 to 100%, respectively.
- Cortical watershed infarcts are thought to be the result of microembolization, either from carotid artery atherosclerosis vulnerable plaque or from artery-to-artery emboli precipitated by an episode of systemic arterial hypotension. Internal watershed infarcts are caused by a combination of hypoperfusion of the internal border zone, severe carotid disease, and a hemodynamic event.
- The sensitivity and specificity of DWI for the diagnosis of acute lacunar infarction are 94.9% and 94.1%, respectively.
- It is important to diagnose transient ischemic attack (TIA) because the short-term risk of stroke following TIA is greatest within the first 48 hours (5.3%).
- Cytotoxic edema in cerebral venous thrombosis (CVT) is thought to be due to reduced cerebral blood flow (CBF) below the penumbra level, which in turn leads to failure of the sodium-potassium-adenosine triphosphate–dependent pump.

6.1 Introduction

Diffusion weighted imaging (DWI) is an advanced imaging technique that allows noninvasive evaluation of water diffusibility in the brain tissue. It is sensitive to the random translational motion of water molecules due to brownian motion. This property of DWI has revolutionized the imaging of vascular pathologies, stroke in particular.

Diffusion weighted images (DWIs) are generated by adding an opposing pair (first tagging and then second untagging) of diffusion gradients to spin-echo or echo planar sequences. For stationary molecules (e.g., stroke), the effects of the tagging and the untagging gradient pulses cancel each other out. This "restricted diffusion" appears hyperintense to normal tissue on DWI. In normal brain tissue, where the molecules are mobile, there is

incomplete rephrasing resulting in a net phase shift, which leads to a signal loss. The degree of signal loss is proportional to the exponent of the diffusion coefficient and to the duration, distance, and strength of the applied diffusion gradients (the so-called b value). The diffusion coefficient measured by DWI is referred to as the apparent diffusion coefficient (ADC) rather than the true diffusion coefficient.

With the advent of intravenous and intra-arterial thrombolytic therapy, the definition of hyperacute stroke has gained significant popularity. As per various trials across the globe, a therapeutic window (4–6 h) has been identified for the treatment of stroke, emphasizing the importance of early diagnosis. The concept of "time is brain" forced us to look at the avenues that can diagnose the early changes in the brain following stroke. DWI has revolutionized the imaging of stroke by identifying cytotoxic edema within minutes of the onset of a stroke. As such, DWI has become the driving force for the diagnosis of the vascular pathologies. Besides diagnosing large territorial strokes, DWI allows for the differentiation of acute stroke from chronic stroke and from nonspecific white matter lesions. DWI also facilitates the detection of very small ischemic lesions, small lacunar infarcts, punctate cortical infarcts, and even small lesions in patients with transient ischemic attacks (TIAs), which are difficult to diagnose on computed tomographic (CT) scans and the T2 and fluid-attenuated inversion recovery (FLAIR) sequences of magnetic resonance imaging (MRI). Multiplicity distribution and other ancillary findings on MRI might help in identifying the underlying etiology of the stroke. This chapter discusses the application of DWI in the diagnosis of various vascular pathologies and their mimics.

6.2 Acute Stroke and Diffusion Weighted Imaging

6.2.1 Introduction

Diagnosing hyperacute stroke or differentiating stroke from its mimics is of vital importance for the appropriate therapy. Two main imaging techniques employed in evaluation of hyperacute stroke include CT-CT perfusion and MR-MR perfusion.

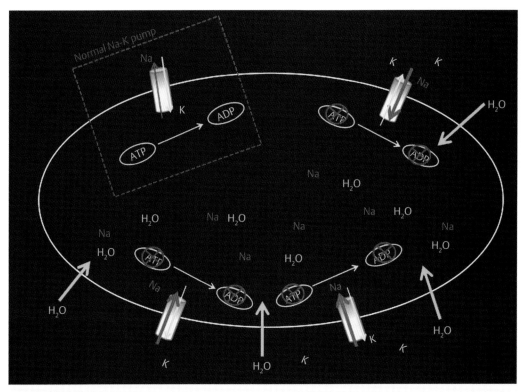

Fig. 6.1 Schematic illustration of sodium-potassium (Na-K) pump failure. The white dotted box shows normal Na-K pump function across the cell membrane. Decrease in adenosine triphosphate (ATP) at the cellular level causes failure of the sodium-potassium-ATP pump, which causes passive diffusion of Na and H_2O inside the cell, leading to intracellular (cytotoxic) edema. A higher level of extracellular K causes depolarization. ADP adenosine diphosphate.

Both techniques have their own advantages and disadvantages. CT perfusion is faster and quantitative but has limitations in the diagnosis of small stroke or lacunar infarctions. A limited MR stroke protocol with DWI and FLAIR sequences can diagnose territorial and lacunar infarcts and their mimics and thus provide the vital information needed for the clinicians.

Pathophysiology of Stroke

Brain damage after infarction is caused by a plethora of complex mechanisms that lead to the accumulation of toxic metabolites causing cellular and architectural damage of brain parenchyma. Within minutes of vascular occlusion, an ischemic cascade begins that includes energy and sodium-potassium pump failure, an increase in intracellular calcium, depolarization, spreading depression, generation of free radicals, disruption of the blood–brain barrier (BBB), inflammation, and apoptosis.[1] These events may not occur strictly in order and can show overlap.

Pump Failures and Metabolic Changes

Cerebral blood flow (CBF) of < 10 mL/100 g of brain tissue causes severe depletion of oxygen and glucose, leading to a severe decrease in adenosine triphosphate (ATP) at the cellular level. This decrease in ATP leads to the failure of the sodium-potassium pump. This failure causes passive diffusion of Na^+ ions inside the cells along with large amounts of fluid. This causes a decrease in the extracellular fluid volume and a decrease in the brownian motion, which is the underlying principle behind DWI imaging in stroke[2,3] (▶ Fig. 6.1).

Depolarization of the cells leads to a large release of excitotoxic amino acids, especially glutamate, into the extracellular compartment. In addition to having primary neurotoxicity, glutamate also causes activation of glutamate receptors, such as N-methyl-d-aspartate (NMDA), α-amino-3-hydroxy-5-methyl-4-isoxazole propionate acid receptor (AMPA), metabotropic glutamate, receptor-operated channels, voltage-gated calcium

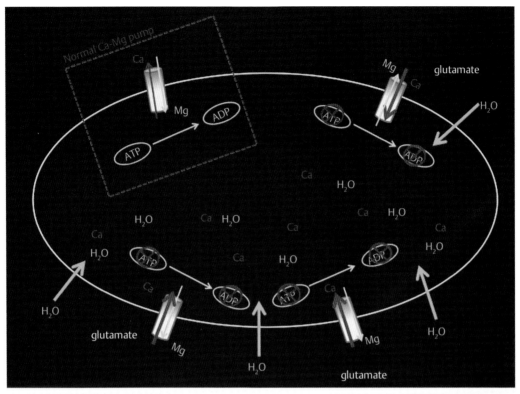

Fig. 6.2 Schematic illustration of calcium pump failure. The white dotted box shows normal calcium–magnesium (Ca-Mg) pump function across the cell membrane. Depolarization of the cell after infarction leads to a release of glutamate, which, in turn, leads to the opening of Ca channels and thus a large influx of Ca inside the cell. Higher levels of intracellular Ca cause mitochondrial damage and cellular rupture. ATP, adenosine triphosphate; ADP, adenosine diphosphate.

channels, and store-operated channels, leading to a large influx of Ca^{2+} into the cells[2,3] (▶ Fig. 6.2). A high concentration of intracellular Ca^{2+} is toxic and leads to irreversible mitochondrial damage, inflammation, necrosis, and apoptosis. Oxygen radicals (superoxide [O_2^-], hydrogen peroxide [H_2O_2], and hydroxyl radicals [^-OH]) produced during the process lead to lipid peroxidation membrane damage, dysregulation of cellular processes, promotion of tissue injury, and disruption of the cellular powerhouse (mitochondrial membranes), leading to mitochondrial burst and cell death.[4,5] The combination of hypoxic damage to the vascular endothelium, toxic damage of inflammatory molecules and free radicals, and destruction of the basal lamina by mitochondrial membrane permeabilization (MMP) damages the BBB. Proteolysis of the neurovascular matrix leading to disruption of the BBB is mainly seen after reperfusion. This destruction of the BBB leads to vasogenic edema, inflammation, and hemorrhagic transformation.[4,6]

Cell Death

Three fundamental mechanisms[6] leading to cell death during ischemic brain injury include excitotoxicity and ionic imbalance, oxidative and nitrosative stresses, and apoptotic-like cell death. These mechanisms have some overlap. Excitotoxicity and ionic imbalance and oxidative and nitrosative stresses lead to the loss of membrane integrity; organelle failure; and, eventually, coagulation necrosis, the most prominent mechanism of cell death in the central core.[6,7] Selective cell death is a well-identified phenomenon after cerebral infarction. Neurons and oligodendrocytes are more vulnerable to cell death than astroglial or endothelial cells.[4,6] Capillary endothelium is quite resistant compared with other central nervous system (CNS) cells, and damage to capillary endothelium begins 4 to 6 hours after infarction. Disruption of the capillary endothelium leads to a break in the BBB.

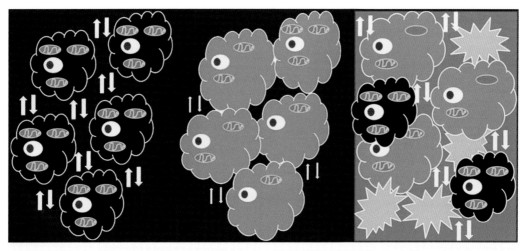

Fig. 6.3 Schematic illustrations of diffusion weighted imaging (DWI) and apparent diffusion coefficient (ADC) basics. (**a**) Arrows show normal brownian motion in extracellular space with normal-sized cells. (**b**) Failure of sodium-potassium-adenosine triphosphate (ATP) pump leads to intracellular edema, swelling of cells (cytotoxic edema), decreased extracellular fluid, and hence a decrease in brownian motion. (**c**) A large influx of Ca^{2+} inside the cells leads to mitochondrial damage and cellular wall disruption, which, in turn, leads to cell rupture and increase in extracellular fluid (vasogenic edema).

6.2.2 Large Vessel Acute Stroke and Diffusion Weighted Imaging Evolutionary Changes

Hyperacute Stage: Less Than 12 Hours

With the advent of intravenous and intra-arterial thrombolytic therapy for stroke, the definition of hyperacute stroke has gained significant importance. As described under pathogenesis, multiple events take place within the infarcted and surrounding parenchyma at the cellular level. Imaging findings in this stage are mainly due to diagnoses of cytotoxic edema by DWI–ADC and of thrombus within the vessels. DWI has revolutionized the imaging of stroke by identifying cytotoxic edema within minutes of stroke.[8,9] Normally there is free motion of molecules within the extracellular space (brownian motion)[8,9] (▶ Fig. 6.3a). A decrease in ATP, failure of the sodium-potassium-ATPase, and anoxic depolarization lead to an intracellular shift of fluid, causing cell swelling (cytotoxic edema) and contraction of the extracellular space (▶ Fig. 6.3b). These changes cause a decrease in brownian motion, which is seen on the DWI sequence as restricted diffusion. Cytotoxic edema is seen within minutes to hours on DWI with sensitivity and specificity of 88 to 100% and 86 to 100%, respectively.[9,10] The regional decrease of

diffusion is visible as hyperintensity on DWI images and as hypointensity on quantitative maps of the ADC (▶ Fig. 6.3c).

The term *operationally defined penumbra* is used to describe the volume of tissue contained within the region of cerebral blood flow-cerebral blood volume (CBF-CBV) mismatch on perfusion CT maps and of CBF–DWI mismatch on perfusion MRI maps. The region of CT–CBV or MR–DWI abnormality represents the core of infarcted tissue, and the CBF–CBV mismatch on CT and CBF–DWI mismatch on MRI represents the surrounding region of tissue that is hypoperfused but salvageable (penumbra) (▶ Fig. 6.4).

Acute Stage: 12 to 24 Hours

During the acute stage, there are further increases in cytotoxic edema and intracellular Ca^{2+}. Activation of a wide range of enzyme systems (proteases, lipases, and nucleases) and production of oxygen-free radicals leads to damage of cell membranes, DNA, and structural neuronal proteins, ultimately leading to cell death. Increased tissue water results in prolongation of T1 and T2 relaxation times on MRI. During this stage there is a combination of cytotoxic and vasogenic edema, with dominance of cytotoxic edema. T2 changes due to vasogenic edema are seen around 6 to 8 hours and are more sensitive than those on T1.

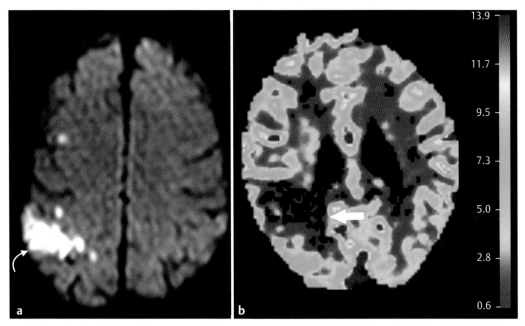

Fig. 6.4 Diffusion perfusion mismatch in a hyperacute stroke in a 56-year-old man. Axial diffusion weighted image (**a**) shows an area of restricted diffusion in the left frontal lobe (curved arrow). Cerebral blood flow (CBF) image (**b**) from perfusion magnetic resonance imaging shows an area of decreased perfusion in the corresponding region (arrow), which is smaller than the diffusion defect, suggestive of penumbra. Penumbra = diffusion weighted imaging defect – CBF. There is viable tissue, and the patient will benefit from thrombolytic therapy.

Subacute Stage: 2 Days to 2 Weeks

Because of a breakdown in the BBB and rupture of swollen cells, there is an increase in extracellular fluid (i.e., vasogenic edema) (▶ Fig. 6.5). This takes about 18 to 24 hours to develop and reaches a maximum by 48 to 72 hours. In this phase, imaging shows increased edema, mass effect, and possible herniation, depending on the size and location of the infarct. Gyral and parenchymal enhancement may be seen on contrast-enhanced T1-weighted imaging and is maximal at the end of the first week. Note that signal intensity in the infarcted area remains increased on DWI for almost 1 week and decreases thereafter, whereas reduced ADC values peak around 3 to 5 days, increase thereafter, and return to normal by 1 to 4 weeks.[8,9]

Chronic Stage: 2 Weeks to 2 Months

The chronic stage begins with restoration of the BBB, resolution of vasogenic edema, and the clearing up of necrotic tissue. Pathologically and on imaging, this phase is characterized by local brain atrophy, gliosis, cavity formation, and ex vacuo dilatation of the adjacent ventricle.[9] DWI can show changes of encephalomalacia with hypointensity in the infarcted area. ADC shows increased signal intensity and prominence of convexity sulci due to loss of parenchyma. Calcification and deposition of blood products (hemosiderin) may be seen on T2 and gradient-recalled echo (GRE) sequences.

6.2.3 Time Course of Diffusion Changes in Acute Stroke

Decreased diffusion in ischemic brain tissue is observed as early as 30 minutes after vascular occlusion[10] (▶ Fig. 6.6 and ▶ Fig. 6.7). This decrease in diffusion is markedly hyperintense on DWI and hypointense on ADC images. The ADC continues to decrease with peak signal reduction at 1 to 4 days (▶ Fig. 6.8a,b). The ADC returns to baseline at 1 to 2 weeks. As the vasogenic edema peaks up, the infarcted area remains mildly hyperintense on the DWI images, due to the T2 component, and isointense on the ADC images (▶ Fig. 6.8c,d and ▶ Fig. 6.9). The ADC is elevated secondary to increased extracellular water, tissue cavitation, and gliosis.

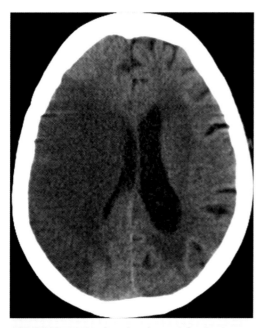

Fig. 6.5 Vasogenic edema in subacute infarction in a 71-year-old woman. An unenhanced computed tomographic scan of the brain shows a large hypodensity in the right middle cerebral artery (MCA) territory with loss of gray matter–white matter differentiation and effacement of convexity sulci with mass effect on surrounding brain parenchyma and the ipsilateral lateral ventricle.

The time course is influenced by a number of factors, including size of the infarct, infarct type, therapy administered, and patient age. Minimum ADC is reached more slowly and the transition from decreasing to increasing ADC is later in lacunar infarctions as compared to large strokes. Early reperfusion causes pseudonormalization as early as 1 to 2 days in humans who receive intravenous recombinant tissue plasminogen activator (rtPA) within 3 hours after stroke onset.

6.2.4 Hemorrhagic Transformation Prediction and Diffusion Weighted Imaging

Hemorrhagic transformation (HT) refers to hemorrhage in an infarcted area. The incidence of HT varies greatly between 10 and 43% (mean 18%)[11] and is highest during the subacute stage. The severity of hemorrhage may range from a few petechiae to a large hematoma with mass effect. Predisposing factors include stroke etiology (HT is

more frequent with embolic strokes), reperfusion, good collateral circulation, hypertension, anticoagulant therapy, and thrombolytic therapy. HT is thought to be due to a combination of vascular injury, reperfusion, and altered permeability. There is alteration in the integrins and disruption of basal lamina, collagen IV, and laminin by free radicals and matrix metalloproteinases (MMPs).[6,12,13] Exposure of this disrupted endothelium to the normal vascular pressure after clot lysis leads to reperfusion injury and extravasation of blood. HT is two to three times more likely in patients treated with thrombolysis. Although CT is commonly used for follow-up of stroke, MRI, especially susceptibility-weighted images (SWI) and GRE imaging, is very sensitive in the diagnosis of early HT (▶ Fig. 6.10).

Because ADC values can mark the severity and extent of ischemia, they may be useful in predicting HT. Selim et al[14] documented that the absolute number of voxels with ADC value $\leq 550 \times 10^{-6}$ mm^2/s correlated with HT of infarctions treated with intravenous tissue plasminogen activator (tPA). Oppenheim et al[15] demonstrated 100% sensitivity and 71% specificity for predicting hemorrhagic transformation when they divided infarcts into those where the mean ADC value of the infarct core was $< 300 \times 10^{-6}$ mm^2/s versus those where the mean ADC value of the infarct core was 300×10^{-6} mm^2/s. Other imaging parameters predictive of HT include hypodensity in greater than one-third of the middle cerebral artery (MCA) territory on CT, early parenchymal enhancement on gadolinium-enhanced MRI, CBF ratio < 0.18 on MR perfusion imaging, and microbleeds detected on T2* gradient echo on initial study.

6.2.5 Reliability of Diffusion Weighted Imaging in Imaging of Stroke

It is an undisputed fact that DWI has revolutionized the imaging of stroke. For routine CT and conventional MRI (without diffusion imaging), sensitivity would largely depend on the time of imaging. For infarctions imaged within 6 hours after stroke onset, reported sensitivities are 38 to 45% for CT and 18 to 46% for MRI.[10,16] This would be significantly higher, 58% for CT and 82% for MRI, when imaged within 6 to 24 hours. DWI is highly sensitive and specific in the detection of hyperacute and acute infarctions, with sensitivity

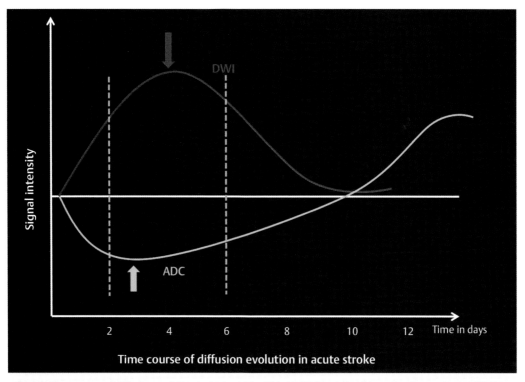

Fig. 6.6 Time course of diffusion evolution in acute stroke. The graph shows signal intensity changes in the diffusion and apparent diffusion coefficient (ADC) in respect to time in an infarcted area. Changes in diffusion weighted imaging (DWI) and ADC appear within 30 minutes of infarction. Decreased ADC values peak up between 2 and 4 days, become isointense between 9 and 11 days, and then become hyperintense by 12 to 14 days. Hyperintensity in the DWI is seen at maximum between 2 and 6 days. This hyperintensity remains for 8 to 10 days and then becomes iso- to hypointense by 12 to 14 days.

ranging from 88 to 100% and specificity between 86 and 100%.[17]

Most false-negative DWI images are seen with punctate lacunar brainstem or deep gray nuclei infarctions, especially under the background of chronic microangiopathic changes. False-positive DWI is seen mostly due to the T2 shine-through effect in subacute or chronic infarction. However, interpreting DWIs along with ADC maps can avoid this pitfall. False-positive DWI may also be seen with other pathologies with restricted diffusion, such as cerebritis/abscess, highly cellular neoplasms, venous infarctions, demyelinating lesions, hemorrhage, herpes encephalitis, and diffuse axonal injury. These lesions are discussed in detail in the Vascular Lesion Mimics section of this chapter. When these lesions are reviewed in combination with routine T1, FLAIR, T2, and gadolinium-enhanced T1-weighted images, they are usually readily differentiated from acute infarctions.

6.2.6 Watershed Infarction

Watershed infarctions are seen at the junction of the distal fields of the two major vascular territories.[11] Watershed infarctions may be cortical/external or subcortical/internal infarcts.[18] Anterior cortical watershed infarcts are between the anterior cerebral artery (ACA) and MCA territories, whereas posterior watershed infarctions develop between the ACA, MCA, and posterior cerebral artery junctional zones (▶ Fig. 6.11). On the basis of imaging, internal watershed infarcts can be further classified into confluent internal watershed infarction or partial internal watershed infarction. Confluent internal watershed infarctions are confluent lesions running parallel to the lateral ventricle (▶ Fig. 6.12). These lesions are usually unilateral, are due to extensive involvement of white matter, and typically present with stepwise onset of contralateral hemiplegia with poor recovery. Partial internal watershed infarction appears

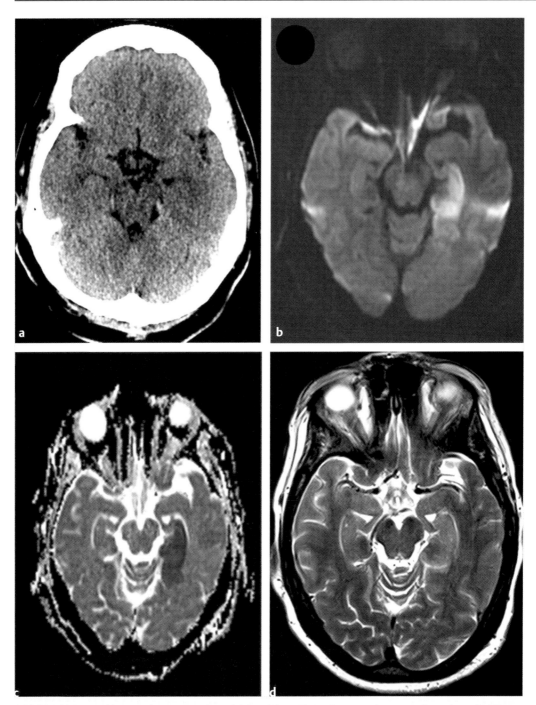

Fig. 6.7 A 47-year-old man with acute neurological deficit. (**a**) Unenhanced computed tomography performed within 4 hours of onset of symptoms does not show any abnormality. Magnetic resonance imaging performed within 5 hours of deficit shows an area of restricted diffusion in the left hippocampus on (**b**) axial diffusion weighted imaging and (**c**) apparent diffusion coefficient map. There was no corresponding abnormality seen on (**d**) axial T2-weighted image.

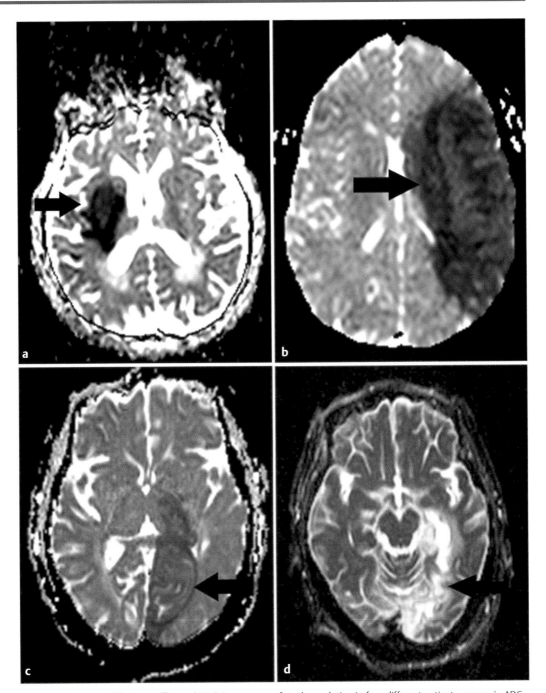

Fig. 6.8 Apparent diffusion coefficient (ADC) time course of stroke evolution in four different patients as seen in ADC maps. (**a**) At 24 hours, hypointensity (arrow) in the right deep gray matter nuclei due to hyperacute stroke. (**b**) At 3 days, pronounced ADC hypointensity (arrow) secondary to increased cytotoxic edema. (**c**) In a 10-day-old left Posterior Cerebral Artery (PCA) infarction (arrow), ADC is almost isointense secondary to a decrease in the cytotoxic edema, cell lysis, and development of vasogenic edema. (**d**) At 12 months, ADC shows hyperintensity in the left stroke (arrow) secondary to the development of gliosis and tissue cavitation.

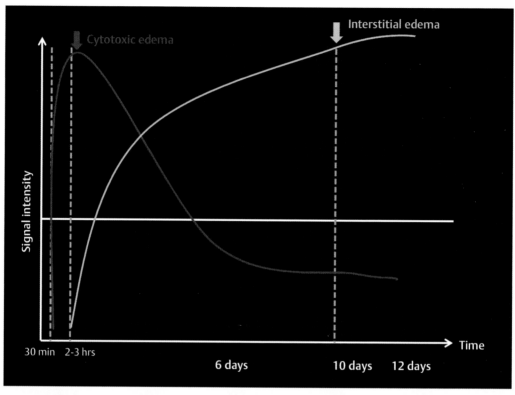

Fig. 6.9 Time course of types of edema in acute stroke. The graph shows the appearance of the cytotoxic edema in a hyperacute stroke within 30 minutes, which peaks within 2 to 3 hours. Vasogenic edema (interstitial) may appear by 2 to 3 hours but peaks at 6 to 10 days.

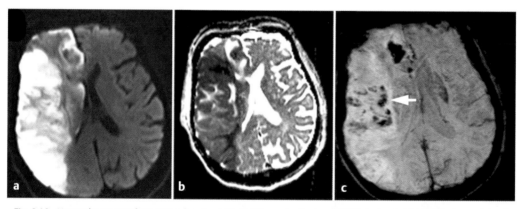

Fig. 6.10 Hemorrhagic transformation of acute right middle cerebral artery (MCA) stroke. Axial (a) diffusion weighted imaging and (b) apparent diffusion coefficient map show a large acute stroke in the right MCA territory. (c) Susceptibility-weighted imaging shows hypointensities (arrow) within the infarcted area due to hemorrhagic transformation.

as a single or multiple discrete rounded lesions in the same distribution as a confluent internal watershed infarction and usually presents as episodes of brachiofacial sensory and motor deficit with good recovery.[18] Although rare, watershed infarctions can also be seen in the posterior fossa between the superior cerebellar artery and the posteroinferior cerebellar artery (PICA) or between

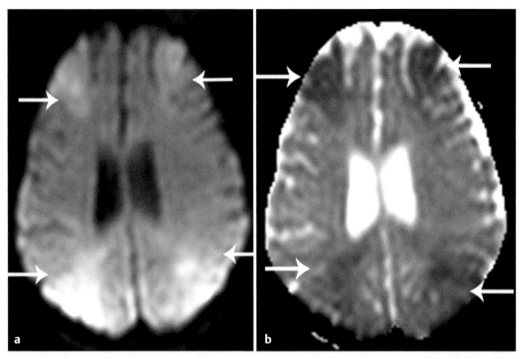

Fig. 6.11 Cortical watershed infarcts. (**a**) Axial diffusion weighted imaging and (**b**) apparent diffusion coefficient map show wedge-shaped lesions that restrict diffusion in regions between major arterial vascular territories. Note the characteristic appearance and distribution of infarcts in the anterior cerebral artery–middle cerebral artery watershed (top arrows) and in the middle cerebral artery–posterior cerebral artery watershed (bottom arrows).

PICA, superior cerebellar artery, and anteroinferior cerebellar artery territories.

The pathogenesis of watershed infarction remains debatable and is thought to be multifactorial. Cortical watershed infarcts are thought to be the result of microembolization, either from carotid artery atherosclerosis or vulnerable plaque or from artery-to-artery emboli precipitated by an episode of systemic arterial hypotension. Internal watershed infarcts are caused by a combination of hypoperfusion of the internal border zone, severe carotid disease, and a hemodynamic event. It occurs at junctions between the white matter perforating arteries (e.g., lenticulostriate) and the major cerebral arteries.

In acute events, DWI is very sensitive for the diagnosis of both cortical watershed infarct and internal watershed infarct. Classically cortical watershed infarcts appear as fan- or wedge-shaped hyperintensities extending from the lateral margins of the lateral ventricle toward the cortex (see ▶ Fig. 6.11). Complete internal border zone infarcts produce confluent, elongated, deep white matter lesions (see ▶ Fig. 6.12), whereas partial

infarction is characterized by a "string of beads" appearance.

6.2.7 Lacunar Infarct

Lacunae are small-vessel deep infarcts < 1.5 cm,[11] which represent 20 to 25% of all strokes. Initially they were thought to be due to intrinsic disease of the small vessels, called lipohyalinosis, resulting from hypertension and diabetes. However, now they are thought to be the result of focal ischemic infarcts caused by thrombi or emboli composed of platelets or fibrin (often with incorporated red blood cells), in a background of diffuse atherosclerotic narrowing of small vessels.[19] Ipsilateral high-grade carotid stenosis and aortic arch atheroma have been shown to be risk factors for lacunar stroke.

Asymptomatic ("silent") lacunar infarcts are at least five times more common than symptomatic infarcts.[19] When symptomatic, lacunar infarcts may present with classic lacunar syndromes: pure motor stroke, pure sensory stroke, sensorimotor stroke, ataxic hemiparesis, and dysarthria. It is important to diagnose lacunae because many

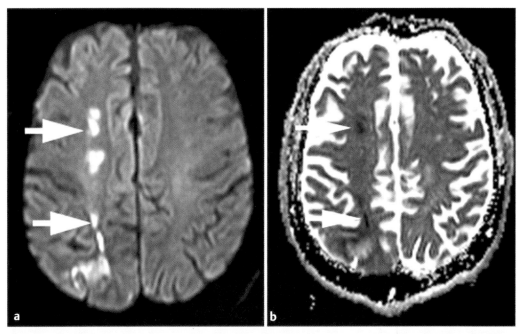

Fig. 6.12 Internal watershed zone infarcts. (**a**) Axial diffusion weighted imaging and (**b**) apparent diffusion coefficient maps showing elongated deep white matter lesions which restrict diffusion, consistent with internal border zone infarcts. Note the difference in appearance between internal watershed infarcts (straight arrows) and the wedge-shaped appearance of cortical watershed infarcts (curved arrows).

neurologists believe that patients with lacunar infarcts need further workup to evaluate for the source of thrombi. Conventional MRI does not reliably identify the acute lacunar infarction related to the clinical symptoms because many patients with lacunar infarctions have preexisting chronic white matter lesions with signal characteristics that do not differ from those of acute lesions. DWI is more sensitive than CT and T2-weighted MRI for the diagnosis of acute lacunar infarctions.[11,19] The sensitivity and specificity of DWI for the diagnosis of acute lacunar infarction are 94.9% and 94.1%, respectively. Acute lacunae show focal areas of restricted diffusion on DWI (▶ Fig. 6.13), most commonly in the deep white matter, whereas chronic lacunae are hyperintense on T2-weighted and FLAIR images. A common differential diagnosis includes prominent Virchow–Robin spaces, which follow cerebrospinal fluid (CSF) signal on all MRI sequences.

6.2.8 Isolated Punctate Cortical Infarctions

Small cortical infarctions may cause monoparesis and other symptoms limited to a single limb. They may occur in the motor or sensory strips but may also involve any part of the cortex, leading to various clinical syndromes. T2-weighted images are limited by their inability to outline lesions neighboring the CSF. Even when they are identified on conventional images, such as T2 or FLAIR sequences, linkage of these small dots to the clinical syndrome is difficult because successful differentiation between acute and chronic lesions cannot be made reliably. Bright cortical dots on DWI indicate isolated punctate cortical infarctions (▶ Fig. 6.14). From the clinical point of view, monoparesis and other symptoms limited to a single limb are the best, perhaps the only, indicator of isolated cortical infarctions.

6.2.9 Transient Ischemic Attack

TIA is defined as a sudden, focal neurological deficit due to focal brain or retinal ischemia that completely resolves within 24 hours. This time limit is somewhat arbitrary, and in actual clinical practice the usual duration is < 2 to 3 hours and often only 5 to 10 minutes. It is important to diagnose TIAs because the short-term risk of stroke following TIAs is greatest within the first 48 hours (5.3%).[20,]

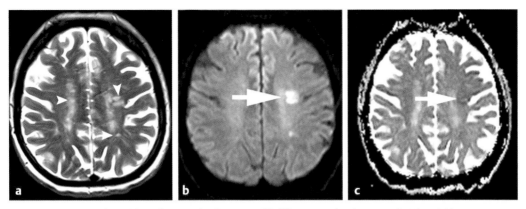

Fig. 6.13 Lacunar infarct. (a) Axial T2-weighted imaging, (b) diffusion weighted imaging (DWI), and (c) apparent diffusion coefficient (ADC) map. Periventricular white matter hyperintensities on (a) T2-weighted imaging (white arrowheads) may be mistaken for chronic microvascular changes or Virchow–Robin spaces. DWI (b) and ADC map (c) show acute lesions (arrow) that may be obscured by chronic changes, especially in locations where benign findings are typical. DWI thus increases sensitivity and specificity of the diagnosis of lacunar infarcts.

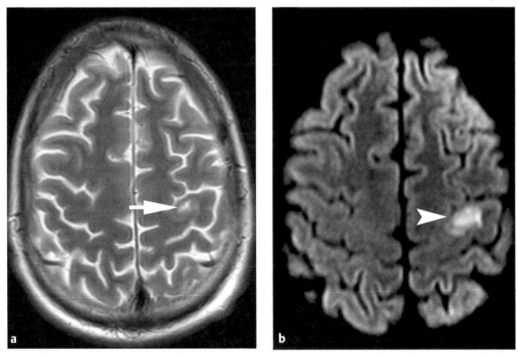

Fig. 6.14 Isolated punctate cortical infarction. (a) Axial T2-weighted imaging (arrow) and (b) diffusion weighted imaging (DWI) (arrowhead) show a focal region of restricted diffusion in the postcentral gyrus. This lesion is very difficult to appreciate on T2-weighted imaging and may be mistaken for prominent sulci. The etiology is difficult to pinpoint in the absence of the DWI sequence. Restricted diffusion, together with the clinical picture, can help solidify the diagnosis.

[21] Up to 20% of TIA patients may suffer stroke within 3 months.[20,21] TIA patients with DWI lesions have a higher stroke risk than DWI-negative TIA patients, thus underscoring the importance of DWI–ADC imaging in evaluation of TIA patients.

Imaging plays an important role because 45 to 62% of referrals to TIA clinics are nonvascular mimics.[22] Because of its sensitivity for tiny ischemic lesions, DWI remains the sequence of choice for diagnosis of TIA. The demonstration of these punctate lesions on DWI supports the ischemic pathophysiology of TIA. DWI helps improve diagnosis of TIA and predict short-term stroke risk. Hyperintense lesions, consistent with small infarctions, usually < 15 mm in size, in the clinically appropriate vascular territory, are seen in 21 to 48% of patients with TIAs.[23] Twenty percent of these lesions may not be seen at follow-up. This could be either due to reversibility or to lesions being too small to see on follow-up conventional MRI due to atrophy. The positivity of the DWI findings largely depends on the clinical presentation. The incidence of having DWI-positive lesions is higher in patients with symptoms lasting between 12 and 24 hours. Also, symptoms such as dysphasia, dysarthria, or motor weakness in the context of atrial fibrillation or carotid stenosis are associated with a higher likelihood of DWI lesions.

6.2.10 Capillary Leak Syndromes

Due to its role in differentiating vasogenic from cytotoxic edema, DWI plays an important role in the evaluation of capillary leak syndrome. Contrary to cytotoxic edema, vasogenic edema is hyperintense on ADC maps and shows iso- to hypointensity on DWI.

Posterior Reversible Encephalopathy Syndrome

Clinically, posterior reversible encephalopathy syndrome (PRES) typically presents with headaches, decreased alertness, altered mental status, seizures, and visual loss, including cortical blindness. Symptoms may develop over several days or may present as an acute encephalopathy.

The exact cause of PRES is not yet understood. Hypertension with loss of cerebral autoregulation and capillary leakage remains a popular theory for the development of cerebral edema. Alternatively, endothelial dysfunction/injury, hypoperfusion, and vasoconstriction may lead to altered integrity of the BBB, leading to extravasation of fluid and the development of vasogenic edema. In 70 to 80% of patients, moderate-to-severe hypertension is observed, whereas blood pressure may be normal to mildly elevated in 20 to 30% of patients.[24] PRES may be seen in a variety of other clinical entities, such as treatment with immunosuppressive agents (e.g., cyclosporin and tacrolimus), treatment with chemotherapeutic agents (e.g., intrathecal methotrexate, cisplatin, and interferon alpha), and hematologic disorders (e.g., hemolytic uremic syndrome, thrombotic thrombocytopenic purpura, acute intermittent porphyria, and cryoglobulinemia).

The posterior circulation predominance is thought to be more prone to PRES due to less protective (vasoconstrictive) sympathetic innervation compared to the anterior circulation. Imaging with CT and MR may show either focal or holohemispheric edema. T2- and FLAIR-weighted sequences typically demonstrate bilateral symmetric hyperintensity and swelling in subcortical white matter and overlying cortex in the occipital, parietal, and posterior temporal lobes as well as the posterior fossa. Patchy areas of vasogenic edema may also be seen in the basal ganglia, brainstem, and deep white matter. Cytotoxic edema may be seen in 11 to 26% and may be associated with adverse outcomes[25] (▶ Fig. 6.15). Types of edema in PRES can be differentiated using DWI and FLAIR sequences. Vasogenic edema is thought to be due to excessive hypertension, leading to hyperperfusion and subsequent vasogenic edema in susceptible vessels. Cytotoxic edema is thought to be due to systemic proinflammatory processes (elevated cytokines such as interleukin [IL]-1, IL-6, interferon-α, and tumor necrosis factor), vasospasm, and microinfarctions. Hemorrhage (focal hematoma, or subarachnoid hemorrhage) is seen in approximately 15% of patients.

Hyperperfusion Syndrome following Carotid Endarterectomy

Hyperperfusion syndrome is thought to be similar to PRES, due to increased pressure leading to damage of endothelial tight junctions, capillary leak, and development of vasogenic edema. Following carotid endarterectomy, patients may present with seizures with or without focal neurological deficits mimicking a stroke.[26,27] On MRI, T2-weighted images demonstrate hyperintensity in the frontal and parietal cortex and subcortical white matter that may mimic arterial infarction. However, DWI

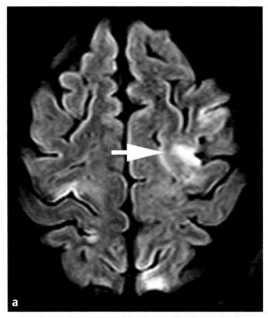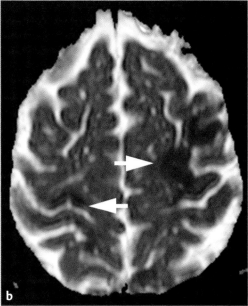

Fig. 6.15 Posterior reversible encephalopathy syndrome (PRES). (**a**) Axial diffusion weighted imaging (arrow) and (**b**) apparent diffusion coefficient map (arrows) show areas of restricted diffusion located in the gyral and subcortical white matter due to cytotoxic edema in a patient with PRES.

does not show any areas of restricted diffusion. There may be peripheral cytotoxic edema due to mass effect and capillary compression.[26,27] Rarely there may be cytotoxic edema in the whole lesion. However, perfusion studies show increased rather than diminished flow-related enhancement in the ipsilateral MCA.

6.2.11 Venous Infarction

Cerebral venous thrombosis (CVT) accounts for 0.5% of all strokes.[28] Clinical presentation of CVT is nonspecific (headache, seizures, vomiting, focal deficit, and papilledema). Predisposing factors for CVT include protein C and S deficiencies; malignancies; pregnancy; medications such as oral contraceptives, steroids, and hormone replacement therapy; collagen vascular diseases; infection; trauma; surgery; and immobilization. For early diagnosis of CVT, a high index of clinical suspicion with the use of appropriate imaging (MRI, MR venography, and CT venography) is a must.

The pathophysiology of venous infarction is multifactorial. It is mainly caused by pressure changes within the vascular tree.[28,29,30] Venous flow obstruction causes back pressure leading to a decrease in CBF. This decrease in CBF causes reduced cerebral perfusion pressure (CPP) that, in

turn, causes venous congestion, disruption of the BBB, and an increase in net capillary filtration leading to vasogenic edema. Areas of restricted diffusion (cytotoxic edema) are frequently seen within the infarcted region.[28,30] Cytotoxic edema in CVT is thought to be due to reduced CBF below the penumbral level, which in turn leads to failure of the sodium-potassium-ATP-dependent pump.

A wide spectrum of parenchymal changes may be seen on imaging. On CT, venous infarction is seen as diffuse low-attenuating subcortical lesions adjacent to white matter with edematous overlying gyri in a nonarterial distribution. On CT these changes may mimic other pathologies, such as encephalitis. MRI is more sensitive and more specific than CT for the diagnosis of venous infarction. MRI shows a combination of vasogenic and cytotoxic edematous changes in the cortical and subcortical parenchyma with areas of hemorrhage (► Fig. 6.16). In contrast to arterial stroke, changes of cytotoxic edema in venous infarction are shown to be reversible on follow-up imaging. This resolution of lesions with decreased diffusion has been related to better drainage of blood through collateral pathways.

Direct signs of sinus thrombosis may be identified on CT or MRI. On CT, an acute blood clot may be seen within the dual sinus (delta sign in the

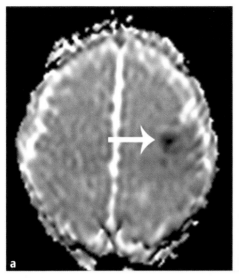 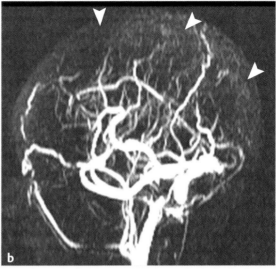

Fig. 6.16 Venous infarction. (**a**) Apparent diffusion coefficient map shows hypointensity (arrow), due to restricted diffusion, in the left frontal lobe due to venous infarction. (**b**) Magnetic resonance venography shows a loss of flow signal in the superior sagittal sinus (arrowheads).

superior sagittal sinus), cortical veins (cord sign), or both. The appearance of signal suggestive of sinus thrombosis on MRI is variable and time dependent.[30] A thrombosed sinus appears isointense on T1 and hypointense on T2 during the first 3 to 5 days (due to the presence of deoxyhemoglobin). Sinus thrombosis shows hyperintensity in the subacute stage on T1 and T2 images. During the acute stage, hypointense thrombus on T2-weighted images may be mistaken for normal flow. An SWI/GRE sequence is more sensitive and shows hypointensity within the thrombosed sinus in the acute stage.

6.2.12 Septic Infarction

Septic infarctions are caused by infected emboli that are most commonly due to an infected cardiac valve, septicemia, or intravenous drug abuse. The source is usually bacterial; however, in immunocompromised patients, the source can be fungal (e.g., aspergillosis).[11] Septic emboli can lead to cerebrovascular occlusion causing septic infarction, abscess, or septic aneurysm. Clinically patients with septic infarction present with focal cerebral or cerebellar signs that do not resolve.

Brain damage is caused by the release of inflammatory mediators, such as lipopolysaccharide and endotoxin, resulting in reduced CBF and reduced oxygen extraction, cerebral edema, disruption of the BBB, impaired astrocyte function, and neuronal death.[31] On imaging, hyperacute or acute septic infarctions cannot be distinguished from bland infarct. The late subacute stage may show increasing vasogenic edema with parenchymal and leptomeningeal enhancement.[11] There may be changes of cerebritis or abscess formation that show restricted diffusion on DWI. Enhancing mycotic aneurysms may be seen within the infarcted bed.

6.3 Vascular Lesion Mimics on Diffusion Weighted Imaging

A number of nonvascular conditions may show decreased diffusion, which may mimic infarctions or vascular pathologies. The most common clinically encountered entities include acute demyelinating lesions with decreased diffusion due to myelin vacuolization; some products of hemorrhage (oxyhemoglobin and extracellular methemoglobin); herpes encephalitis with decreased diffusion due to cytotoxic edema from cell necrosis; diffuse axonal injury with decreased diffusion due to cytotoxic edema or axotomy with retraction ball formation; abscess with decreased diffusion due to the high viscosity of pus; tumors, such as lymphoma and small round cell tumors, with decreased diffusion due to dense cell packing; and Creutzfeldt–Jakob disease with decreased

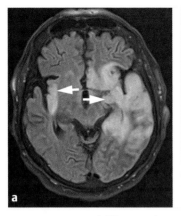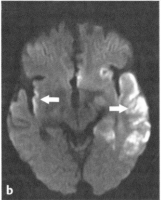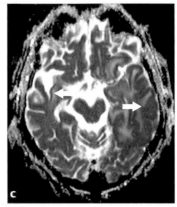

Fig. 6.17 Restricted diffusion in herpes encephalitis. (**a**) Axial fluid-attenuated inversion recovery image shows hyperintensities in a classic bilateral temporal and left frontal lobe distribution (arrows). (**b**) Axial diffusion weighted imaging and (**c**) apparent diffusion coefficient sequences show patchy areas of restricted diffusion in the left temporal lobe (right arrow in (**b**) and (**c**)) and right insular cortex (left arrow in (**b**)) due to cytotoxic edema from perivascular cuffing and inflammation.

diffusion from myelin vacuolization. When these lesions are reviewed in combination with routine T1-, FLAIR-, T2-, and gadolinium-enhanced T1-weighted images, they are usually readily differentiated from acute infarctions. However, occasionally diffusion and conventional imaging cannot distinguish between the mimics and stroke, and in such cases molecular imaging techniques, such as MR spectroscopy, perfusion, and DTI, and further follow-up studies are useful.

6.3.1 Infection: Herpes Encephalitis

Herpes simplex encephalitis (HSE) is one of the most common cerebral viral infections. The clinical presentation of acute encephalitis is nonspecific. Typical T2 hyperintensity in the temporal and frontal localization with petechial hemorrhage are characteristic MR findings.[32] In the acute stage of HSE due to marked perivascular cuffing with inflammatory cells, part of the lesion may show restricted diffusion due to cytotoxic edema. The DWI appearance may mimic a subacute infarct (▶ Fig. 6.17). DWI sequences are found to be significantly better for lesion conspicuity in comparison to T2-weighted sequences and are slightly better than FLAIR sequences. Areas of cytotoxic edema correspond to a worse outcome compared to areas of vasogenic edema. In the chronic stages there is neuronal death and necrosis, and lesions are less conspicuous on DWI than T2-weighted images or FLAIR.

6.3.2 Metabolic Hypoglycemia

Hypoglycemia can present with diverse neurological manifestations ranging from focal neurological deficits to permanent dysfunction. Pathological changes are mainly seen in the cerebral cortex, hippocampus, and basal ganglia.[33,34] In the acute phase these areas may show restricted diffusion, which is thought to be due to energy failure, excitotoxic edema, and asymmetric CBF. DWI changes are usually transitory, and abnormalities normalize with time or following removal of the causative pathological factors. Unlike with hypoxic damage, the occipital cortex, dorsofrontal cortex, and hippocampus are less frequently involved.

6.3.3 Tumor: Lymphoma

Cerebral lymphomas are hypercellular tumors consisting of large lymphoid cells. On T2-weighted images, lesions are slightly hyperintense compared to normal brain tissue with ring-shaped or diffuse enhancement. Tightly packed cells change the composition and microarchitecture of cerebral tissue leading to a decrease in extracellular water and resultant restriction in diffusion. The ADC values of the primary CNS lymphomas may be lower than the surrounding brain parenchyma, mimicking acute infarct (▶ Fig. 6.18). The key imaging findings to differentiate CNS lymphomas include the hypercellularity sign (low signal on T2-weighted images), large perifocal edema, contrast enhancement, and often close contact with the leptomeningeal and/or ependymal space.

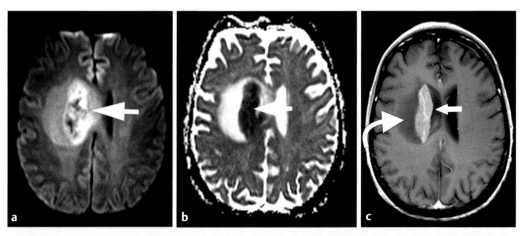

Fig. 6.18 Primary central nervous system (CNS) lymphoma mimicking acute infarct. (a) Axial diffusion weighted imaging and (b) apparent diffusion coefficient map in a patient with primary CNS lymphoma show a region of restricted diffusion in the right periventricular white matter due to hypercellularity of the tumor. (arrow in (a) and (b)) (c) Contrast-enhanced T1-weighted image shows intense enhancement of the periventricular mass (arrow) with surrounding hypointense vasogenic edema (curved arrow).

6.3.4 Multiple Sclerosis

Multiple sclerosis is an inflammatory demyelinating disorder that may clinically mimic stroke. In the acute phase, patients may present with sudden-onset aphasia, dysarthria, hemiplegia, or hemisensory deficits. Diagnosis is easy when the typical MRI findings of multiple periventricular, deep, and juxtacortical hyperintensities are seen on T2-weighted or FLAIR images. Many of these patients can be accurately diagnosed by considering the patient history, clinical findings, associated MRI findings, and CSF examination for oligoclonal bands. However, acute demyelinating lesions may show prominent restricted diffusion that could be confused with acute ischemia/lacunar infarction[35] (▶ Fig. 6.19). In such cases, a combination of clinical features and short-term follow-up imaging allows accurate diagnosis.

6.3.5 Transient Global Amnesia

Transient global amnesia (TGA) is a clinical syndrome characterized by the sudden onset of profound memory impairment resulting in both retrograde and anterograde amnesia, without other neurological deficits.[36,37] The symptoms typically resolve in 3 to 4 hours. Clinically, TGA needs to be differentiated from stroke or TIA. The majority of these patients are negative on imaging. However, numbers of studies have reported punctate or diffuse lesions with decreased diffusion in the medial hippocampus, the parahippocampal gyrus, and the splenium of the corpus callosum that resolved on follow-up imaging.[36,37] Lesions measure 1 to 3 mm in size and are most often unilateral. It is currently unclear whether the TGA patients with DWI abnormalities have a different prognosis or a different etiologic mechanism, or whether they should be managed differently compared to TGA patients without DWI abnormalities.

6.4 Summary

DWI uses the principle of brownian motion to evaluate dynamic microstructural tissue properties in an effort to help characterize vascular pathology. DWI is useful in the diagnosis of hyperacute stroke because it can reflect the immediate changes that begin upon failure of cellular mechanisms to regulate intra- and extracellular fluid volumes and result in subtle biochemical changes not readily apparent on other MRI sequences. This in turn can facilitate more rapid treatment decisions with greater certainty in the setting of acute stroke. The information obtained from DWI and ADC sequences can also help predict various other vascular pathologies, such as watershed and lacunar infarcts, cerebral hyperperfusion, and venous infarction, with increased accuracy and precision. DWI and ADC must be used in the context of the clinical picture and other available imaging; however, vascular mimics, such as infection, tumor,

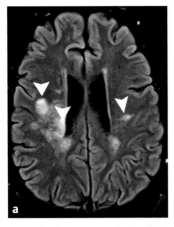 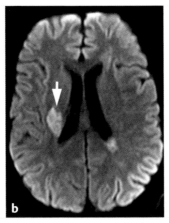 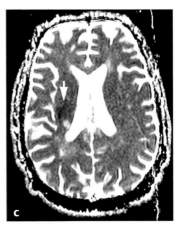

Fig. 6.19 Acute demyelinating lesions mimicking acute vascular pathology. (**a**) Axial fluid-attenuated inversion recovery (FLAIR) image shows classical multiple periventricular and deep white matter demyelinating plaques (arrowheads). (**b**) Diffusion weighted imaging and (**c**) apparent diffusion coefficient map show area of restricted diffusion in an active plaque (arrow). This lesion may be confused for a lacunar infarct. The classical distribution of lesions on FLAIR/T2-weighted images, CSF examination, and follow-up imaging can help in clinching the diagnosis.

demyelinating lesions, and metabolic abnormalities, can be confused for vascular infarcts if appropriate context is not taken into account. The addition of DWI and ADC provides a valuable tool in the expeditious diagnosis of cerebral vascular infarcts and helps complement previous technology in the management of various cerebral pathologies.

References

[1] Durukan A, Tatlisumak T. Acute ischemic stroke: overview of major experimental rodent models, pathophysiology, and therapy of focal cerebral ischemia. Pharmacol Biochem Behav 2007; 87(1): 179–197

[2] Mergenthaler P, Dirnagl U, Meisel A. Pathophysiology of stroke: lessons from animal models. Metab Brain Dis 2004; 19(3–4): 151–167

[3] Dirnagl U, Iadecola C, Moskowitz MA. Pathobiology of ischaemic stroke: an integrated view. Trends Neurosci 1999; 22(9): 391–397

[4] Chan PH. Reactive oxygen radicals in signaling and damage in the ischemic brain. J Cereb Blood Flow Metab 2001; 21 (1): 2–14

[5] Fiskum G. Mitochondrial participation in ischemic and traumatic neural cell death. J Neurotrauma 2000; 17(10): 843–855

[6] Lo EH, Dalkara T, Moskowitz MA. Mechanisms, challenges and opportunities in stroke. Nat Rev Neurosci 2003; 4(5): 399–415

[7] Nicotera P, Leist M, Fava E, Berliocchi L, Volbracht C. Energy requirement for caspase activation and neuronal cell death. Brain Pathol 2000; 10(2): 276–282

[8] Provenzale JM, Jahan R, Naidich TP, Fox AJ. Assessment of the patient with hyperacute stroke: imaging and therapy. Radiology 2003; 229(2): 347–359

[9] Schaefer PW, Grant PE, Gonzalez RG. Diffusion weighted MR imaging of the brain. Radiology 2000; 217(2): 331–345

[10] González RG, Schaefer PW, Buonanno FS, et al. Diffusion weighted MR imaging: diagnostic accuracy in patients imaged within 6 hours of stroke symptom onset. Radiology 1999; 210(1): 155–162

[11] Marks MP. Cerebral ischemia and infarction. In: Atlas SW, ed. Magnetic Resonance Imaging of the Brain and Spine. Vol 1. 4th ed. Philadelphia, PA: Williams & Wilkins; 2009:772–825

[12] Montaner J, Alvarez-Sabín J, Molina C, et al. Matrix metalloproteinase expression after human cardioembolic stroke: temporal profile and relation to neurological impairment. Stroke 2001; 32(8): 1759–1766

[13] Slivka A, Pulsinelli W. Hemorrhagic complications of thrombolytic therapy in experimental stroke. Stroke 1987; 18(6): 1148–1156

[14] Selim M, Fink JN, Kumar S, et al. Predictors of hemorrhagic transformation after intravenous recombinant tissue plasminogen activator: prognostic value of the initial apparent diffusion coefficient and diffusion weighted lesion volume. Stroke 2002; 33(8): 2047–2052

[15] Oppenheim C, Samson Y, Dormont D, et al. DWI prediction of symptomatic hemorrhagic transformation in acute MCA infarct. J Neuroradiol 2002; 29(1): 6–13

[16] Mohr JP, Biller J, Hilal SK, et al. Magnetic resonance versus computed tomographic imaging in acute stroke. Stroke 1995; 26(5): 807–812

[17] Bryan RN, Levy LM, Whitlow WD, Killian JM, Preziosi TJ, Rosario JA. Diagnosis of acute cerebral infarction: comparison of CT and MR imaging. AJNR Am J Neuroradiol 1991; 12 (4): 611–620

[18] Momjian-Mayor I, Baron JC. The pathophysiology of watershed infarction in internal carotid artery disease: review of cerebral perfusion studies. Stroke 2005; 36(3): 567–577

[19] Ay H, Oliveira-Filho J, Buonanno FS, et al. Diffusion weighted imaging identifies a subset of lacunar infarction associated with embolic source. Stroke 1999; 30(12): 2644–2650

[20] Eliasziw M, Kennedy J, Hill MD, Buchan AM, Barnett HJ North American Symptomatic Carotid Endarterectomy Trial Group. Early risk of stroke after a transient ischemic attack

in patients with internal carotid artery disease. CMAJ 2004; 170(7): 1105–1109

[21] Daffertshofer M, Mielke O, Pullwitt A, Felsenstein M, Hennerici M. Transient ischemic attacks are more than "ministrokes". Stroke 2004; 35(11): 2453–2458

[22] Giles MF, Rothwell PM. Substantial underestimation of the need for outpatient services for TIA and minor stroke. Age Ageing 2007; 36(6): 676–680

[23] Purroy F, Montaner J, Rovira A, Delgado P, Quintana M, Alvarez-Sabín J. Higher risk of further vascular events among transient ischemic attack patients with diffusion weighted imaging acute ischemic lesions. Stroke 2004; 35 (10): 2313–2319

[24] McKinney AM, Short J, Truwit CL, et al. McKinneyAM. Posterior reversible encephalopathy syndrome: incidence of atypical regions of involvement and imaging findings. AJR Am J Roentgenol 2007; 189(4): 904–912

[25] Donmez FY, Basaran C, Kayahan Ulu EM, Yildirim M, Coskun M. MRI features of posterior reversible encephalopathy syndrome in 33 patients. J Neuroimaging 2010; 20(1): 22–28

[26] Kuroda H, Ogasawara K, Hirooka R, et al. Prediction of cerebral hyperperfusion after carotid endarterectomy using middle cerebral artery signal intensity in preoperative single-slab 3-dimensional time-of-flight magnetic resonance angiography. Neurosurgery 2009; 64(6): 1065–1071, discussion 1071–1072

[27] Cho A-H, Suh D-C, Kim GE, et al. MRI evidence of reperfusion injury associated with neurological deficits after carotid revascularization procedures. Eur J Neurol 2009; 16(9): 1066–1069

[28] Bousser MG, Ferro JM. Cerebral venous thrombosis: an update. Lancet Neurol 2007; 6(2): 162–170

[29] Stam J. Thrombosis of the cerebral veins and sinuses. N Engl J Med 2005; 352(17): 1791–1798

[30] van den Bergh WM, van der Schaaf I, van Gijn J. The spectrum of presentations of venous infarction caused by deep cerebral vein thrombosis. Neurology 2005; 65(2): 192–196

[31] Finelli PF, Uphoff DF. Magnetic resonance imaging abnormalities with septic encephalopathy. J Neurol Neurosurg Psychiatry 2004; 75(8): 1189–1191

[32] Bulakbasi N, Kocaoglu M. Central nervous system infections of herpesvirus family. Neuroimaging Clin N Am 2008; 18(1): 53–84, viii

[33] Lo L, Tan ACH, Umapathi T, Lim CC. Diffusion weighted MR imaging in early diagnosis and prognosis of hypoglycemia. AJNR Am J Neuroradiol 2006; 27(6): 1222–1224

[34] Ma J-H, Kim Y-J, Yoo W-J, et al. MR imaging of hypoglycemic encephalopathy: lesion distribution and prognosis prediction by diffusion weighted imaging. Neuroradiology 2009; 51(10): 641–649

[35] Rosso C, Remy P, Creange A, Brugieres P, Cesaro P, Hosseini H. Diffusion weighted MR imaging characteristics of an acute strokelike form of multiple sclerosis. AJNR Am J Neuroradiol 2006; 27(5): 1006–1008

[36] Enzinger C, Thimary F, Kapeller P, et al. Transient global amnesia: diffusion weighted imaging lesions and cerebrovascular disease. Stroke 2008; 39(8): 2219–2225

[37] Sedlaczek O, Hirsch JG, Grips E, et al. Detection of delayed focal MR changes in the lateral hippocampus in transient global amnesia. Neurology 2004; 62(12): 2165–2170

7 Diffusion Weighted Imaging in the Evaluation of Brain Tumors

Fernanda C. Rueda-Lopes, Celso Hygino da Cruz Jr., and Emerson Leandro Gasparetto

Key Points

- Diffusion weighted imaging is an important tool for evaluating brain tumors and can be used for diagnosis, follow-up, and determining the prognosis.
- Apparent diffusion coefficients (ADCs) are inversely correlated with high cellularity.
- A reduced extracellular to intracellular space ratio and a high nuclear to cytoplasm ratio are correlated to reduced ADC.
- In atypical meningiomas there is an inverse correlation between ADC (lower ADCs are markers of high cellularity) and Ki-67 expression (high Ki-67 expression is a marker of high cell proliferation).
- Primary central nervous system lymphoma usually demonstrates restricted diffusion due to its histology: the high degree of cellularity and the high nuclear to cytoplasm ratio.
- Diffusion imaging sequences can be used to assess posttreatment changes and may serve as an early biomarker tool for predicting treatment outcomes, monitoring treatment response, and detecting recurrent cancer.

7.1 Introduction

Conventional magnetic resonance imaging (MRI) has some limitations when used to evaluate brain tumors. Differential diagnoses between cystic lesions, primary or secondary (metastasis) brain tumors, and glioma grading usually demand the use of advanced MRI techniques.[1,2,3,4] Diffusion weighted imaging (DWI) is an important tool for the evaluation of brain tumors. It can be used for diagnosis, follow-up, and determining the prognosis. Diffusion tensor imaging (DTI) parameters such as fractional anisotropy (FA), radial diffusivity (RD) and axial diffusivity (AD) are also used for brain tumor evaluation.[2]

Tumor cell density increases with tumor grade and impedes membranes, thereby causing the apparent diffusion coefficient (ADC) values to decrease. Thus an inverse correlation has been proposed between tumor cellularity and ADC

values that can be helpful to noninvasively distinguish low- and high-grade gliomas.[3,4] Moreover, some specific neoplasms, such as lymphoma and medulloblastoma, have higher nucleus to cytoplasm ratios and are characterized by low ADC values.[5,6] The location of the restricted diffusion (in the central core or in the peripheral tissue) helps to differentiate tumors from cystic lesions.[1,2] ADC may serve as a prognostic tool for patients with neoplasm. Low ADC values before treatment correlate with poor survival in malignant astrocytomas.[3] Alternatively, low ADC values along the surgical cavity may indicate good prognoses.[7,8] In posttreatment evaluation, differentiating between pseudoresponse, pseudoprogression, and tumor recurrence is critical for follow-up.[8] DWI and DTI parameters are based on water diffusion within the microstructure of brain tissue and can be of great clinical importance in the posttreatment follow-up.

7.2 Clinical Applications

7.2.1 Differentiation between Cystic Brain Lesions

Glioblastoma multiforme, cystic/necrotic metastasis, and abscesses may appear quite similar on conventional MRI. They appear mostly as peripherally enhancing expansive lesions surrounded by a perilesional hyperintensity on T2-WI. DWI can be helpful to differentiate tumors from abscesses because fluid-filled abscesses have high signal intensity on DWI with reduced ADC values in their centers (▶ Fig. 7.1). The restricted diffusivity in abscesses is due to the high viscosity of the fluid inside the cavity, which leads to reduced water diffusion,[2] whereas the enhancing ring is a fibrous capsule formed by organized collagen fibres.[1] On the other hand, the cavity of a tumor is necrotic and usually not associated with restricted diffusion. Likewise, the enhancing portion of a tumor is due to viable tumor cells,[1] which may demonstrate restricted diffusion secondary to high cell density. Nevertheless, DTI can help to differentiate brain abscesses from necrotic neoplasms.[1,2] Depending on the organization of viable inflammatory cells inside abscesses, the FA values

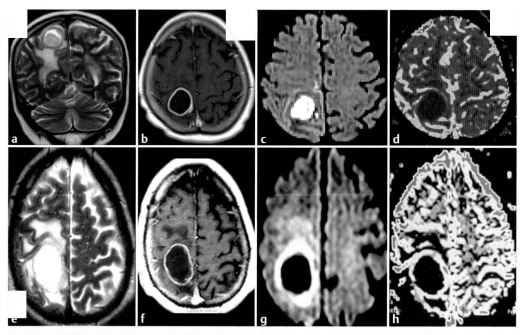

Fig. 7.1 (**a**) T2-weighted image (T2-WI), (**b**) enhanced T1-weighted image (T1-WI), (**c**) diffusion weighted image (DWI), and (**d**) relative cerebral blood volume (CBVr) map in a case of pyogenic abscess, which has restricted diffusion on the center of the lesion due to the pus. In another case (**e**) T2-WI, (**f**) enhanced T1-WI, (**g**) DWI, and (**h**) CBVr map show a glioblastoma multiforme with similar signal characteristics on conventional sequences, showing restricted diffusion at the periphery of the lesion on DWI and areas of high perfusion in the tumor wall on the CBVr map.

can be higher in abscesses than in the cystic/necrotic cavities of tumors. Higher FA values in abscess walls are due to the presence of concentric layers of collagen fibers rather than neoplastic cells in the tumor wall.[1]

7.2.2 Tumor Grading and Infiltration

Tumor grading is essential for treatment decisions and prognosis. Conventional MRI sequences enable exact anatomical localization, treatment planning, and follow-up, but do not provide substantial information regarding cellular composition of tumors, grade, or tumor infiltration, which are better addressed by advanced MRI techniques.[4] Identifying the boundaries between tumors, infiltrating cells, peritumoral edema, and normal brain parenchyma is crucial for preoperative planning. DWI and DTI are widely used techniques for these purposes due to their capabilities to image the brain microstructures.[2,4,9] Generally, tumor cell proliferation increases tumor cellularity, whereas apoptosis reduces tumor cellularity. Both affect the

extracellular space surrounding tumors.[9] Some local factors, such as high cellularity, the shape of the extracellular space characterized by reduced ratios of extracellular to intracellular space,[9] as well as high nuclear to cytoplasmic ratios, affect diffusion.[2] ADC is inversely correlated with high cellularity, and the changes in the intra- and extracellular spaces already mentioned restrict diffusion of water molecules.[2,3]

The meta-analysis conducted by Chen et al[9] to evaluate correlations between ADC and cellularity in all cancer types suggested that DWI can be used as a biomarker for tumor cellularity. Malignant tumors have larger nuclei, richer stroma, and higher cell numbers. These features restrict diffusion and reduce ADC values compared with benign tumors. DWI can also differentiate between high- and low-grade gliomas in most cases. Lower ADC values are measured in high-grade gliomas (World Health Organization [WHO] grades III and IV) due to their higher cellularity compared with low-grade gliomas (WHO grade II).[2,4,10] Nevertheless, some overlap can happen and is probably due to the high histopathological heterogeneity in gliomas (▶ Fig. 7.2).[2,10]

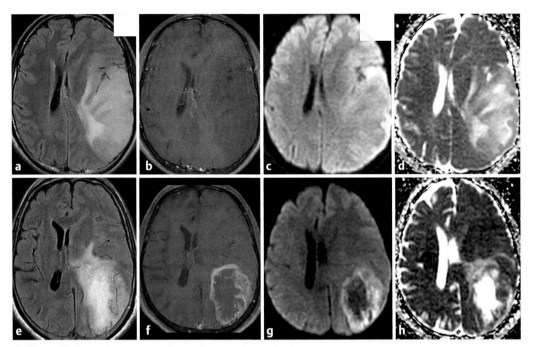

Fig. 7.2 (**a**) Fluid-attenuated inversion recovery (FLAIR) and (**b**) enhanced T1-weighted image (T1-WI) show an infiltrating low-grade glioma, which has no restricted diffusion (**c**) DWI and (**d**) ADC map. In another case, a high-grade glioma (**e**) FLAIR and (**f**) enhanced T1-W with peripheral areas of restricted diffusion and a necrotic center with facilitate diffusion (**g**) DWI and (**h**) ADC map

DTI parameters have also been used to differentiate high- and low-grade gliomas. The most controversial findings regarding this differentiation are for fractional anisotropy (FA). No differences in FA values have been observed in some studies, which is consistent with disorganization of fiber tracts in the tumor center. However, some studies have made the unlikely observation of increased FA values in high-grade gliomas compared to low-grade gliomas. The possible mechanisms remain controversial, including different methodologies employed by these studies and the potential for hypercellularity to reduce the extracellular space and thus increase the directionality of water diffusion, leading to increased FA values.[10,11] Although FA is not yet a reliable tool for grading gliomas, other DTI parameters may be more useful.[10] Radial Diffusivity (RD) and Axial Diffusivity (AD) are higher in low-grade gliomas than in high-grade gliomas, reflecting an inverse relationship between AD and RD, and glial tumors of WHO grades II through IV.[10]

Differentiating a solitary metastasis from a primary brain tumor may be challenging in some clinical scenarios. ADC values in metastases are lower than in low-grade gliomas, but ADC values measured at the peritumoral hyperintensity area are higher in metastases. The higher ADC in the periphery of metastases is likely explained by increased vasogenic edema,[4] increased extracellular space, which has a linear correlation with diffusivity.[12] The intratumoral FA values are greater in low-grade gliomas compared to metastases, explained by less cellular proliferation and vascularization in low-grade tumors.

On the other hand, the evaluation of peritumoral brain tissue reveals higher ADC values in metastases due to vasogenic edema compared to peritumoral cell infiltration described in high-grade gliomas.[4,11,13] A previous study suggested a cutoff value of 1.302×10^{-3} mm^2/s for the minimum peritumoral ADC to optimize sensitivity and specificity for distinguishing between glioblastoma multiforme and metastases.[11] However, other studies considered ADC values $< 1.200 \times 10^{-3}$ mm^2/s to suggest cell infiltration and that ADC values $> 1.600 \times 10^{-3}$ mm^2/s are suggestive of vasogenic edema.[13] The values in between these correspond to a combination of cell infiltration and edema and thus cannot be used to distinguish these lesions.[13]

The width of the tumor infiltration in high-grade gliomas can also be evaluated by ADC values. Lower ADC values were measured closest to the tumor border. Alternatively, ADC values measured in the abnormal hyperintensity surrounding metastatic lesions on T2-weighted images (T2-WIs) remain constant.[13]

DTI analysis of the peritumoral region demonstrated higher FA values in high-grade gliomas when compared to metastases. This observation may be explained by the fact that gliomas have infiltrating tumor cells in their surrounding parenchyma, restricting water diffusivity and increasing FA. Alternatively, the area surrounding the metastases is composed of vasogenic edema and white matter (WM) tract displacement, which reduces FA.[4,11] Previous reports have, however, demonstrated the utility of FA analysis of the perilesional region to distinguish metastases from primary brain tumors, but these results are still controversial.[4,11,12] Because tumor cell infiltration is known to damage myelinated neurofibers, this could reduce FA values.[12] The culmination of the effects of histological abnormalities that occur in the peritumoral brain tissue will ultimately determine FA values. Overlap between FA values from infiltration and edema may occur.[12] Indeed, AD and RD may help to distinguish these. The rapid increase of RD values in the tumor-infiltrated area may be associated with myelin sheath destruction when compared to the stable AD and RD increases associated with vasogenic edema in the extracellular space.[12]

7.2.3 Patterns of Peritumoral White Matter Tracts

Maximal resection is a goal of brain tumor treatment. Identifying tumor borders and peritumoral brain tissue is crucial to surgery success, but difficult to establish in high-grade gliomas. Previous reports have demonstrated that DWI and DTI measurements may play an important role in the assessment of the peritumoral area. These techniques, especially color-coded FA maps and tractography, can identify different patterns of WM tract involvement.[2,14]

The first pattern described consists of normal or only slightly decreased FA values with an abnormal location or direction resulting from bulk mass displacement. This pattern suggests that the main WM tract is intact and thus could be preserved during resection. The tract can also be better identified on tractography and on color-coded FA maps. The second pattern is probably related to vasogenic edema. FA is substantially decreased, but the main fiber tracts remain with normal locations and have normal directionality that is represented by normal colors on directional color maps, whereas color intensity is reduced. The following pattern is characterized by substantially decreased FA values with abnormal colors on directional color maps. The color change cannot be attributed to a bulk effect as with disrupted tracts most frequently seen in infiltrating gliomas. The last pattern described consists in an isotropic or almost isotropic diffusivity within the lesion. In this pattern, the tracts cannot be identified on directional color maps and is observed when some portion of the tract is completely destroyed by the tumor and is commonly observed in high-grade gliomas. This pattern may be useful in preoperative planning, relying on the notion that the main WM tracts are already disrupted so no special care is required to avoid damage during ressection.[14]

Although these are classical patterns of WM tracts, disturbances in the peritumoral area better illustrates their involvement. A combination of patterns may occur, such as displacement, infiltration, and edema, and these may limit the clinical application of these patterns for tumor grading and differential diagnoses.[2,14] As a result, the main clinical application of DTI and tractography in brain tumors is presurgical planning (▶ Fig. 7.3).

7.3 Special Cases

7.3.1 Meningioma

Meningiomas represent 14 to 20% of all intracranial brain tumors, and 10% have an atypical behavior that requires different therapeutic approaches. Differentiating typical from atypical meningiomas with conventional MRI is still a challenge. Heterogeneous appearances and enhancement, surrounding edema, and irregular cerebral surfaces are more commonly detected in atypical meningiomas, but they are not unique to these tumors. Atypical meningiomas have high cellularity and therefore may have restricted diffusion, although this is not a hallmark for these tumors. Some typical meningiomas may demonstrate abnormally increased ADC values that are probably secondary to increased fluid within the tumor or even a microcystic component. The high *b* values measured, explained later in this chapter, also corroborate these findings (▶ Fig. 7.4).[15] The atypical meningiomas express the proliferation marker Ki-67. There is an inverse correlation between ADC

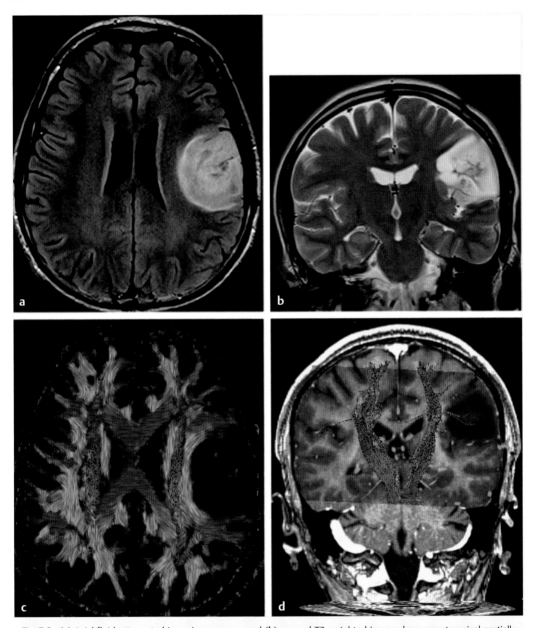

Fig. 7.3 (a) Axial fluid-attenuated inversion recovery and (b) coronal T2-weighted image show a postsurgical partially removed World Health Organization grade II oligodendroglioma. After deciding to reoperate the tumor, the surgeon was in doubt regarding the relationship between the lesion and the corticospinal tract and the superior longitudinal fasciculus. (c) Fractional anisotropy color map shows the deviation of the superior longitudinal fasciculus due to the mass effect of the lesion. The tractography fused with (d) T1-weighted image demonstrates minimal deviation of the left corticospinal tract, as well as a surgical plane between the tract and the tumor.

values (lower ADC values correlate to high cellularity) and Ki-67 expression (marker of high cell proliferation), and an ADC cutoff of 0.70×10^{-3} mm²/s can be considered an important statistical point to differentiate atypical and typical meningiomas.[16]

7.3.2 Lymphoma

Primary central nervous system lymphoma (PCNSL) is usually represented by an infiltrating lesion with low signal intensity on T2-WI that

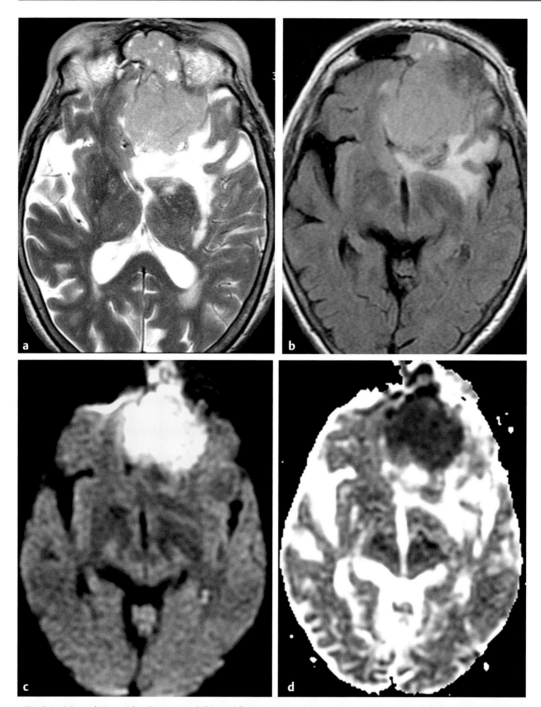

Fig. 7.4 (a) Axial T2-weighted image and (b) axial fluid-attenuated inversion recovery show a left frontal extra-axial mass, with isointense signal, surrounded by vasogenic edema. The lesion demonstrates hyperintensity on (c) diffusion weighted imaging and low signal intensity on (d) apparent diffusion coefficient map, characterizing restricted diffusion. The histological diagnosis was atypical meningioma.

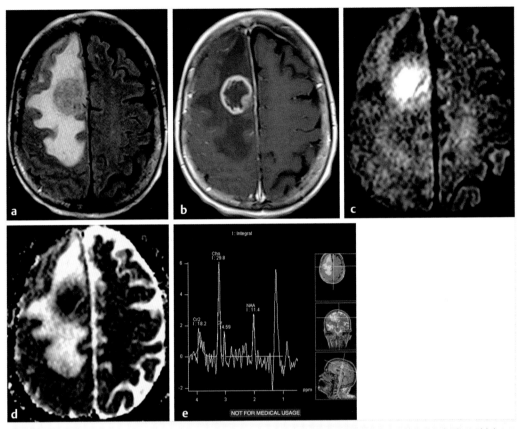

Fig. 7.5 (a) Fluid-attenuated inversion recovery and enhanced (b) T1-weighted image in a case of right frontal lobe primary central nervous system lymphoma after kidney transplantation. (c) Diffusion weighted imaging and (d) apparent diffusion coefficient map show restricted diffusion on the lesion. (e) The proton magnetic resonance spectroscopy demonstrates high choline/N-acetyl aspartate (CHo/NAA) ratio, as well as peak of lipids/lactate.

enhances after intravenous contrast administration. Nevertheless, differential diagnoses with enhancing high-grade gliomas may be difficult. A previous report demonstrated restricted diffusion in lymphoma compared to glioblastoma multiforme that is likely due to the morphology of lymphoma, its higher degree of cellularity, and higher nucleo-to-cytoplasma ratio, when compared to glioblastoma (▶ Fig. 7.5).[5]

ADC values in PCNSL may also be used as a prognostic tool in the assessment of these patients. A study has suggested that lower pretreatment ADC values (cutoff of 0.384×10^{-3} mm^2/s) can predict worse clinical outcomes in immunocompetent patients treated with methotrexate-based chemotherapy. The studies concluded that the lower the ADC is at baseline, the shorter the progression-free time and overall survival will be. If these findings were combined with perfusion evaluation, the presence of low cerebral blood volume could identify the PCNSL cases with the worst prognoses.[17]

7.3.3 Epidermoid Tumors

The major differential diagnosis consideration in an epidermoid cyst is arachnoid cyst because both lesions have signal intensity similar to the cerebrospinal fluid (CSF) on T1- and T2-WI and usually do not enhance after intravenous contrast administration. Although fluid-attenuated inversion recovery (FLAIR) sequences can be an important tool in the evaluation of these lesions and contribute to their differentiation, DWI evaluation is even more characteristic. On DWI, the epidermoid tumor has a hyperintense signal, whereas the arachnoid cysts are hypointense and demonstrate high diffusivity. The ADC of the epidermoid is similar to the brain parenchyma or may also be slightly reduced due to

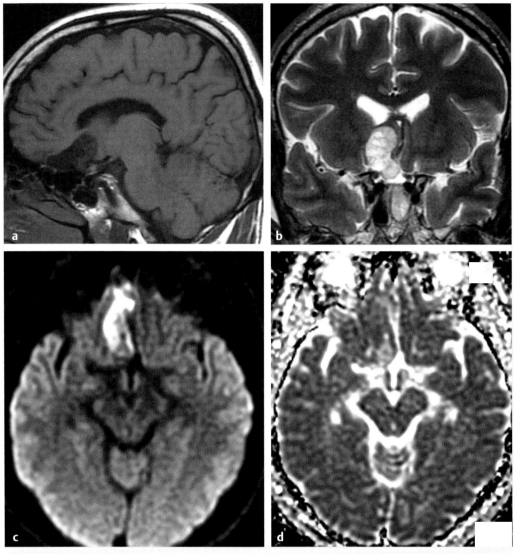

Fig. 7.6 (a) Sagittal T1-weighted image and coronal (b) T2-weighted image show a right anterior fossa epidermoid tumor. The lesion was high signal intensity on (c) diffusion weighted imaging and heterogeneous signal intensity, predominantly isointense to brain parenchyma, on (d) apparent diffusion coefficient map.

the tumor contents, and the ADC within the arachnoid cyst is similar to the CSF (▶ Fig. 7.6).[2,6]

7.3.4 Pediatric Intracranial Tumors

Central nervous system tumors are the most common type of solid tumors in the pediatric population and are the major cause of death from cancer in children. The age of patients, imaging characteristics, and tumor location are essential for the diagnosis. Supratentorial tumors are more common in neonates and infants, whereas infratentorial tumors are more common in children older than 2 years.[6]

The primitive neuroectodermal tumor (PNET), which arises from undifferentiated brain cells, is composed of small round cells with scant cytoplasm. The ADC of PNET, mostly in the medulloblastoma, is decreased because of high cellularity and high nucleus to cytoplasm ratios.[6] Restricted diffusion is one of the most important indicators of infratentorial lesions because ADC values are significantly lower in medulloblastomas than in other tumors, such as ependymomas, brainstem

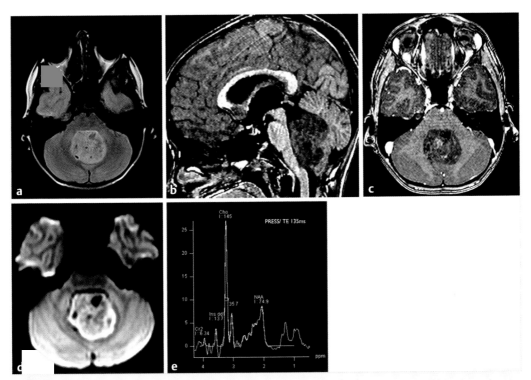

Fig. 7.7 (a) Axial fluid-attenuated inversion recovery, (b) sagittal T1-weighted image (T1-WI), and (c) enhanced axial T1-WI show a fourth ventricle lesion with mass effect in the cerebellar vermis. (d) The lesion has hyperintensity on (e) diffusion weighted imaging and very high choline/N-acetil aspartate ratio at the proton magnetic resonance spectroscopy. The histological diagnosis was typical medulloblastoma.

gliomas, and juvenile pilocytic astrocytoma (▶ Fig. 7.7).[6,18]

Diffusion on pineal masses, including germinomas and pinealoblastomas, is restricted due to the high cellularity of these tumors. DWI is also helpful in the differential diagnosis of these lesions. Low- and high-grade astrocytomas in the pediatric population behave similarly to those in adults. The higher the cellularity is (usually representing high-grade gliomas), the lower the ADC values will be.[6]

7.4 Posttreatment Evaluation

Diffusion imaging can be used to assess posttreatment changes. DWI may serve as an early biomarker tool for predicting treatment outcomes, monitoring treatment response, and detecting recurrent cancer.[9] In a tumor that demonstrated restricted diffusion before treatment, an increased ADC is a good indicator of treatment response. Treatment will lead to a reduction in tumor cellularity and a consequent increase in the ADC values, which may also precede changes in tumor size and patterns of contrast enhancement.

7.4.1 Immediate Postoperative Evaluation

The most widely used method to assess therapeutic response after surgery for high-grade gliomas has been to examine changes in contrast enhancement.[8] Subsequent MRI 24 to 48 hours after surgery is performed to reveal the extent of tumor resection.[2,7] Weeks or months after the treatment is ended, additional imaging is used to evaluate tumor size, mostly based on the MacDonald criteria evaluation.[2,8] Nevertheless, the MacDonald criteria are limited when evaluating low-grade gliomas, which usually do not enhance, and new therapeutic approaches, such as chemoradiation with temozolomide and antiangiogenic agents, pseudoprogression, and pseudoresponse alter the way conventional MRI scans must be interpreted.[8]

DWI should be performed during the postoperative MRI for its prognostic value. Areas of restricted diffusion may be detected adjacent to the resected tumor.[2,7] The perioperative abnormalities observed on DWI may represent impaired blood flow due to injury to normal vessels or cytotoxic edema with contusion caused by mechanical stimuli during surgery. DWI may be classified as a thin linear lesion next to the tumor cavity that represents a brain contusion and corresponds to vascular regions extending outward from the tumor cavity and likely results from interrupted vascular perfusion of the underlying WM.[7] The DWI abnormalities correspond to contrast-enhanced areas in follow-up imaging, and the enhancement subsequently regresses to form an area of encephalomalacia.[2,7] This fact should not be misdiagnosed as tumor recurrence,[2] and it is reasonable to expect that the tumor will not recur where blood flow was disrupted at surgery.[7] Thus restricted diffusion in the postoperative MRI within 24 to 48 hours represents infarction and/or contusion and also represents complications induced by surgery. This abnormality may paradoxically benefit patients with high-grade gliomas and serve as a prognostic factor.[7]

7.4.2 Pseudoprogression

Enhancing lesions that arise on routine follow-up brain MRI at the site of a previously identified and treated high-grade glioma might present a significant diagnostic dilemma. MRI cannot reliably discriminate tumor recurrence/progression from inflammatory or necrotic changes resulting from chemoradiation.[19] Radiation necrosis and pseudoprogression are forms of treatment-related enhancement following chemoradiation with temozolomide.[8] Pseudoprogression usually refers to an increase in contrast enhancement within the first 3 to 6 months after chemoradiation that occurs earlier than radiotherapy damage alone in about 30% of cases. It is generally self-limiting and represents a combination of treatment effects on residual tumor cells and disruption of the blood–brain barrier. Pseudoprogression has been reported to be correlated with O6-methylguanine-DNA methyltransferase (MGMT) promoter methylation status.[8] The diagnosis is primarily based on routine follow-up conventional MRI exams. The Response Assessment in Neuro-Oncology (RANO) criteria are currently used to assess posttreatment changes in brain tumor patients and are based on conventional MRI findings. Evidence regarding the use of DWI and DTI to differentiate pseudoprogression from recurrent tumors is currently limited and conflicting.[8,19]

The ADC value of the contrast-enhancing portion of the new lesion can be measured. Higher ADC values were identified in patients with recurrences relative to patients without recurrences.[19] This fact is supported by histopathological findings of increased extracellular spaces and micronecrosis in the tumor area. In enhancing nonrecurrent lesions, fibrosis, gliosis, macrophage invasion, vascular changes, and demyelination predominate, and restricted diffusion is seen.[19] However, there is some disagreement in interpreting ADC values in recurrent lesions. It would be expected that the high cellularity of the tumor would reduce ADC values. Thus the ADC will be influenced by the predominant histopathological alterations within the area of tumor recurrence. Changes in ADC would correspond with tumor progression; thus ADC changes would not be considered a favorable prognostic factor.[8] Furthermore, no differences in FA values were observed between recurrence and nonrecurrence lesions.[19,20] AD and RD parameters may, however, be more sensitive, especially in the surrounding lesion tissue.[19]

7.4.3 Pseudoresponse

The unregulated angiogenesis characterized by dilated and hyperpermeable vessels allows tumor growth. These vessels promote inefficient tumor perfusion that leads to necrosis. Novel antiangiogenic agents for tumor treatment, including bevacizumab, act directly against vascular endothelial growth factor (VEGF) or its receptor on vessel walls to inhibit vascularization. Normalization of vasculature causes a reduction in the diameter and permeability of the vessels and often causes a rapid decrease in contrast enhancement (within 24 hours) without a true antitumoral effect.[8] Changes to the RANO criteria have been proposed to address the evaluation of these new conditions related to the use of novel drugs. The nonenhancing portion of the lesion is now evaluated by FLAIR sequences. Pseudoresponse is demonstrated when the nonenhancing portion of the tumor increases in addition to the enhancing portion. In some cases, DWI can depict restricted areas adjacent to the lesion that, in some cases, may correspond to tumor progression in the follow-up MRI examinations (▶ Fig. 7.8).[8]

However, the importance of a new diffusion restricted area in patients with high-grade gliomas during therapy is unclear. In some cases, this

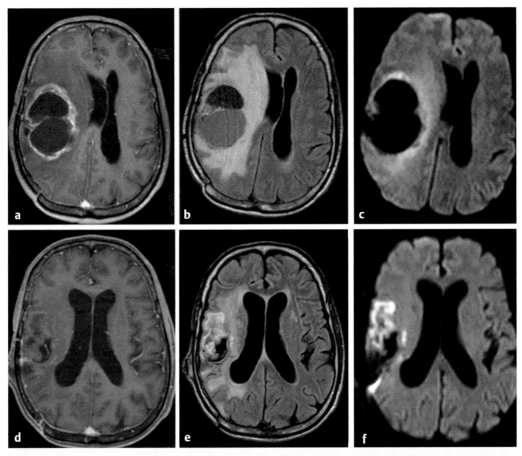

Fig. 7.8 (a) Enhanced T1-weighted image, (b) fluid-attenuated inversion recovery (FLAIR), and (c) diffusion weighted imaging (DWI) of a postsurgical high-grade glioma that presented failure of the concomitant radio- and chemotherapy. (d) Antiangiogenic drug was initiated, and, besides a reduction in the enhancing portion of the lesion, (e) an expansion and tumor infiltration are observed in the FLAIR. (f) DWI demonstrates areas of restricted diffusion that may correspond to tumor dissemination.

region may remain stable over time instead of evolving into a region of enhancing tumor, which may not represent tumor progression but rather vascular cooption by tumors or even atypical necrosis.[8] A trend of decreasing ADC in both contrast-enhanced MRI and FLAIR-hyperintense regions is shown in tumors that ultimately progress, whereas stable/nonrecurrent tumors show small progressive increases in ADC during follow-up.[21]

7.5 Future Applications

7.5.1 High b Value Diffusion Weighted Imaging (HBDWI)

The use of increased b values on DWI (HBDWI) (e.g., 3,000/4,000 mm^2/s) may be useful for evaluating pseudoprogression and pseudoresponse.[22,23] The hypothesis is that the kinetics of signal decay in heterogeneous voxels can be evaluated with multiple b factor acquisitions to allow characterization of the various water diffusivity compartments within a single voxel.[24] There are several models for interpreting multiple b values, including kurtosis, biexponential models, stretched exponential models, and the most common two-compartmental model.[24] At HBDWI, there is more contrast of the tissues of interest than at regular b values[22,23] and less T2 shine-through effect.[23] The two-compartmental model detects slow and fast diffusion components, representing intra- and extracellular diffusion, respectively. The slow component is more sensitive at HBDWI, suggesting that ADC values based on higher *b* values reflect changes in cellularity more accurately than at lower *b* values.[22,23] ADC values acquired at higher *b* values are lower than those acquired at standard *b* values due to the predominance of the slow diffusion component on HBDWI.[23] HBDWI is limited by an inferior signal-to-noise ratio than regular *b* value DWI, and optimal *b* values have not yet established.[22]

HBDWI can be considered superior to RANO criteria and MacDonald criteria for pseudoresponse evaluation.[22] Areas of high signal intensity on HBDWI represent tumor recurrence similar to regular DWI *b* value images.[22] Lower ADC values are also detected in tumor recurrence compared to pseudoprogression. However, the fifth percentile value of the cumulative ADC histogram obtained with HBDWI is a promising parameter to distinguish this.[23] The distinction between vasogenic edema and tumoral infiltration surrounding the tumor lesion can also be made using DWI with multiple *b* values.[24]

7.5.2 Functional Diffusion Maps

The functional diffusion maps (fDMs) display changes in ADC that occur over time and can be a biomarker for glioma follow-up. The fDM requires image registration between a current ADC map and the baseline map. After the appropriate registration, a voxel-by-voxel subtraction is performed to compare different time points, including postsurgical and pretreatment points.[8,22,25] Each voxel is then categorized based on the change in ADC relative to the baseline values. Red voxels represent increased ADC above baseline (considered hypocellular voxels), blue voxels represent decreased ADC values compared to the baseline (hypercellular voxels), and green voxels represent no ADC change. Edema, gliosis, infection, and ischemia are other tissue conditions that may influence ADC values, and care should be taken during map interpretation. In practice, a threshold of 0.4×10^{-3} mm^2/s is used based on the 95% confidence limit of normal-appearing white and gray matter and allows optimal sensitivity and specificity to distinguish stable from progressive disease.[25] The rate of change in fDM hypercellular volumes compared to FLAIR hypersignal abnormalities may predict tumor progression, time to progression, and overall survival for antiangiogenic and cytotoxic treatments because the ADC changes precede changes in standard anatomical images.[25]

7.5.3 Diffusion Tensor Imaging Outcomes

The future of DTI is to move beyond the tensor representation of diffusion and improve the well-known obstacles that include cases of fiber intersection and dispersion in the same voxel. The supertensor representations will be a useful technique to overcome the crossing fibers obstacle, and a possible approach is diffusion spectrum imaging (DSI).[2]

Diffusion kurtosis (DK) imaging allows the characterization of nongaussian water diffusion and is complementary to ADC and FA. The mean kurtosis (MK) can be used to evaluate the gray and white matter, resolve the crossing fiber tracts, and grade tumors[2] (see Chapter 15).

7.5.4 Tractography

Distinguishing normal tissue from disrupted WM tracts is essential before resection of brain tumors.[26] The patterns of WM involvement in the peritumoral area are based on FA maps from DTI acquisitions.[14] However, the diffusion tensor model is ideal only for describing a single fiber population within a given voxel and does not accurately describe the microstructure in complex WM voxels that contain more than one fiber population arising from intersecting tracts or to partial volume averaging of adjacent pathways that have different fiber orientations.[27] To overcome these problems, it is desirable to use the information derived from high angular resolution diffusion imaging (HARDI), which is reconstructed by the q-ball, providing an orientation distribution function (ODF) that can better resolve multiple fiber populations within a single voxel.[27] The probabilistic q-ball fiber tracking approach surpasses standard fiber tracking methods for tumor presurgical planning[26,27] because it is more sensitive and better delineates the involved fiber tracts, notably in the spinal cord.[27]

7.6 Summary

DWI and DTI are advanced MRI techniques that help brain tumor evaluation. Primary tumor grading and invasion, differential diagnosis between other intracranial lesions, and treatment prognosis may be assessed by such techniques. New postprocessing and acquisition methods for DWI and DTI will further improve them as tools for tumor evaluation.

References

[1] Toh CH, Wei KC, Ng SH, Wan YL, Lin CP, Castillo M. Differentiation of brain abscesses from necrotic glioblastomas and cystic metastatic brain tumors with diffusion tensor imaging. AJNR Am J Neuroradiol 2011; 32(9): 1646–1651

[2] Hygino da Cruz LC, Jr, Vieira IG, Domingues RC. Diffusion MR imaging: an important tool in the assessment of brain tumors. Neuroimaging Clin N Am 2011; 21(1): 27–49, vii

[3] Zulfiqar M, Yousem DM, Lai H. ADC values and prognosis of malignant astrocytomas: does lower ADC predict a worse prognosis independent of grade of tumor?—a meta-analysis. AJR Am J Roentgenol 2013; 200(3): 624–629

[4] Svolos P, Tsolaki E, Kapsalaki E, et al. Investigating brain tumor differentiation with diffusion and perfusion metrics at 3 T MRI using pattern recognition techniques. Magn Reson Imaging 2013; 31(9): 1567–1577

[5] Kickingereder P, Wiestler B, Sahm F, et al. Primary central nervous system lymphoma and atypical glioblastoma: multiparametric differentiation by using diffusion-, perfusion-, and susceptibility-weighted MR imaging. Radiology 2014; 272(3): 843–850

[6] Borja MJ, Plaza MJ, Altman N, Saigal G. Conventional and advanced MRI features of pediatric intracranial tumors: supratentorial tumors. AJR Am J Roentgenol 2013; 200(5): W483–W503

[7] Furuta T, Nakada M, Ueda F, et al. Prognostic paradox: brain damage around the glioblastoma resection cavity. J Neurooncol 2014; 118(1): 187–192

[8] Shiroishi MS, Booker MT, Agarwal M, et al. Posttreatment evaluation of central nervous system gliomas. Magn Reson Imaging Clin N Am 2013; 21(2): 241–268

[9] Chen L, Liu M, Bao J, et al. The correlation between apparent diffusion coefficient and tumor cellularity in patients: a meta-analysis. PLoS ONE 2013; 8(11): e79008

[10] Server A, Graff BA, Josefsen R, et al. Analysis of diffusion tensor imaging metrics for gliomas grading at 3 T. Eur J Radiol 2014; 83(3): e156–e165

[11] Lee EJ, Ahn KJ, Lee EK, Lee YS, Kim DB. Potential role of advanced MRI techniques for the peritumoural region in differentiating glioblastoma multiforme and solitary metastatic lesions. Clin Radiol 2013; 68(12): e689–e697

[12] Min ZG, Niu C, Rana N, Ji HM, Zhang M. Differentiation of pure vasogenic edema and tumor-infiltrated edema in patients with peritumoral edema by analyzing the relationship of axial and radial diffusivities on 3.0 T MRI. Clin Neurol Neurosurg 2013; 115(8): 1366–1370

[13] Pavlisa G, Rados M, Pavlisa G, Pavic L, Potocki K, Mayer D. The differences of water diffusion between brain tissue infiltrated by tumor and peritumoral vasogenic edema. Clin Imaging 2009; 33(2): 96–101

[14] Jellison BJ, Field AS, Medow J, Lazar M, Salamat MS, Alexander AL. Diffusion tensor imaging of cerebral white matter: a pictorial review of physics, fiber tract anatomy, and tumor imaging patterns. AJNR Am J Neuroradiol 2004; 25(3): 356–369

[15] Bano S, Waraich MM, Khan MA, Buzdar SA, Manzur S. Diagnostic value of apparent diffusion coefficient for the accurate assessment and differentiation of intracranial meningiomas. Acta Radiol Short Rep 2013; 2(7): 2047981613512484

[16] Tang Y, Dundamadappa SK, Thangasamy S, et al. Correlation of apparent diffusion coefficient with Ki-67 proliferation index in grading meningioma. AJR Am J Roentgenol 2014; 202(6): 1303–1308

[17] Valles FE, Perez-Valles CL, Regalado S, Barajas RF, Rubenstein JL, Cha S. Combined diffusion and perfusion MR imaging as biomarkers of prognosis in immunocompetent patients with primary central nervous system lymphoma. AJNR Am J Neuroradiol 2013; 34(1): 35–40

[18] Rodriguez Gutierrez D, Awwad A, Meijer L, et al. Metrics and textural features of MRI diffusion to improve classification of pediatric posterior fossa tumors. AJNR Am J Neuroradiol 2014; 35(5): 1009–1015

[19] Sundgren PC, Fan X, Weybright P, et al. Differentiation of recurrent brain tumor versus radiation injury using diffusion tensor imaging in patients with new contrast-enhancing lesions. Magn Reson Imaging 2006; 24(9): 1131–1142

[20] Alexio GA, Zikou A, Tsiouris S, et al. Comparison of diffusion tensor, dynamic susceptibility contrast MRI and (99m)Tc-Tetrofosmin brain SPECT for the detection of recurrent high-grade glioma. Magn Reson Imaging 2014; 32(7): 854–859

[21] Jain R, Scarpace LM, Ellika S, et al. Imaging response criteria for recurrent gliomas treated with bevacizumab: role of diffusion weighted imaging as an imaging biomarker. J Neurooncol 2010; 96(3): 423–431

[22] Yamasaki F, Kurisu K, Aoki T, et al. Advantages of high b-value diffusion weighted imaging to diagnose pseudo-responses in patients with recurrent glioma after bevacizumab treatment. Eur J Radiol 2012; 81(10): 2805–2810

[23] Chu HH, Choi SH, Ryoo I, et al. Differentiation of true progression from pseudoprogression in glioblastoma treated with radiation therapy and concomitant temozolomide: comparison study of standard and high-b-value diffusion weighted imaging. Radiology 2013; 269(3): 831–840

[24] Vandendries C, Ducreux D, Lacroix C, Ducot B, Saliou G. Statistical analysis of multi-b factor diffusion weighted images can help distinguish between vasogenic and tumor-infiltrated edema. J Magn Reson Imaging 2014; 40(3): 622–629

[25] Schmainda KM. Diffusion weighted MRI as a biomarker for treatment response in glioma. CNS Oncol 2012; 1(2): 169–180

[26] Zhang H, Wang Y, Lu T, et al. Differences between generalized q-sampling imaging and diffusion tensor imaging in the preoperative visualization of the nerve fiber tracts within peritumoral edema in brain. Neurosurgery 2013; 73(6): 1044–1053, discussion 1053

[27] Bucci M, Mandelli ML, Berman JI, et al. Quantifying diffusion MRI tractography of the corticospinal tract in brain tumors with deterministic and probabilistic methods. Neuroimage Clin 2013; 3: 361–368

8 Diffusion Weighted and Diffusion Tensor Imaging in Infectious Diseases

Claudia da Costa Leite, Maria da Graça Morais Martin, and Mauricio Castillo

Key Points

- Diffusion weighted imaging (DWI) is a useful diagnostic tool for central nervous system (CNS) infectious disease, among other pathologies.
- Meningitis, regardless of its cause, can present subarachnoid hyperintensities on DWI. Complications of meningitis, such as infarctions, venous thrombosis, empyema, ventriculitis, and abscess also present characteristic findings on DWI.
- Pyogenic abscess usually presents as a hypointense rim on T2-weighted imaging, a peripheral enhancement after contrast administration, and a hyperintense core on DWI with reduced apparent diffusion coefficient (ADC). Fungal or tuberculous abscesses may present variable signal intensities on DWI and are not always hyperintense as pyogenic abscesses are. Fungal abscesses are commonly multiple, and their borders are loculated or crenated.
- DWI can identify early findings of herpesvirus infection with areas of restricted diffusion on the temporal and frontal lobes, insula, and cingulate gyrus.
- In immunocompromised patients, progressive multifocal leukoencephalopathy (PML) can present as a leading edge of hyperintensity on DWI, sometimes with restricted diffusion. Toxoplasmosis lesions do not present with restricted diffusion.
- DWI is very useful in patients with Creutzfeldt–Jakob disease because the lesions present as hyperintense signal on DWI and are better seen than with other imaging sequences.

8.1 Clinical Applications

8.1.1 Introduction

Neuroimaging is an essential tool in the diagnosis and therapeutic planning of central nervous system (CNS) infectious disease. The introduction of diffusion weighted imaging (DWI) has improved the diagnosis of certain infectious process. DWI can provide additional information to conventional magnetic resonance imaging (MRI) sequences that allows a better understanding of the pathophysiology as well as more precise and early diagnosis in many infectious diseases. DWI is an important imaging tool for the diagnosis of many infectious lesions, such as encephalitis, abscess, ventriculitis, empyema and other complications of infectious processes, such as infarcts due to vasculitis or venous thrombosis. In some instances diffusion tensor imaging (DTI) may help follow up lesion response after proper treatment is initiated, and may better evaluate its sequelae. This chapter discusses the main groups of etiologic agents: bacterial, viral, fungal, parasitic, and prion diseases, and the contributions of DWI and DTI in their diagnosis, therapeutic strategies, and follow-up.

8.1.2 Brief Overview of Infectious Diseases and DWI and DTI

Bacterial Infections

Bacterial infections require prompt diagnosis and treatment. The infectious process can be restricted to the meninges and cerebrospinal fluid (CSF) compartment (meningitis, ventriculitis) or can spread to the brain parenchyma (cerebritis, brain abscess). It can also be located within the meningeal layers (empyema).

Meningitis is defined as the inflammation of the membranes surrounding the brain and spinal cord. Usually the diagnosis is based on clinical findings and CSF analysis. Imaging can be required before lumbar puncture to rule out increased intracranial pressure and to detect complications of meningitis.[1]

In meningitis, computed tomography (CT) is the most commonly used imaging diagnostic tool, regardless of underlying bacteria. Magnetic resonance imaging (MRI) is not usually required for uncomplicated meningitis, but MRI is superior to CT for depicting meningitis complications, such as vasculitis and empyema. MRI can show meningeal abnormalities on fluid-attenuated inversion recovery (FLAIR) or postcontrast T1-weighted images (the authors reserve the use of postcontrast FLAIR imaging for specific conditions, such as infectious and carcinomatous meningitis). DWI

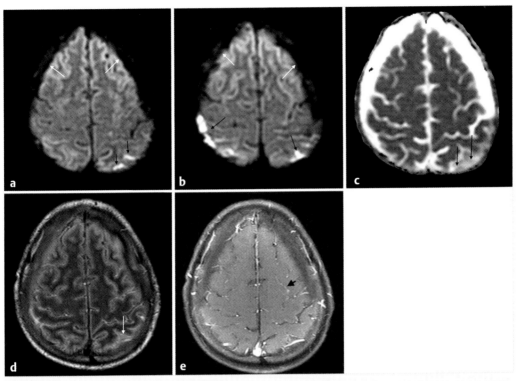

Fig. 8.1 *Streptococcus pneumoniae* meningitis with hyperintensity on diffusion weighted imaging (DWI). (**a,b**) Axial DWI shows hyperintense parietal sulci (black arrows) and hypointense subdural effusions bilaterally (white arrows). On the apparent diffusion coefficient (ADC) map, (**c**) the parietal sulci ADC (black arrows) is reduced compared to CSF, although not reduced compared to the parenchyma. In the subdural collections the ADC is close to cerebrospinal fluid (CSF). (**d**) The axial enhanced fluid-attenuated inversion recovery image also shows hyperintensity in parietal sulci (white arrow) and the bilateral subdural effusion similar to CSF. (**e**) The contrast-enhanced axial T1-weighted image shows subtle leptomeningeal enhancement in some sulci (black arrow).

can demonstrate subarachnoid hyperintensities as well as complications of meningitis, such as acute infarcts due to septic vasculitis and venous thrombosis. Subarachnoid DWI hyperintensity in meningitis is attributed to proteinaceous exudate with inflammatory cells and debris (▶ Fig. 8.1).[2]

MRI is an excellent tool for the diagnosis of extra-axial collections associated with meningitis, which can be sterile (effusion/hygroma) or infected (empyema). These complications are more common in pneumococcal meningitis affecting children under 2 years of age. Effusion/hygroma tends to be bilateral, large, and located in the frontal or temporal regions (▶ Fig. 8.2). On the other hand, empyemas can be located in the subdural or epidural spaces and are usually hyperintense to CSF on precontrast T1-weighted images, hyperintense on T2-weighted images, and show peripheral contrast enhancement and hyperintensity on DWI with reduced diffusion coefficients (▶ Fig. 8.3).[1]

The diagnosis of pyogenic abscess is crucial for proper and prompt therapeutic management. The main etiologic agents associated with bacterial abscesses are *Staphylococcus aureus* and *Streptococcus* species.

Classically the evolution of brain abscess consists of four stages: early cerebritis, late cerebritis, early capsule formation, and late capsule formation. Regardless of the etiologic agent the MRI findings of the brain abscess are very similar.[3] The first phase of cerebritis is characterized by vascular congestion, petechial hemorrhages, and edema, causing a poorly demarcated parenchymal softening. The MRI findings are nonspecific, with hyperintensity on T2-weighted images and little or no contrast enhancement. The capsular stage may begin approximately during the second week and can last for months, being characterized by a central zone of necrosis encircled by a collagen capsule. The abscess capsule can present as a smooth or

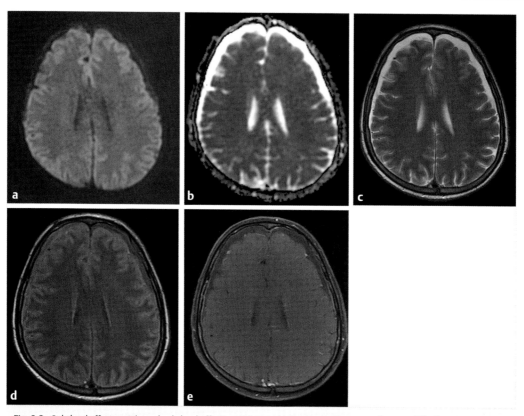

Fig. 8.2 Subdural effusion. Bilateral subdural effusion with signal intensity similar to cerebrospinal fluid (CSF), low signal on (**a**) axial diffusion weighted imaging and high signal on (**b**) apparent diffusion coefficient map, high signal on (**c**) T2, just more hyperintense to CSF on (**d**) fluid-attenuated inversion recovery, probably due to proteinaceous content, and no enhancement on postcontrast (**e**) T1-weighted image.

lobulated hyperintense rim on T1-weighted and a hypointense rim on T2-weighted images with smooth and thin contrast enhancement. Because abscesses are ring-enhancing lesions many other differential diagnoses should be included, especially necrotic tumor. On DWI an abscess usually presents as hyperintensity with reduced apparent diffusion coefficients (ADCs) within the center of the abscess. In ring-enhancing lesions, if the ADC is low, the accuracy of the diagnosis of a capsular phase abscess versus necrotic tumor is high, and it is even higher when a complete T2-hypointense rim is present (▶ Fig. 8.4).[3] The reduced ADC that occurs in the center of the lesion is attributable to pus that contains microorganisms, macromolecules, debris, proteins, amino acids, and inflammatory cells that bind, obstruct, and prevent the normal random motion of water.[4] Even though low ADC in the center of a ring enhancing lesion is a sign of high accuracy for the diagnosis of bacterial abscess, some fungal abscesses and even necrotic

tumors (especially metastases) can occasionally present restricted diffusion in its central portion, and, also, some bacterial abscesses may not have restricted diffusion. Brain abscess has a higher ADC (less restricted) after treatment than before treatment; thus DWI is a tool to evaluate treatment response (▶ Fig. 8.5 and ▶ Fig. 8.6). Relapse of a brain abscess decreases ADC values again.[6]

Gupta et al,[7,8] using DTI, found increased fractional anisotropy (FA) in the cavity of the bacterial abscess (▶ Fig. 8.4f), which had a positive correlation with neuroinflammatory molecules, suggesting that FA elevation reflects upregulation of various adhesion molecules in brain abscess inflammation. Nath et al[6] showed in 20 patients with abscesses that the FA in the cavities decreased following a successful 4 week treatment period.

Ventriculitis is a rare intracranial infection, associated with abscess rupture into the ventricular system, extension of basal cistern meningitis to

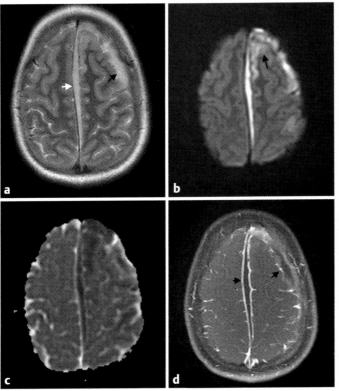

Fig. 8.3 This patient had a sinusitis and suffered a facial trauma, evolving to meningitis complicated with empyema, cerebritis and/or vasculitis and infarct in the left hemisphere. **(a)** The axial T2-weighted image shows a left frontal (black arrow) and parafalcine (white arrow) subdural collections, **(b)** which also show hyperintensity on diffusion weighted imaging (DWI) **(c)** and hypointensity on the apparent diffusion coefficient (ADC) map, typical of a subdural empyema. **(b)** Note also DWI hyperintensities in the left frontal gyri (arrow), which correlated with hypointensities on the ADC map and could be attributable to cerebritis or infarct. **(d)** The enhanced axial T1-weighted image shows contrast enhancement along the margins of the infected collections (arrows).

the ventricles, and ventricular empyema extension, or it may be iatrogenic. It is a potential fatal CNS infection. The ventricles are enlarged on MRI scans; the ependyma shows hyperintensity on fluid attenuated inversion recovery (FLAIR) and T2-weighted images, and there is contrast enhancement of the ventricular lining. Within the ventricles debris/suppurative content can sometimes be seen as -fluid levels, with sediments deposited in the depent parts. The debris/suppurative content presents hyperintensity on FLAIR images and on DWI with reduced ADC (▶ Fig. 8.7).[9]

Other complications associated with meningitis are vascular, such as acute infarcts and venous thrombosis (▶ Fig. 8.8). DWI is a helpful diagnostic tool for the diagnosis of acute arterial infarcts but is less useful in venous infarcts, which may present as a variety of findings.

In intracranial bacterial infections, neurotuberculosis (neurotb) must be emphasized because it has increased prevalence in immunocompromised patients, such as those with acquired immunodeficiency syndrome (AIDS) and organ transplants and those from endemic regions. The main presentation of neurotb is meningitis (up to 95% of cases) affecting mainly the basal meninges. Brain parenchyma involvement can be seen as a complication of meningeal involvement and includes infarcts or abscess/granuloma.[10] DWI is useful for the diagnosis of acute ischemic infarcts, differentiating acute from subacute or chronic infarcts, and detecting vasculitis.[11] Tuberculomas can present a T2-hypointense or T2-hyperintense core, and usually these lesions present with DWI hypointensity and ADC map hyperintensity (no restriction of diffusion) (▶ Fig. 8.9). However, DWI hyperintensity and ADC map hypointensity have also been described for tuberculomas.[12] Both tuberculomas and tuberculous abscess can present as ring enhancement, central hyperintensity, or hypointensity on DWI, with or without reduced ADC, making differentiation between solid and necrotic caseation difficult on conventional MRI sequences and DWI (▶ Fig. 8.10).[13] ▶ Table 8.1 summarizes the main DWI findings on bacterial infections.

Viral Infectious

The diffuse and generalized infection of the brain known as encephalitis is most often the result of viruses. CNS viral infection can present as meningitis, encephalitis, and chronic encephalopathy.

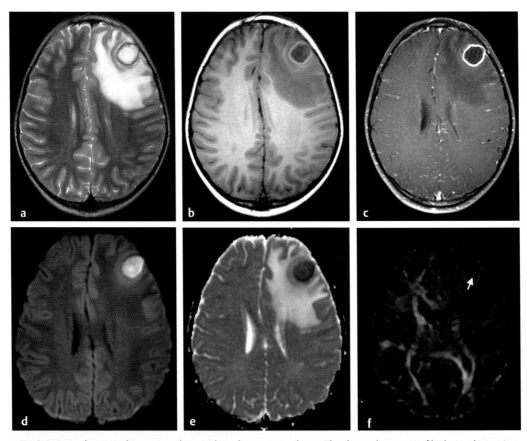

Fig. 8.4 Brain abscess and extensive edema within adjacent parenchyma. The abscess has a core of high signal intensity on the axial T2-weighted image (**a**), low signal on T1-weighted image pre-(**b**) and postgadolinium (**c**) and restricted diffusion with hyperintensity on the axial diffusion weighted imaging (**d**) and hypointensity on the apparent diffusion coefficient (ADC) map (**e**), whereas the adjacent edema has a facilitated diffusion (hyperintensity on the ADC map). There is a halo of hypointensity on the T2-weighted image (**a**) and hyperintensity on the T1-weighted image (**b**), with regular peripheral enhancement (**c**). The diffusion tensor imaging (**f**) usually shows a high fractional anisotropy value compared to other cystic lesions, and the color coded map may show an internal heterogeneous pattern (arrow), suggesting some organization that is typical of pus.

Table 8.1 Main presentations of cranial bacterial infections on diffusion weighted imaging

Lesions	DWI findings
Meningitis	normal or CSF hyperintensity on DWI with no ADC restriction compared to parenchyma, but restricted compared to CSF
Effusion/hygroma	Isointense or slightly hyperintense to CSF on DWI, no restricted diffusion on ADC maps
Empyema	Hyperintense to CSF with low ADC
Brain abscess	Hyperintense core on DWI with low ADC
Successfully treated abscess	Increase ADC compared to untreated abscess
Ventriculitis	Hyperintense intraventricular content on DWI with restricted ADC

Abbreviations: ADC, apparent diffusion coefficient; CSF, cerebrospinal fluid; DWI, diffusion weighted image.

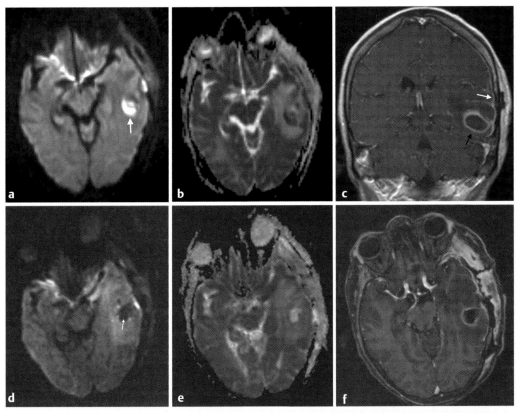

Fig. 8.5 Abscess **(a)** Axial diffusion weighted imaging (DWI) shows a hyperintense lesion in the left temporal lobe (arrow). **(b)** The apparent diffusion coefficient (ADC) of the lesion is reduced. **(c)** The coronal contrast-enhanced T1-weighted image shows peripheral enhancement of the lesion (black arrow) associated with meningeal involvement (white arrow). The diagnosis was a bacterial abscess. **(d)** After surgical drainage note reduction of the lesion size, with hypointensity of its core on DWI (arrow), **(e)** increased ADC, and persistent enhancement of the borders of the surgical cavity and adjacent meninges on **(f)** enhanced axial T1-weighted images. The lack of high DWI signal indicates that all pus has been drained.

The most common viral CNS infection is herpes encephalitis type 1, or oral herpesvirus, that carries a significant morbidity and mortality. The histopathology on herpes encephalitis is a fulminating necrotizing and, many times, hemorrhagic meningoencephalitis, predominantly in the temporal lobes, basal frontal lobes, insula, and cingulate gyri.[14] The diagnosis of herpes encephalitis is made by polymerase chain reaction (PCR) techniques in the CSF, but this test can be negative within the first 72 hours of the disease. In such cases, DWI may play an important role in the detection of the characteristic lesions because early treatment is crucial. DWI shows hyperintensity in the affected regions with areas of decreased ADC, suggesting cytotoxic or excitotoxic edema (▶ Fig. 8.11). T2-weighted and FLAIR images show unilateral or bilateral hyperintense lesions in the temporal lobes, basal frontal lobes, insula, and/or cingulate gyri, with gyral edema, meningeal or cortical enhancement, and sometimes hemorrhagic foci. DWI shows the same abnormalities, but these are detected earlier and are easier to be identified than on other MRI sequences. Furthermore, DWI shows more extensive brain involvement than T1- or T2-weighted images, providing better mapping of the degree of brain involved.

In the chronic stage of herpes encephalitis there is increased ADC in the affected areas. Grydeland et al[15] used DTI to study five patients that presented chronic unilateral medial temporal lobe lesions due to herpes encephalitis and manifested both verbal and visuospatial memory deficits. Besides the abnormalities in the affected side, the unaffected side also showed decreased FA and increased mean diffusivity (MD) and radial

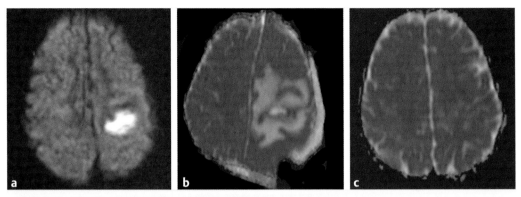

Fig. 8.6 Improvement of abscess postsurgery. (**a**) Axial diffusion weighted imaging shows a hyperintense lesion in the left hemisphere. (**b**) Three days following surgical drainage an axial apparent diffusion coefficient (ADC) map shows reduction of the lesion volume, increased peripheral edema, and an extra-axial postoperative collection. (**c**) One-month follow-up axial ADC map shows almost complete resolution of the lesion.

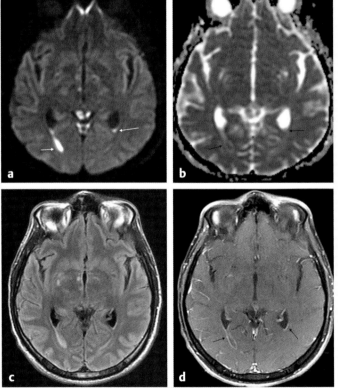

Fig. 8.7 Patient with pneumococcal meningitis and ventriculitis with restricted diffusion in the lateral ventricles, which can be seen as (**a**) hyperintense fluid levels (arrows) on diffusion weighted imaging and (**b**) hypointensity (arrows) on the apparent diffusion coefficient map. (**c**) The fluid-attenuated inversion recovery image shows hyperintensity in those locations, and (**d**) there is subependymal enhancement (arrows) on the enhanced T1-weighted image.

diffusivity (RD) in tracts connecting the medial temporal lobes with other parts of the brain. The involvement of the dominant medial temporal lobe (usually the left) explains the impairment of verbal memory, and the involvement of the right medial temporal lobe explains visuospatial memory compromise. Thus these findings explain how unilateral herpes encephalitis can produce either visuospatial and verbal memory impairments.

Cytomegalovirus (CMV) is a herpesvirus that most often affects the CNS of immunocompromised patients. The most common presentation of CMV CNS infection is ventriculoencephalitis. In such cases FLAIR and DWI can show abnormal

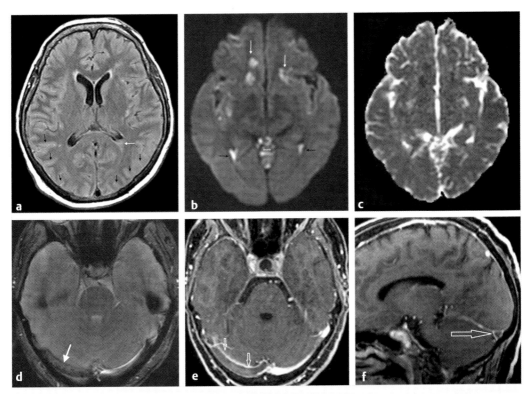

Fig. 8.8 Venous thrombosis due to meningitis. (**a**) Axial fluid-attenuated inversion recovery showing subtle hyperintensities in the sulci (black arrows) and in the posterior horn of the left lateral ventricle (white arrow). (**b**) The diffusion weighted imaging highlights the abnormalities in the lateral ventricles (ventriculitis) (black arrows), the meningitis in the cerebellar sulci (asterisks) and in the sylvian fissures, and also shows areas of restricted diffusion in subcortical areas (white arrows), also dark on apparent diffusion coefficient map (**c**), due to infarcts. (**d**) The T2 gradient-recalled echo shows hypointensity in the right transverse venous sinus (white arrow) that presents as a filling defect (open arrows) on the enhanced (**e**) axial and (**f**) sagittal images due to venous thrombosis.

hyperintensity on subependymal/periventricular lining and septum pellucidum, whereas enhanced T1-weighted images can show ependymal enhancement. On DWI the previously described areas show reduced (restricted) ADC (▶ Fig. 8.12).[16]

Progressive multifocal leukoencephalopathy (PML) is a disease associated with replication of the JC virus in oligodendrocytes of immunocompromised patients and usually affecting the white matter. The diagnosis is based on PCR of JC virus DNA in CSF. PML lesions usually have a scalloped appearance affecting the subcortical u-fibers, without mass effect and typically without contrast enhancement. On DWI the leading edge presents hyperintensity (▶ Fig. 8.13) which is attributed to active demyelination and inflammation. The lesion periphery may present as decreased ADC and MD.[17,18] On follow-up studies, the DWI hyperintense rim loses its signal intensity while sustaining its hyperintensity on T2-weighted images.[17] After

highly active antiretroviral therapy Buckle and Castillo[19] found higher maximal ADC values in the initial evaluation of patients with rapid versus slow clinical progression.

The direct effect of human immunodeficiency virus (HIV) in the CNS is associated with the late stages of acquired immunodeficiency syndrome (AIDS) and the AIDS dementia complex. Chen et al[20] used DTI in a study of HIV + patients with and without dementia and found that the white matter involvement is widespread, more severe in the HIV patients with dementia than in the HIV patients without dementia (changes in FA, MD, radial and axial diffusivity) and that radial diffusivity (RD) is the most affected parameter, suggesting an important component of demyelination in this disease.

Other viral infections that less commonly affect the CNS include influenza virus and Epstein–Barr virus that can also present with DWI changes that precede and/or are more extensive than those on

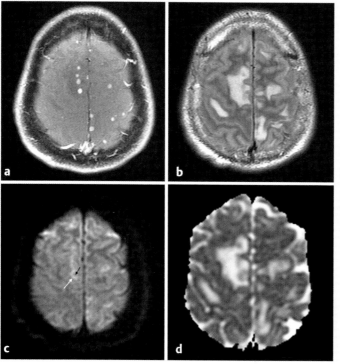

Fig. 8.9 Miliary tuberculosis. (a) Patient with multiple small contrast-enhancing nodules on T1-weighted image, (b) and edema on fluid-attenuated inversion recovery images. (c) The diffusion weighted imaging shows mild hyperintensity in the periphery (white arrow), and hypointensity in the core of the lesions (black arrow), (d) with no restricted diffusion on a corresponding apparent diffusion coefficient map.

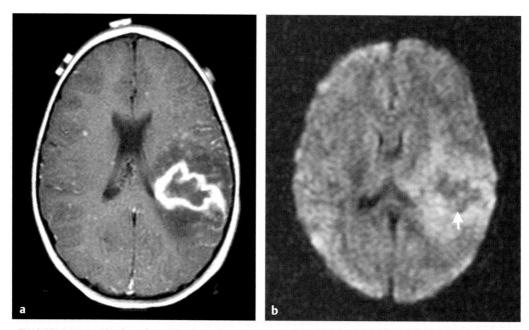

Fig. 8.10 Patient with tuberculosis. (a) Enhanced axial T1-weighted image shows a lesion with peripheral enhancement and perilesional edema. (b) Axial diffusion weighted imaging shows hypointensity on its central portion (arrow).

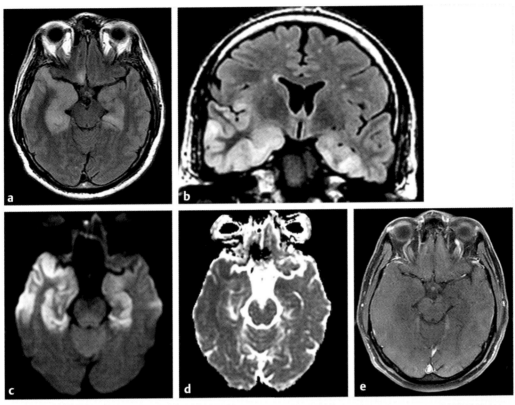

Fig. 8.11 Patient with herpes encephalitis. (**a**) Studies show bilateral temporal corticosubcortical involvement characterized by hyperintensity on axial and (**b**) coronal fluid-attenuated inversion recovery images, extending to frontal and insular areas. (**c**) There is hyperintensity on diffusion weighted imaging, (**d**) hypointensity on apparent diffusion coefficient map, and (**e**) no enhancement on enhanced T1-weighted image.

T2-weighted images. The hyperintense DWI lesions can present as restricted diffusion, probably related to encephalitis and cytotoxic edema.[21] The cytotoxic edema as the explanation of ADC restriction in these cases is still controversial; some patients present with complete resolution of the lesions in the follow-up studies or important clinical recovery both of which would not be expected in cytotoxic edema.[22]

Subacute sclerosing panencephalitis (SSPE) is a rare progressive degenerative/inflammatory disease that occurs several years following measles infection. Correlation between clinical staging of the disease and MRI findings is poor, and sometimes MRI examinations show normal findings in severely compromised patients. The regions most affected are the periventricular and subcortical white matter and corpus callosum, which present as hyperintensity on T2-weighted and FLAIR images, generally with no contrast enhancement. Areas with decreased and increased ADC have been described in very early SSPE. In the most advanced stages of the disease, ADC of diverse regions of the brain is increased, and these values become higher with disease progression.[23]

Fungal Infections

Fungal infections are rare in the general population, except in diabetic and immunocompromised patients. CNS involvement in fungal disease may be secondary to paranasal sinus infections (▶ Fig. 8.14) or due to hematogenous dissemination from other sites such as the lung.[24] In the same manner as bacterial infections, fungal infections can present as meningitis, cerebritis, abscesses, and granulomas. Vascular complications can also ensue and include acute infarctions and mycotic (infectious) aneurysms. CNS involvement depends on the size of the fungal agent: yeast, which are small unicellular fungi, more commonly tend to cause meningitis and microabscesses,

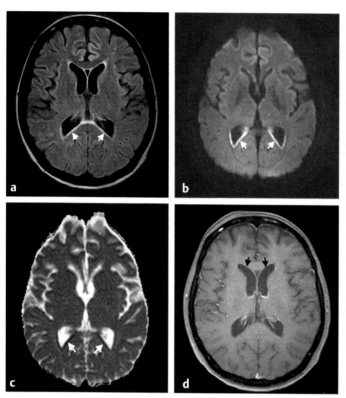

Fig. 8.12 Patient with cytomegalovirus. (**a**) Axial fluid-attenuated inversion recovery and (**b**) diffusion weighted image at the atrium level shows a curvilinear hyperintensity (arrows) along the ventricular wall with (**c**) definite low apparent diffusion coefficient value (arrows), along with subtle ependymal enhancement on (**d**) postcontrast T1-weighted image (arrows).

whereas the large hyphal organisms tend to involve the brain parenchyma.[25]

The most common fungal agents resulting in meningitis are *Cryptococcus neoformans* and *Candida albicans*. Besides the meningeal contrast enhancement, DWI can demonstrate subarachnoid hyperintensity in cryptococcal meningitis (▶ Fig. 8.15). When fungal meningitis is associated with paranasal sinus infection, the characteristic findings of the fungal sinus infection should be searched for and include sinonasal mucosal nodular thickening, typically without air-fluid levels, presenting hyperintensity on CT and hypointensity on T1 and T2-weighted images.[25]

MRI findings of fungal cerebritis are nonspecific with T2-weighted and FLAIR hyperintensity and variable DWI findings and contrast enhancement. DWI can show a heterogeneous hyperintense lesion with foci of restricted diffusion, and contrast enhancement can be subtle or absent.[25,26]

Both pyogenic and fungal abscesses in immunocompetent patients can present as ring-enhancing lesions. In the immunocompromised patient the lack of enhancement may be related to the host immune system not working properly.[25] A T2-hypointense rim is also described for both fungal and bacterial abscesses. The differentiation of fungal from pyogenic abscess should be based on the numbers of lesions wherein fungal abscesses are usually multiple as well as on the lesion borders characteristics usually fungal abscesses presenting lobulated or crenulated borders. On DWI, the walls of fungal abscesses may present as restricted diffusion, but its central portion usually has no restricted diffusion (▶ Fig. 8.16). Rarely restricted diffusion of the core of fungal abscesses similar to pyogenic abscesses have been described (▶ Fig. 8.17 and ▶ Fig. 8.18).[24,25]

Fungal granulomas are rare and usually related to *Aspergillus* or *Cryptococcus* infections. They present intermediate to low signal intensity on T2-weighted images with surrounding T2-hyperintense edema.[25]

Cryptococcus neoformans is a yeastlike fungus that affects immunocompromised as well as immunocompetent patients. Cryptococcosis can affect the CNS as mentioned before and most commonly presents as meningitis, but it can also present as parenchymal involvement (gelatinous pseudocysts or cryptococcomas). Parenchymal involvement can be secondary to dissemination through the Virchow–Robin spaces, forming gelatinous pseudocysts. The gelatinous pseudocysts do not present restricted diffusion (▶ Fig. 8.19), and their enhancement varies

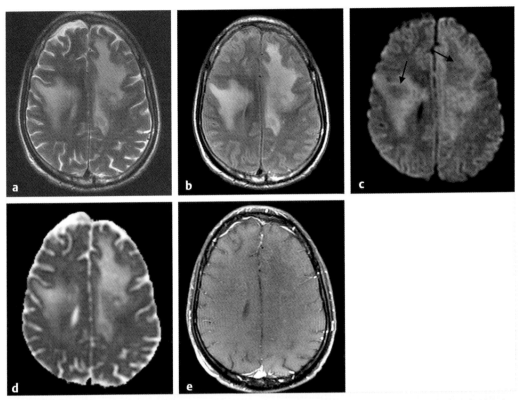

Fig. 8.13 Patient with acquired immunodeficiency syndrome with progressive multifocal leukoencephalopathy (PML). PML lesions involve the subcortical white matter bilaterally and assymetrically. There are hyperintensity lesions on (**a**) T2, (**b**) fluid-attenuated inversion recovery, (**c**) diffusion weighted imaging (DWI), and (**d**) apparent diffusion coefficient map images. On DWI, the periphery of the lesions is hyperintense when compared to their central portions (arrows). (**e**) No contrast enhancement is seen on T1-weighted images postgadolinium.

depending on the immune status of the patient. Cryptococcomas usually occur in immunocompetent patients, and they can be located in perivascular spaces or in the cortical regions.[27]

Aspergillus fumigatus is the most common fungus to result in CNS parenchymal involvement. CNS invasive aspergillosis can present as encephalitis with or without abscess, granulomas, and dural-based masses. MRI findings of *Aspergillus* abscess are the same as already described for other fungal abscesses, but hemorrhagic foci can occur and DWI findings vary (▶ Fig. 8.20). Aspergillosis can also manifest as extra-axial dural-based lesions that can show hypointensity on T2-weighted images and homogeneous contrast enhancement. Other characteristics of CNS aspergillosis are the occurrence of vascular invasion with vasculitis, secondary brain infarction, and, rarely, mycotic aneurysms or parenchymal hemorrhages. DWI can detect early infarctions that can later be complicated by cerebral abscesses.[24]

Parasitic Diseases

The most common parasitic diseases of the CNS are neurocysticercosis (NCC) and toxoplasmosis, which most commonly affect immunocompetent and immunosuppressed patients, respectively.

NCC is a pleomorphic disease in its clinical and imaging presentations. The main location in the CNS is the brain parenchyma, followed by the CSF spaces. Brain lesions present four different stages: vesicular, colloidal, granular nodular, and nodular calcified. The coexistence of different stages in various locations is frequent. In the vesicular stage the cysticercus is viable, there is no inflammation, and the lesion has CSF signal intensity with the scolex as an eccentric mural nodule.[28] On DWI the scolex shows as a hyperintense dot/comma-shaped structure (▶ Fig. 8.21), and, due to its small size, its ADC cannot be accurately measured in many cases. The scolex can also be identified in the colloidal vesicular stage lesions.

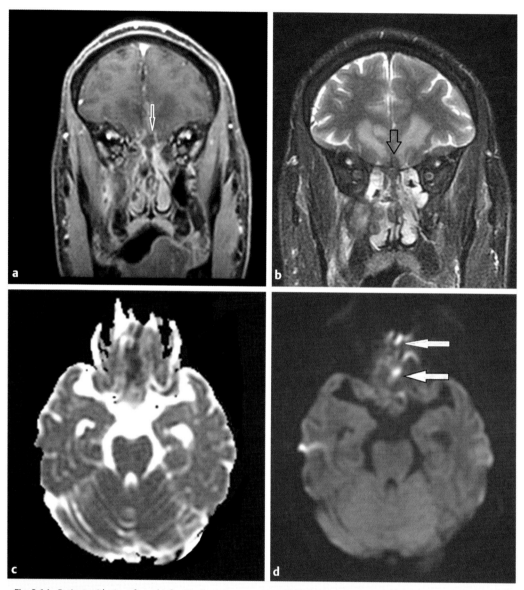

Fig. 8.14 Patient with sinus fungal infection (mucormycosis). Study showes intracranial extension to the anterior fossa (open arrow) as seen on the (a) coronal enhanced T1-weighted image as a peripherally enhancing lesion, hypointensity (arrow) on (b) T2-weighted image with perilesional edema. (c) There is restricted diffusion better characterized as hypointensity on the apparent diffusion coefficient map, (d) but also visible as high signal on diffusion weighted imaging (arrows).

Detection of the scolex has an important diagnostic role because its presence is nearly pathognomonic of NCC.[29] In the colloidal stage there is perilesional edema and peripheral contrast enhancement as degeneration begins and an inflammatory process ensues. The signal intensity of the lesion is becames higher than CSF on FLAIR images as the scolex starts to degenerate.

In the granular nodular stage, the parasite is dead, the lesion retracts, and the edema and contrast enhancement progressively subside. On DWI, NCC in the colloidal vesicular or granular nodular phases may appear hyperintense with restriction of diffusion (▶ Fig. 8.22), which may be related to cyst degeneration. In the nodular calcified stage there is mineralization of the

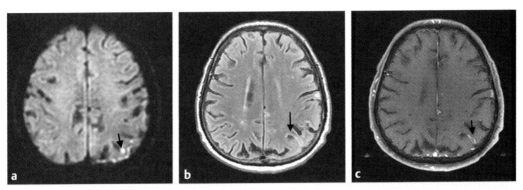

Fig. 8.15 Cryptococcal meningitis. (a) Magnetic resonance imaging shows enlarged parietal sulci and some foci of hyperintensity on diffusion weighted imaging (arrow) throughout the frontal and parietal lobes. (b) Note also peripheral lesion and sulcal hyperintensities on fluid-attenuated inversion recovery (arrow) and (c) enhancement in the same regions on the post-contrast T1-weighted image (arrow).

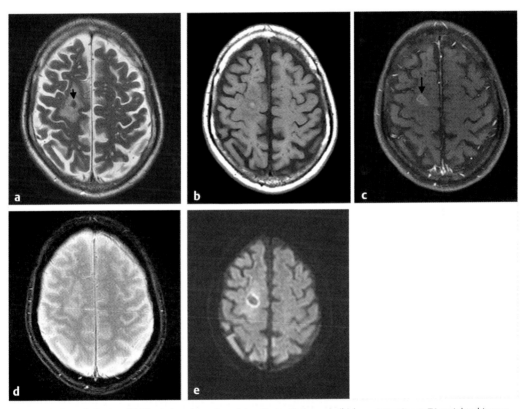

Fig. 8.16 Fungal abscess. (a) The lesion shows hypointensity on T2 (arrow), (b) hyperintensity on T1-weighted image, (c) subtle contrast enhancement (arrow), and (d) no susceptibility effect on the T2 gradient-recalled echo. There is perilesional edema. (e) Diffusion weighted imaging shows peripheral hyperintensity and hypointensity in the core.

lesion.[30] Gupta et al[31] used DTI in a study of 25 patients with NCC and found decreased MD during evolution of NCC lesions from vesicular to granular. FA presented higher values in the calcified stage compared to the other stages, explained by a decrease of water content from vesicular to granular forms and more organized appearance in the calcified lesion.

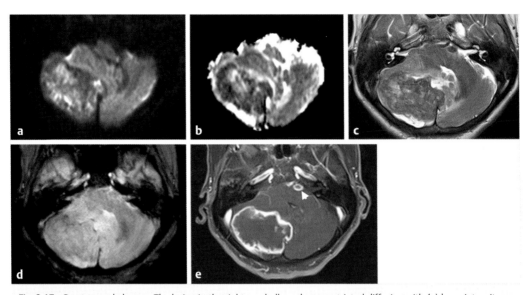

Fig. 8.17 Cryptococcal abscess. The lesion in the right cerebellum shows restricted diffusion with (**a**) hyperintensity on diffusion weighted imaging, and (**b**) hypointensity on apparent diffusion coefficient. There is hypointensity on (**c**) T2-weighted image, but not on (**d**) T2 gradient-recalled echo, confirming that its T2 appearance is not due to hemorrhage or calcifications. (**e**) Predominantly peripheral contrast enhancement is seen on postgadolinium T1-weighted image. Note that there is a smaller lesion with the same characteristics in the left anterior pons (white arrow).

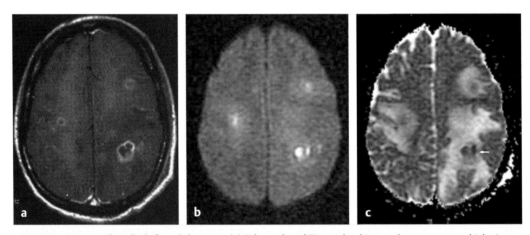

Fig. 8.18 Patient with multiple fungal abscesses. (**a**) Enhanced axial T1-weighted image demonstrates multiple ring-enhancing lesions. (**b**) Axial diffusion weighted image shows that some of these lesions present central hyperintensities with reduced apparent diffusion coefficient (arrow) in the (**c**) ADC map.

Toxoplasmosis is an opportunistic disease whose prevalence has increased since the AIDS epidemic. Its etiologic agent is an intracellular protozoan, *Toxoplasma gondi*. PCR of serum or CSF has a high sensitivity and specificity for the diagnosis of toxoplasmosis. The basal ganglia, thalamus, and cortico–white matter junctions are affected most commonly. The lesions are usually multiple.

Toxoplasma lesions are most commonly seen as ring-enhancing lesions with an eccentric target sign that corresponds to a nodule along the wall of the enhancing rim, a finding that is highly suggestive of toxoplasmosis but is seen in < 30% of cases. On DWI the lesion core is iso- to slight hypointense to normal white matter with increased ADC (no restriction of diffusion) (▶ Fig. 8.23). The fact

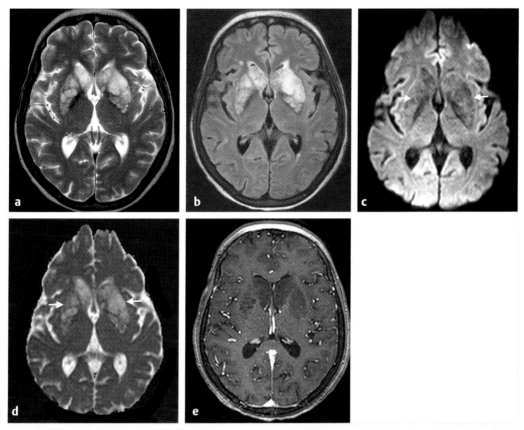

Fig. 8.19 Cryptococcal gelatinous pseudocysts. Mucinous cryptococcal material filling and dilating perivascular spaces within the basal ganglia, known as gelatinous pseudocysts, (**a**) tend to mirror cerebrospinal fluid signal intensity on T2-weighted image, and (**b**) show hyperintensity on fluid-attenuated inversion. There is no restricted diffusion on (**c**) DWI and (**d**) ADC map (arrows on both images) neither (**e**) contrast enhancement.

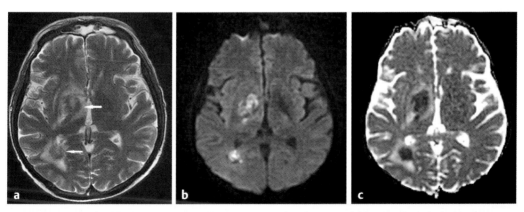

Fig. 8.20 Patient immunosuppressed after bone marrow transplant due to myelofibrosis with cerebral and pulmonary aspergillosis. (**a**) Axial T2-weighted image shows two lesions with hypointense rim (arrows), central hyperintensity and peripheral edema. (**b**) Axial diffusion weighted image shows hyperintensity on the central core and on the borders of the lesions with restricted diffusion on (**c**) apparent diffusion coefficient map.

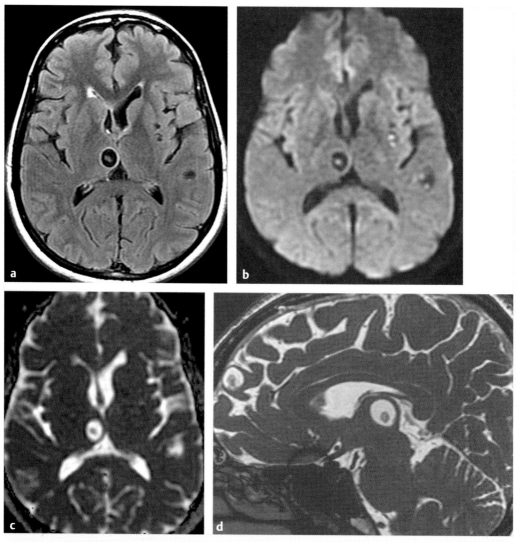

Fig. 8.21 Multiple neurocysticercosis lesions are identified on (**a**) fluid-attenuated inversion recovery (FLAIR), (**b**) diffusion weighted imaging (DWI), (**c**) apparent diffusion coefficient (ADC) map, and, most accurately, on (**d**) Fast Imaging Employing Steady-State Acquisition (FIESTA imaging) (GE Healthcare, Waukesha, WI). The scolex is identified as a hyperintense dot on the (**b**) DWI sequence and (**a**) FLAIR, and low signal on the (**c**) ADC map and (**d**) FIESTA images. It is particularly easy to see it in the vesicule located in the right thalamus.

that the wall of a *Toxoplasma* abscess has intracellular and extracellular tachyzoites with no collagenous capsule and that its core consists primarily of necrotic tissue without any viscous, proteinaceous, and inflammatory debris may explain its presentation on DWI.[32] Unfortunately ADC values of lymphoma and toxoplasmosis lesions may present a significant overlap in patients with AIDS; thus the use of DWI to differentiate among these lesions is limited.[33]

Prion Infections

Prion infections are caused by self-replicating proteins that induce lethal neurodegenerative diseases. The most common human prion infection is the sporadic Creutzfeldt–Jakob disease (sCJD) that causes dementia in younger patients.[34]

DWI has an important role in the diagnosis of prion infections that usually affect cortical and deep gray matter. Restricted diffusion is the typical finding, although its pathological substrate is still

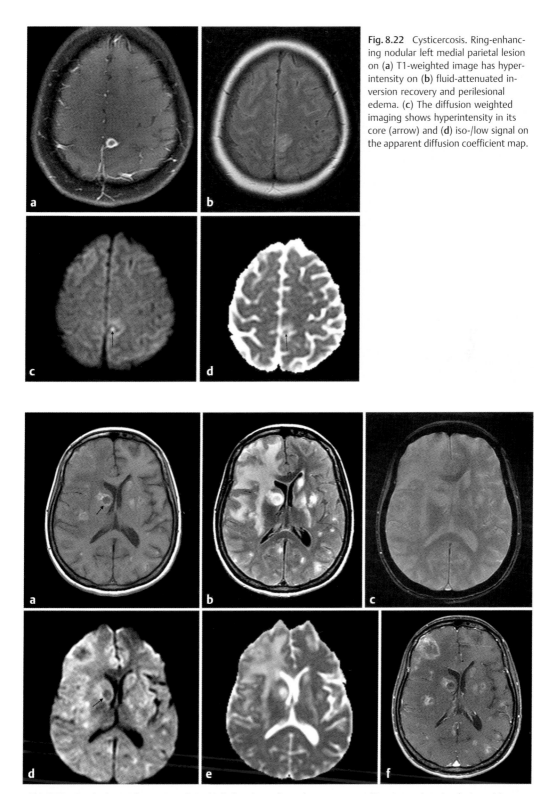

Fig. 8.22 Cysticercosis. Ring-enhancing nodular left medial parietal lesion on (**a**) T1-weighted image has hyperintensity on (**b**) fluid-attenuated inversion recovery and perilesional edema. (**c**) The diffusion weighted imaging shows hyperintensity in its core (arrow) and (**d**) iso-/low signal on the apparent diffusion coefficient map.

Fig. 8.23 Cerebral toxoplasmosis with multiple basal ganglia and gray matter–white matter junction lesions. (**a**) Unenhanced T1-weighted image shows hyperintense borders (arrow) in some lesions, which have a somewhat irregular and "shaggy" appearance and hypointensity of their central portions. (**b**) Axial fluid-attenuated inversion recovery and (**c**) T2 gradient-recalled echo magnetic resonance images show hyperintense lesions and marked perilesional edema but no susceptibility effects. (**d**) Diffusion weighted imaging shows hyperintensity rims (arrow) and hypointensity core in the lesions, (**e**) with no restriction on the apparent diffusion coefficient map. (**f**) Contrast-enhanced T1-weighted image shows predominantly peripheral but also some internal enhancement of the lesions.

controversial (▶ Fig. 8.24). It seems that reduced ADC in the deep gray matter correlates with spongiform changes, whereas restricted diffusion in the cortex correlates to spongiform changes, gliosis, and neuronal loss. In the late stages of the disease, ADC may be normal in the affected areas.[34]

In sCJD, DWI has a high sensitivity (83–100%) for lesion detection. Wang et al, in 2013,[35] used DTI in a cohort of nine patients with sCJD and found decreased MD, axial diffusivity, and radial diffusivity, but normal FA within the caudate nuclei and pulvinars in comparison with other patients with progressive dementia and controls. These authors hypothesize that spongiform changes impair water diffusion in all directions with a relative preservation of FA.

8.2 Summary

As stated before, DWI can be a very useful tool in the diagnosis of CNS infectious diseases. Infectious meningitis can present areas of hyperintensity on DWI regardless of its etiology, and when this finding is associated with meningeal enhancement it can suggest the proper diagnosis.

DWI can provide additional information that is useful in the differentiation of the types of abscesses because all may present similar appearances on conventional MRI scans. Pyogenic abscesses present smooth walls, T2-weighted hypointense rims, and a hyperintense core with reduced (restricted) ADC. Tuberculous and fungal abscesses present variable signal intensity on DWI. Fungal abscesses tend to be multiple with crenated or lobulated borders. The diffusion is variable, but restricted diffusion could be seen.

The most common viral CNS infection is herpes encephalitis, which presents as areas of restricted diffusion in the temporal and frontal lobes, insula, and cingulated gyrus. The DWI findings are early findings of herpes encephalitis and can help in instituting prompt treatment.

In immunocompromised patients, PML may show a leading edge with hyperintensity on DWI and restricted diffusion, usually without contrast enhancement. Toxoplasmosis lesions are usually multiple enhancing lesions that do not present with restricted diffusion.

In sporadic Creutzfeldt Jacob disease, DWI is an important diagnostic tool. DWI has a high sensitivity (83–100%) for lesion detection in this disease.

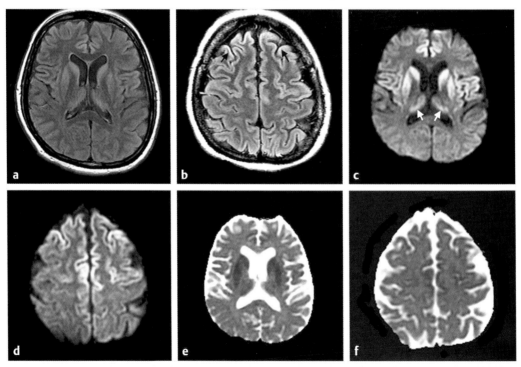

Fig. 8.24 Creutzfeldt–Jakob disease. (a,b) Magnetic resonance images demonstrate basal ganglia, thalamus, and frontal ribbon-like cortical (arrows) signal intensity abnormalities on fluid-attenuated inversion recovery, (c,d) but more striking on diffusion weighted imaging, (e, f) and with low signal on the apparent diffusion coefficient map. Note the typical involvement of the posterior and medial thalami (arrows in (c)).

References

[1] Hughes DC, Raghavan A, Mordekar SR, Griffiths PD, Connolly DJ. Role of imaging in the diagnosis of acute bacterial meningitis and its complications. Postgrad Med J 2010; 86 (1018): 478–485

[2] Kastrup O, Wanke I, Maschke M. Neuroimaging of infections. NeuroRx 2005; 2(2): 324–332

[3] Fertikh D, Krejza J, Cunqueiro A, Danish S, Alokaili R, Melhem ER. Discrimination of capsular stage brain abscesses from necrotic or cystic neoplasms using diffusion weighted magnetic resonance imaging. J Neurosurg 2007; 106(1): 76–81

[4] Ebisu T, Tanaka C, Umeda M, et al. Discrimination of brain abscess from necrotic or cystic tumors by diffusion weighted echo planar imaging. Magn Reson Imaging 1996; 14(9): 1113–1116

[5] Reddy JS, Mishra AM, Behari S, et al. The role of diffusion weighted imaging in the differential diagnosis of intracranial cystic mass lesions: a report of 147 lesions. Surg Neurol 2006; 66(3): 246–250, discussion 250–251

[6] Nath K, Ramola M, Husain M, Kumar M, Prasad K, Gupta R. Assessment of therapeutic response in patients with brain abscess using diffusion tensor imaging. World Neurosurg 2010; 73(1): 63–68, discussion e6

[7] Gupta RK, Hasan KM, Mishra AM, et al. High fractional anisotropy in brain abscesses versus other cystic intracranial lesions. AJNR Am J Neuroradiol 2005; 26(5): 1107–1114

[8] Gupta RK, Nath K, Prasad A, et al. In vivo demonstration of neuroinflammatory molecule expression in brain abscess with diffusion tensor imaging. AJNR Am J Neuroradiol 2008; 29(2): 326–332

[9] Han K-T, Choi DS, Ryoo JW, et al. Diffusion weighted MR imaging of pyogenic intraventricular empyema. Neuroradiology 2007; 49(10): 813–818

[10] Nickerson JP, Richner B, Santy K, et al. Neuroimaging of pediatric intracranial infection—part 1: techniques and bacterial infections. J Neuroimaging 2012; 22(2): e42–e51

[11] Shukla R, Abbas A, Kumar P, Gupta RK, Jha S, Prasad KN. Evaluation of cerebral infarction in tuberculous meningitis by diffusion weighted imaging. J Infect 2008; 57(4): 298–306

[12] Gupta RK, Prakash M, Mishra AM, Husain M, Prasad KN, Husain N. Role of diffusion weighted imaging in differentiation of intracranial tuberculoma and tuberculous abscess from cysticercus granulomas-a report of more than 100 lesions. Eur J Radiol 2005; 55(3): 384–392

[13] Gupta RK, Kumar S. Central nervous system tuberculosis. Neuroimaging Clin N Am 2011; 21(4): 795–814, vii–viii

[14] Sener RN. Herpes simplex encephalitis: diffusion MR imaging findings. Comput Med Imaging Graph 2001; 25(5): 391–397

[15] Grydeland H, Walhovd KB, Westlye LT, et al. Amnesia following herpes simplex encephalitis: diffusion tensor imaging uncovers reduced integrity of normal-appearing white matter. Radiology 2010; 257(3): 774–781

[16] Seok JH, Ahn K, Park HJ. Diffusion MRI findings of cytomegalovirus-associated ventriculitis: a case report. Br J Radiol 2011; 84(1005): e179–e181

[17] Cosottini M, Tavarelli C, Del Bono L, et al. Diffusion weighted imaging in patients with progressive multifocal leukoencephalopathy. Eur Radiol 2008; 18(5): 1024–1030

[18] Barata Tavares J, Geraldo AF, Neto L, Reimão S, Campos JG. Diffusion weighted MR imaging characterization of progressive multifocal leukoencephalopathy (PML) lesions [in Portuguese]. Acta Med Port 2012; 25 Suppl 1: 34–37

[19] Buckle C, Castillo M. Use of diffusion weighted imaging to evaluate the initial response of progressive multifocal leukoencephalopathy to highly active antiretroviral therapy: early experience. AJNR Am J Neuroradiol 2010; 31(6): 1031–1035

[20] Chen Y, An H, Zhu H, et al. White matter abnormalities revealed by diffusion tensor imaging in non-demented and demented HIV+ patients. Neuroimage 2009; 47(4): 1154–1162

[21] Tokunaga Y, Kira R, Takemoto M, et al. Diagnostic usefulness of diffusion weighted magnetic resonance imaging in influenza-associated acute encephalopathy or encephalitis. Brain Dev 2000; 22(7): 451–453

[22] Kim JH, Joo B-E, Koh S-B. Serial diffusion weighted MR imaging findings in a patient with Epstein-Barr virus encephalitis. J Neurol 2007; 254(11): 1616–1618

[23] Abuhandan M, Cece H, Calik M, Karakas E, Dogan F, Karakas O. An evaluation of subacute sclerosing panencephalitis patients with diffusion weighted magnetic resonance imaging. Clin Neuroradiol 2013; 23(1): 25–30

[24] Saini J, Gupta AK, Jolapara MB, et al. Imaging findings in intracranial aspergillus infection in immunocompetent patients [published correction appears in World Neurosurg 2012;78(6):e1. Note: Chandreshekher, Kesavadas corrected to Kesavadas, Chandrasekharan]. World Neurosurg 2010; 74 (6): 661–670

[25] Mathur M, Johnson CE, Sze G. Fungal infections of the central nervous system. Neuroimaging Clin N Am 2012; 22(4): 609–632

[26] Gaviani P, Schwartz RB, Hedley-Whyte ET, et al. Diffusion weighted imaging of fungal cerebral infection. AJNR Am J Neuroradiol 2005; 26(5): 1115–1121

[27] Khandelwal N, Gupta V, Singh P. Central nervous system fungal infections in tropics. Neuroimaging Clin N Am 2011; 21(4): 859–866, viii

[28] Raffin LS, Bacheschi LA, Machado LR, Nóbrega JP, Coelho C, Leite CC. Diffusion weighted MR imaging of cystic lesions of neurocysticercosis: a preliminary study. Arq Neuropsiquiatr 2001; 59(4): 839–842

[29] Del Brutto OH, Rajshekhar V, White AC, Jr et al. Proposed diagnostic criteria for neurocysticercosis. Neurology 2001; 57(2): 177–183

[30] Santos GT, Leite CC, Machado LR, McKinney AM, Lucato LT. Reduced diffusion in neurocysticercosis: circumstances of appearance and possible natural history implications. AJNR Am J Neuroradiol 2013; 34(2): 310–316

[31] Gupta RK, Trivedi R, Awasthi R, Paliwal VK, Prasad KN, Rathore RK. Understanding changes in DTI metrics in patients with different stages of neurocysticercosis. Magn Reson Imaging 2012; 30(1): 104–111

[32] Chong-Han CH, Cortez SC, Tung GA. Diffusion weighted MRI of cerebral toxoplasma abscess. AJR Am J Roentgenol 2003; 181(6): 1711–1714

[33] Schroeder PC, Post MJ, Oschatz E, Stadler A, Bruce-Gregorios J, Thurnher MM. Analysis of the utility of diffusion weighted MRI and apparent diffusion coefficient values in distinguishing central nervous system toxoplasmosis from lymphoma. Neuroradiology 2006; 48(10): 715–720

[34] Letourneau-Guillon L, Wada R, Kucharczyk W. Imaging of prion diseases. J Magn Reson Imaging 2012; 35(5): 998–1012

[35] Wang LH, Bucelli RC, Patrick E, et al. Role of magnetic resonance imaging, cerebrospinal fluid, and electroencephalogram in diagnosis of sporadic Creutzfeldt-Jakob disease. J Neurol 2013; 260(2): 498–506

9 Diffusion Weighted Imaging and Diffusion Tensor Imaging in Demyelination and Toxic Diseases

Celi Santos Andrade, Carolina de Medeiros Rimkus, Claudia da Costa Leite, Alexander M. McKinney, and Leandro T. Lucato

Key Points

- Demyelinating lesions can be pathologically heterogeneous, depending on the degree of inflammation, membrane disruption, and type of cellular damage. Demyelinating lesions are more frequently associated with increased diffusion of water molecules (high apparent diffusion coefficient [ADC]), but may show areas of restricted diffusion (low ADC), depending on the age and size of the lesions.
- Diffusion tensor imaging (DTI) in chronic diseases, such as multiple sclerosis and neuromyelitis optica, is more likely to demonstrate occult microscopic damage, which can be detected by increased mean diffusivity (MD) and decreased fractional anisotropy (FA) in the normal-appearing brain tissue.
- Central nervous system (CNS) toxic diseases can be caused by a wide variety of chemicals, whether due to medications or environmental exposure. Although some neurotoxins may preferentially affect specific CNS structures, the main magnetic resonance imaging (MRI) findings are often nonspecific, with white matter (WM) areas of hyperintensity on T2-weighted and fluid-attenuated inversion recovery (FLAIR) images, and, less commonly, variable changes in the basal ganglia and cerebellar nuclei. Typically, the MRI changes are symmetric and present with reduced diffusion in the acute phase, a finding often described as acute toxic leukoencephalopathy.

9.1 Diffusion Weighted Imaging and Diffusion Tensor Imaging in Demyelinating Diseases

9.1.1 Introduction

Demyelinating lesions are pathologically heterogeneous, depending on the phase of inflammatory activity, the degree of cellular destruction, or their etiological background.[1] The tissue changes associated with demyelination determine variations in water content of the tissue, reflecting variable degrees of cellular swelling and extracellular edema.[2]

Acute demyelinating lesions may show different levels of cytotoxic or intramyelinic edema. Increases in water concentration in the brain tissues demonstrate nonspecific hyperintensity on T2-weighted images, but the abnormal cellular uptake of water or restricted water between myelin membranes reduces its molecular diffusion, showing high signal intensity on diffusion weighted images (DWIs) with decreased apparent diffusion coefficient (ADC).[2]

On the other hand, inflammatory and metabolic changes may cause vasogenic and interstitial edema secondary to increased permeability of small vessels and blood–brain barrier (BBB) disruption, which causes increased ADC values. The superposition of events leading to restricted and facilitated water diffusion may produce variable results in DWI and ADC, from water restriction to mixed findings to T2 shine-through effects.[2]

In chronic phases, demyelinating lesions may show complete resolution, with normalization of T2, DWI, and ADC, but lesions can also present persistent T2 hyperintense foci, representing residual gliosis, and persistent demyelination or axonal loss. In these situations the extracellular space is expanded frequently, resulting in increased ADC values.[3,4] Although DWI is sensitive to lesions with long T2 relaxation times, in the late stages of demyelination this technique is not specific enough to classify or to grade the underlying pathological substrate.

Diffusion tensor imaging (DTI) allows further assessment of the microstructure of brain tissues.[5] Chronic demyelinating lesions frequently show visible foci of decreased fractional anisotropy (FA) with increased mean diffusivity (MD) (▶ Fig. 9.1). Those DTI parameters do not differentiate demyelination, axon disruption, or gliosis. But recently, the analysis of decomposed eigenvalues of DTI showed stronger correlations between radial diffusivity ($\lambda_\perp$) and demyelination, whereas the axial

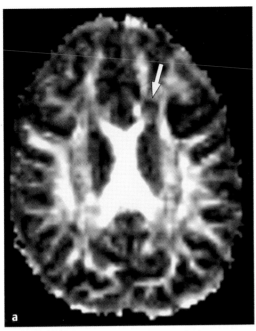 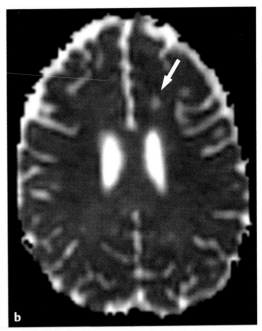

Fig. 9.1 Chronic demyelinating lesion in a patient with multiple sclerosis. (a) The fractional anisotropy (FA) map shows a periventricular focus of decreased FA (arrow), (b) whereas the mean diffusivity image demonstrates high signal (arrow), corresponding to the increased diffusion in a chronic demyelinating lesion.

diffusivity ($\lambda_{||}$) seems to be associated with more profound tissue damage or axonal loss.[5,6]

DTI is also becoming a valuable tool in the differential diagnosis of demyelinating diseases. Chronic demyelinating diseases, such as multiple sclerosis (MS), are known to present extension of microarchitectural damage outside of the macroscopic lesions.[3,7] Even though the white and gray matter abnormalities are not visible in DTI maps, several studies have demonstrated abnormal quantitative parameters, such as FA reduction and MD increase in the normal-appearing white matter (NAWM) and gray matter (NAGM) of patients with demyelinating disorders.[5,7,8,9]

9.1.2 Multiple Sclerosis

MS is the most common chronic demyelinating disease in adults. MS lesions usually appear as hyperintense foci on T2-weighted and fluid-attenuated inversion recovery (FLAIR) images with perivenular distribution, typically affecting the periventricular, juxtacortical, infratentorial, and spinal cord white matter (WM). Acute demyelinating MS lesions present variable DWI and ADC findings, which are time dependent.[10] The ADC values increase by the time gadolinium (Gd)

enhancement appears, then they progressively decrease as enhancement vanishes and increase again with lesion progression to chronic stages.[10]

Most lesions, by the time of a clinical relapse evaluation, have some degree of demyelination, inflammatory infiltrate and/or microstructural damage, and variable cytotoxic and intramyelinic edema,[5,10] which may show mixed diffusion effects, with areas of restricted and facilitated diffusion (▶ Fig. 9.2) or T2 shine-through effects (▶ Fig. 9.3).

As already mentioned, MS lesions show decreased FA and increased MD, with lower FA in the ring of enhancement.[5] In MS, DTI changes can be detected in the NAWM, being more evident in the periplaque regions, corpus callosum (▶ Fig. 9.4), and temporal and parietal lobes,[5,6] which can be helpful in distinguishing MS from other demyelinating disorders.

9.1.3 Acute Disseminated Encephalomyelitis

Acute disseminated encephalomyelitis (ADEM) is a monophasic demyelinating disease with a wide range of clinical manifestations.[3] It is often considered in the differential diagnosis of clinical isolated

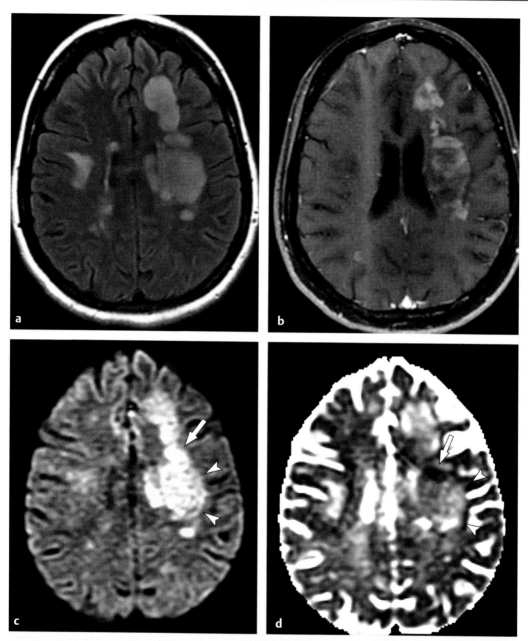

Fig. 9.2 Mixed diffusion effects in a diffuse infiltrating multiple sclerosis lesion. (**a**) Axial fluid-attenuated inversion recovery shows large, hyperintense, confluent cerebral lesions, especially on the left. (**b**) Enhanced axial T1-weighted image shows signs of inflammatory activity characterized by multiple foci of enhancement. (**c**) On diffusion weighted imaging the lesion is hyperintense, but notice a more intense hyperintense portion (arrow), when compared to other areas (arrowheads). (**d**) The corresponding apparent diffusion coefficient map confirms that they present distinct behavior: whereas the former shows restricted diffusion (hypointense, arrow), the latter are associated with increased diffusion (hyperintense, arrowheads).

syndromes (CISs) and other multiphasic demyelinating diseases, such as MS and neuromyelitis optica (NMO).[11]

ADEM lesions affect deep gray matter structures more frequently than MS, and the white matter lesions can be larger, with indistinct borders and

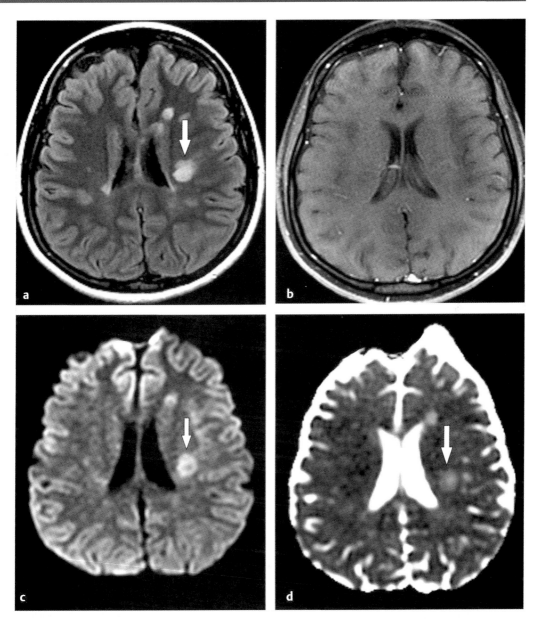

Fig. 9.3 T2 shine-through effect in a chronic multiple sclerosis lesion. (**a**) Axial fluid-attenuated inversion recovery demonstrates a hyperintense lesion (arrow) with no signs of acute inflammatory exacerbation on (**b**) corresponding enhanced axial T1-weighted image. The lesion presents hyperintensity on (**c**) diffusion weighted imaging (DWI) and (**d**) apparent diffusion coefficient map, corresponding to facilitated diffusion (arrows in (**c, d**)). Thus the increased signal intensity seen on DWI more likely represents a T2 shine-through effect, and not true restricted water diffusion.

occasional gadolinium enhancement.[11,12] DWI findings can vary, more frequently showing increased ADC in the central portions of the lesions. When restricted diffusion is seen, it appears in the borders of larger lesions or in the enhancing margins (▶ Fig. 9.5).[12,13]

Although ADEM is usually monophasic, some patients may show both clinical and imaging findings of recurrence, with T2-weighted imaging characteristics that can overlap those of with MS and NMO.[11] Unlike MS, the abnormalities seen on DWI tend to be restricted to the T2-weighted

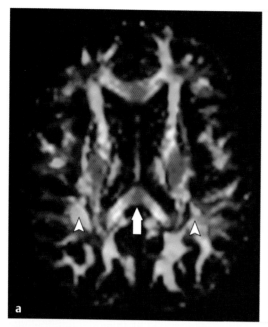 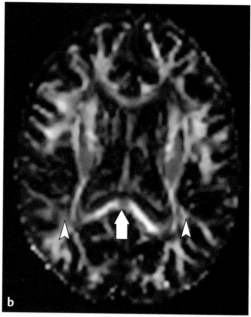

Fig. 9.4 Color fractional anisotropy (FA) maps for a healthy control compared to those for a patient with multiple sclerosis (MS). (**a**) The color FA map of a healthy subject compared to that of (**b**) a patient with MS shows a more intense red color in the splenium of the corpus callosum of the subject when compared to the patient (arrows in (**a,b**)). Areas of decreased color intensity in the MS patient compared to the healthy subject are also observed in the peritrigonal white matter, bilaterally (arrowheads in (**a,b**)).

lesions, and it is unusual to detect increased MD in the NAWM in ADEM outside of the acute phase.[13]

In ADEM the deep gray matter structures show more significant abnormalities on DTI than in MS, even without evidence of T2-weighted detectable lesions, and they present as increased MD in the thalami and basal ganglia.[11] These findings suggest that, not only can the qualitative changes in DTI parameters be helpful but also the pattern of abnormalities can play a role in the differential diagnosis.

9.1.4 Neuromyelitis Optica

NMO is a demyelinating disease characterized by severe, recurrent attacks of optic neuritis and extensive myelitis.[14] The classical presentation of NMO is associated with an autoantibody targeted to the water channel protein aquaporin 4 (NMO–immunoglobulin G [IgG]), which is not only present in the optic nerve and spinal cord but is also commonly found around the ventricles, the hypothalamus, and the subcortical white matter.[15]

NMO does not spare the brain, and NMO-related hyperintense lesions on T2-weighted images tend to be larger than MS lesions and follow the typical distribution of aquaporin 4 channel sites (▶ Fig. 9.6), but may show overlapping characteristics with MS and ADEM, especially in the initial stages.[8]

There are abnormalities in the NAWM in NMO, seen as reduced FA in the pyramidal tracts and optic radiations, presumably associated with wallerian degeneration secondary to optic nerve and spinal cord lesions.[8,15] Recently, a tract-based spatial statistics study showed FA reduction in the genu and body of the corpus callosum, external capsules, uncinate fasciculus, inferior longitudinal fasciculus, and inferior fronto-occipital fasciculus, mostly related to $\lambda_\perp$ (radial diffusion) changes, probably reflecting extensive demyelination.[15]

Furthermore, DTI changes in the corpus callosum in NMO were described as milder and predominantly in its anterior half, whereas in MS DTI changes are more extensive and have a posterior predominance.[6,8]

9.1.5 Tumefactive Demyelinating Lesion

Tumefactive demyelinating lesions (TDLs) are defined as lesions > 2 cm in diameter. They can be

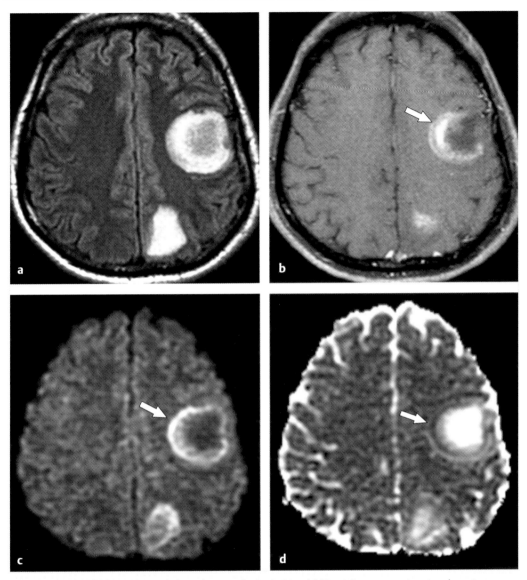

Fig. 9.5 Acute disseminated encephalomyelitis tumefactive lesions. (**a**) Magnetic resonance imaging shows two tumefactive left cerebral subcortical lesions on fluid-attenuated inversion recovery. (**b**) One of the lesions demonstrates incomplete ring enhancement in the corresponding enhanced axial T1-weighted image (arrow). The enhancing area presents peripheral restricted diffusion (arrows in (**c, d**)), (**c**) observed as increased signal on diffusion weighted imaging and decreased signal on the (**d**) apparent diffusion coefficient map.

the first presentation of MS, NMO, ADEM, or idiopathic demyelinating events. On MRI, a TDL is a large white matter lesion with variable mass effect, absence of cortical involvement, a complete or open ring of contrast enhancement, vessel-like structures running through its center, a T2-hypointense ring, and peripheral restricted diffusion on DWI (▶ Fig. 9.7).[16] Conventional MRI findings

overlap between the different demyelinating syndromes and TDL and can mimic high-grade gliomas or other neoplastic lesions.[16,17]

DTI yields additional information to distinguish TDL from high-grade gliomas.[17] High-grade gliomas frequently demonstrate a rim of increased FA in the perilesional edema, which is not usually described in TDLs.[17]

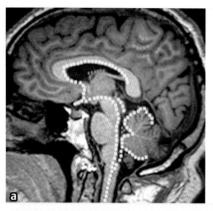
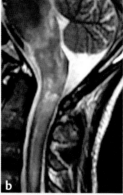
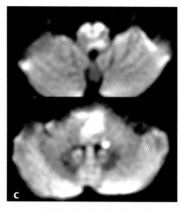

Fig. 9.6 Neuromyelitis optica (NMO) lesions and the aquaporin-4 (AQP-4) channel distribution in the central nervous system. Overlaid to a (**a**) sagittal T1-weighted image there is a schematic view of the main distribution of AQP-4 channel protein sites in the central nervous system. There is a high concentration of AQP-4 channel protein in the central spinal cord, hypothalamus, subependymal white matter, supraoptic nuclei, optic nerve/chiasm, cerebellar cortex (yellow spots), ependymal cells (blue spots) and also in the subcortical white matter (orange spots). (**b**) Acute NMO lesions commonly present as longitudinally extensive or transverse myelitis on sagittal T2-weighted image, commonly affecting the medulla and spinal cord junction. (**c**) Acute lesions may show restricted diffusion, with hyperintensity on diffusion weighted imaging (axial views at the levels of medulla and pons).

9.1.6 Baló Concentric Sclerosis

Baló concentric sclerosis is a rare variant of acute demyelinating diseases, characterized by alternating rings of demyelination and preserved myelin or remyelination.[1] Pathological studies describe edges of active demyelination surrounding demyelinated areas where exacerbated inflammatory activity is present. Interestingly, the active demyelination edges sometimes follow the pattern of hypoxic lesions.[1] In the acute phase, MRI shows concentric bands of demyelination, hyperintense on T2-weighted images and hypointense on T1-weighted images, alternating with rings isointense to white matter thought to be preserved myelin or remyelination. Concentric ring gadolinium enhancement is seen in the bands of active demyelination and progressively disappears in the late acute and chronic stages of the disease. Restricted diffusion is frequently present in the enhancing rings, whereas the nonenhancing bands usually show high ADC values (▶ Fig. 9.8).[1]

9.1.7 Osmotic Myelinolysis

Osmotic demyelination typically occurs after rapid correction of hyponatremia.[18] It refers, more frequently, to central pontine myelinolysis, with acute demyelination of white matter tracts in the pons, sparing peripheral fibers (ventrolateral longitudinal fibers), and the periventricular white matter. Similar lesions can occur outside the pons, affecting the basal ganglia, midbrain, and subcortical white matter, characteristic of the so-called extrapontine myelinolysis.[19]

Osmotic myelinolysis is usually preceded by an initial phase of unspecific encephalopathy attributed to the electrolyte disturbance. Following rapid reversal of this disturbance, a transient improvement is observed, and 2 or 3 days later, the patient progresses to spastic quadriplegia, pseudobulbar palsy, and variable levels of consciousness.[18]

In the hyperacute onset of osmotic demyelination, restricted diffusion is seen in the lesions. Later, there is increasing T2-hyperintensity and T1-hypointensity, symmetrically distributed in the central pons, frequently showing a classic trident appearance (▶ Fig. 9.9) with progressive increases in ADC levels. T1 and T2 changes may take up to 2 weeks to appear after the hyperacute phase when increased diffusion is more often observed.[19]

9.2 Diffusion Weighted Imaging and Diffusion Tensor Imaging in Toxic Diseases

9.2.1 Introduction

Toxic diseases can be secondary to exposure to a wide variety of exogenous agents, including cranial

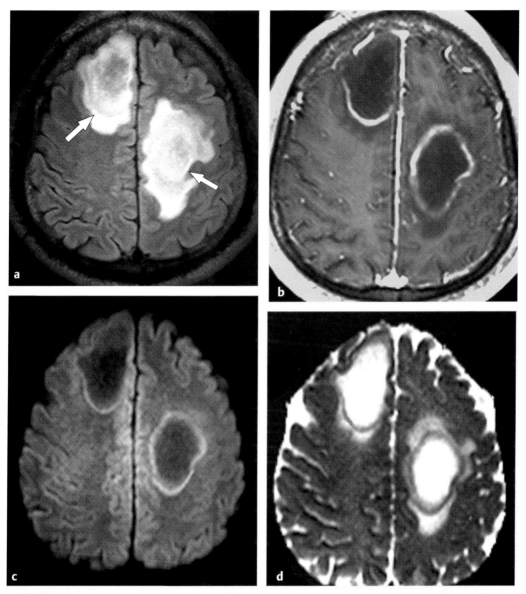

Fig. 9.7 Tumefactive demyelinating lesions (TDLs). TDLs are demyelinating lesions > 2 cm in diameter, frequently showing mass effect and surrounding edema. (a) Axial fluid-attenuated inversion recovery image show two examples (arrows). (b) Axial enhanced T1-weighted image shows the enhancing edges that represent areas of increased inflammatory activity. (c) The lesion periphery frequently shows restricted water diffusion, with hyperintensity on diffusion weighted imaging (d) and hypointensity on the apparent diffusion coefficient map.

irradiation, chemotherapy, antiepileptic agents, drugs of recreational use, and environmental toxins. Although the CNS is naturally protected by the BBB from chemically induced neurotoxicity, a great number of neurotoxins are known to interfere or damage it, allowing them to penetrate neural tissues and exposing the brain to them. Substances that are characteristically lipid soluble have a

facilitated penetration and distribution in the CNS, where they can promote direct neuroglial excitotoxic injury or metabolic disturbances.[20,21]

Toxic leukoencephalopathy (TL) may be acute, and the so-called acute toxic leukoencephalopathy (ATL) may have a dramatic clinical onset. This entity must be placed in perspective with the more common and ubiquitous chronic TL that is

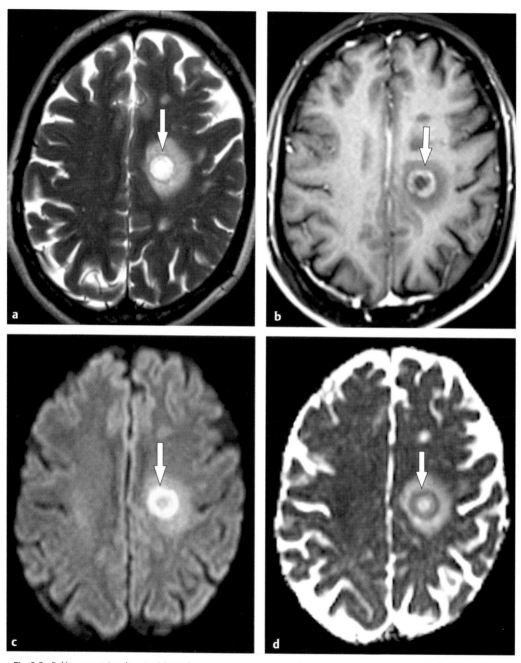

Fig. 9.8 Balό concentric sclerosis. (a) Axial T2-weighted image depicts the layered appearance of a Balό demyelinating lesion (arrow). (b) Rings of active demyelination usually enhance after gadolinium administration (arrow) with surrounding edges of restricted diffusion characterized by hyperintensity on (c) diffusion weighted imaging (arrow) and (d) hypointensity on the apparent diffusion coefficient map (arrow).

present in many patients undergoing chemotherapy or radiation.[21] Clinical presentations are somewhat nonspecific in both, generally characterized by a recent onset of neurological decline, cognitive changes, headache, and other focal neurological signs.[20,22]

The damage generally involves the WM tracts and other high metabolic areas, which are

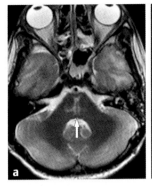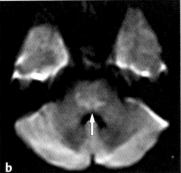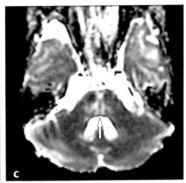

Fig. 9.9 Osmotic myelinolysis. (**a**) Axial T2-weighted image shows a pontine lesion with the typical trident appearance (arrow). T2 and T1 signal changes frequently appear after a few days or weeks, when increased diffusion is usually seen, showing hyperintensity on (**b**) diffusion weighted imaging (arrow) and hyperintensity on (**c**) the apparent diffusion coefficient map (arrow).

particularly susceptible to neurotoxic damage, including the deep gray matter, brainstem, and cerebellar nuclei.[22] Therefore, TL may solely involve the WM, but also may affect the basal ganglia, brainstem, and cerebellum.[21]

Typically, the MRI appearance of ATL is that of symmetric hyperintense WM lesions on T2-weighted and FLAIR images. Restricted diffusion can be seen in areas of acute demyelination and cytotoxic edema. Usually, with drug discontinuation, supportive therapy, or specific treatments, most of these imaging findings are reversible. Therefore, the clinical features and neurological outcome are neither necessarily correlated to the degree of early T2, FLAIR, or DWI abnormalities, nor to their resolution in subsequent imaging studies.[22]

9.2.2 Antineoplastic Treatment

Radiation Therapy

There is a wide range of radiation therapy adverse effects, from minor acute symptoms (headache, fatigue) to life-threatening subacute and late neurological complications (radionecrosis, progressive leukoencephalopathy, radiation-induced tumors).[21] The emphasis here is on subacute leukoencephalopathy.

Although it is not entirely clear which individual characteristics are linked to the development of radiation-induced toxicity, some recognized risk factors are increasing age, diabetes mellitus, systemic hypertension, combined chemotherapy regimens, and the presence of underlying leukoaraiosis.[23]

Regarding subacute leukoencephalopathy, most patients are asymptomatic. Mild or moderate cognitive impairment is more common than severe dementia. Although clinical symptoms stabilize or evolve slowly in most patients, some individuals may develop progressive dementia and eventually die.[23] Imaging findings usually reflect diffuse WM injury. On MRI, periventricular WM lesions are depicted as areas of hyperintensity on FLAIR and T2-weighted images (▶ Fig. 9.10), ADC is usually normal or slightly increased. Brain atrophy may also coexist. No effective treatment is known to revert the clinical and imaging features of radiation-leukoencephalopathy.[23,24]

Chemotherapy

Lately, the so-called chemobrain has been highlighted in several studies that evaluate the effects of chemotherapy in cognition, both during and after treatment. Advanced neuroimaging techniques have reaffirmed the relationship between chemotherapy and cognitive deficits. The use of DTI to probe these patients demonstrates widespread reductions in FA, which correlates with cognitive decline.[25]

On the other hand, some critical complications of chemotherapy may produce more acute and reversible neurological illness, along with striking imaging findings that may be easily recognized on MRI scans. Symptoms are usually nonspecific, and the clinical suspicion should take into account the history of exposure to neurotoxic agents. Imaging findings may be easily recognized and usually subside late in the course of the disease, along with resolution of clinical symptoms, especially if

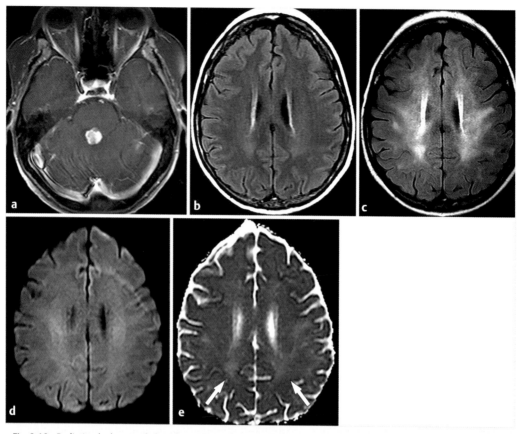

Fig. 9.10 Radiation leukoencephalopathy. A 53-year-old woman presented with metastatic disease secondary to lung cancer. (a) An axial enhanced T1-weighted image demonstrated one secondary lesion in the dorsal pons. (b) At the same time point, an axial fluid-attenuated inversion recovery (FLAIR) image at the plane of the corona radiata was unremarkable. (c) After 4 months, as the patient was treated using total brain radiation, a diffuse, bilateral and symmetric leukoencephalopathy appeared in the follow-up FLAIR image, without significant changes on the (d) corresponding diffusion weighted image. (e) In the apparent diffusion coefficient map, white matter hyperintensity can be seen (arrows).

the administration of the neurotoxic agent is interrupted.

Fluorouracil

5-Fluorouracil (5-FU) is widely used for control of various solid tumors, such as adenocarcinomas of the gastrointestinal tract, prostate, and breast. In one series, almost 6% of patients who received high-dose 5-FU developed an encephalopathy.[26]

In patients with acute/subacute 5-FU leukoencephalopathy, DWI may show marked restricted diffusion in the cerebral WM, especially within the centrum semiovale (▶ Fig. 9.11) and splenium of the corpus callosum. FLAIR images may be normal or show mild to moderate hyperintensity in the periventricular WM.[21] Restricted diffusion may completely revert as soon as 1 week to a few months after drug withdrawal. Effective medical treatments are not well established, but withdrawal of 5-FU is mandatory.[26]

Methotrexate

Methotrexate (MTX) is largely administered to treat solid cancers, acute lymphoblastic leukemia, and non-Hodgkin lymphoma. In addition, it is also an immunomodulator in the treatment of collagen diseases. Because MTX scarcely penetrates the BBB, high doses are usually administered via intrathecal or intravenous routes to eradicate malignant cells from the CNS. Combined therapy with irradiation improves therapy efficacy but also enhances neurotoxicity.[27]

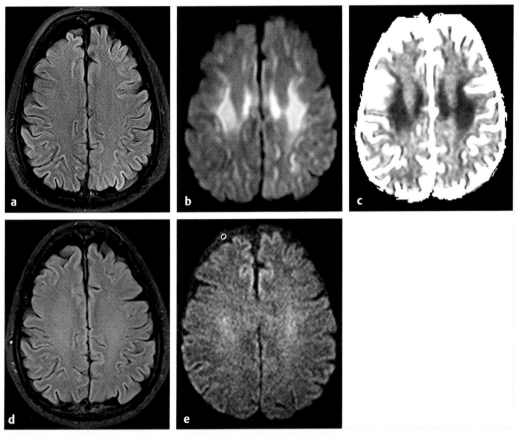

Fig. 9.11 Fluorouracil (5-FU) treatment effects. After 5 days of chemotherapy for esophageal cancer, a 57-year-old woman presented with altered mental status. The initial magnetic resonance imaging (MRI) showed an almost normal (a) fluid-attenuated inversion recovery (FLAIR) image, but signs of restricted diffusion in the periventricular and deep white matter can be appreciated, (b) identified as hyperintense areas in diffusion weighted imaging, (c) with corresponding hypointensity on the apparent diffusion coefficient map. After discontinuation of therapy, 18 days after the initial MRI study, the MRI findings were almost totally reversed on a follow-up examination with (d) FLAIR and (e) diffusion weighted imaging,

Although not always present, imaging findings may be typical and conclusive, avoiding unnecessary biopsy and other potentially harmful interventions. DWI may show focal or multifocal areas of restricted diffusion, more often affecting the periventricular WM (▸ Fig. 9.12). Some atypical sites may be affected, such as the cerebral and cerebellar cortex, subcortical WM, and thalami.[21] These unusual imaging findings are associated with a more severe clinical presentation than that of classic acute leukoencephalopathy. Postcontrast enhancement is usually absent in the lesions.[28] Toxic effects respond well to therapy with folinic acid, high-dose leucovorin, and aminophylline.[29]

Fludarabine

Fludarabine is mainly used in patients with hematologic malignancies, and as an immunosuppressive agent before bone marrow transplantation.[30]

Interestingly, MRI abnormalities are disproportionately mild in comparison to the clinical picture and histopathological findings. T2-weighted and FLAIR images depict slight hyperintensity in the periventricular WM, usually with corresponding restricted diffusion, confirmed by low signal intensity on ADC maps (▸ Fig. 9.13). Typically, there is no associated contrast enhancement.[30]

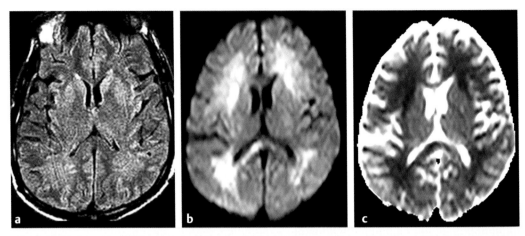

Fig. 9.12 Methotrexate (MTX) leukoencephalopathy. A 50-year-old man underwent intrathecal MTX therapy 2 days before he was found unresponsive. (a) Mild bilateral and symmetric slightly hyperintense areas involved the white matter on a fluid-attenuated inversion recovery image, with severe restricted diffusion, (b) identified as hyperintense areas on diffusion weighted imaging, with (c) corresponding hypointensity on the apparent diffusion coefficient map.

9.2.3 Drugs of Recreational Use

Heroin

The primary neuropathological effect of injected heroin is hypoxic-ischemic leukoencephalopathy, which can be related to prolonged and recurrent heroin-induced respiratory depression or to infections.[31] Heroin abusers may present variable degrees of cerebral atrophy, demyelination, acute and chronic perfusion abnormalities, and decreased nigrostriatal neuronal density.[22,31]

Spongiform leukoencephalopathy is a rare complication of inhalation of heated heroin, known as "chasing the dragon," in allusion to the shape of the heroin fumes after the heating of the drug powder on aluminum foil.[22,32] Generally it has a dramatic evolution, with a 23% mortality rate, and even mild cases may show a significant degree of spongiform degeneration and neurological deterioration. MRI shows symmetric hyperintensity on T2-weighted and FLAIR images in the cerebral and cerebellar WM. Typically, the abnormalities involve the posterior limbs of internal capsules, sparing the anterior limbs. Although there is a predominant change in the periventricular WM, the subcortical WM can also be affected.[22] In the acute phase, there is restricted diffusion in the affected areas (▶ Fig. 9.14), with progressive normalization or increase in the ADC values later.[22,32]

Cocaine

Cocaine is a stimulant drug that increases the intrasynaptic levels of dopamine and interferes in the serotonin transporter protein. In addition, it also stimulates the noradrenergic activity, inducing cardiovascular distress, leading to hypertension and vasoconstriction, which can produce hypoxic-ischemic injury, cerebral hemorrhage, hypertensive encephalopathy, and posterior reversible leukoencephalopathy syndrome (PRES). Cocaine can also have a direct excitotoxic effect with an MRI appearance indistinguishable from the other aforementioned toxic lesions, presenting as increased hyperintensity on T2-weighted images in the cerebral WM, globi pallidi, and splenium of the corpus callosum with variable diffusion in the affected areas.[31]

9.2.4 Other Drugs

Cyclosporine

Cyclosporine-A (CSA) is a potent immunosuppressive agent used in the prophylaxis of graft rejection and graft-versus-host disease after bone marrow transplantation and solid organ transplants. It is also used in the treatment of various immunologic disorders. Secondary neurological symptoms include tremor, headache, seizures, hallucinations, memory deficits, and visual

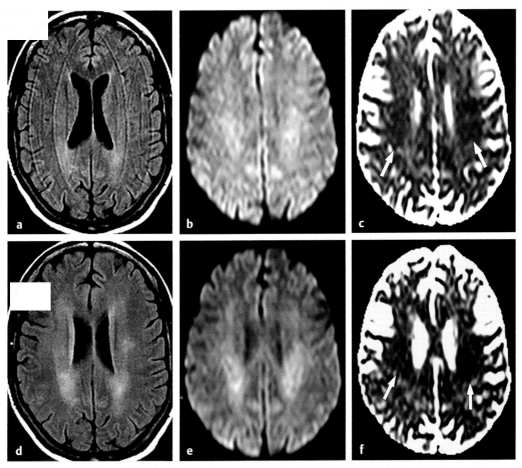

Fig. 9.13 Fludarabine treatment effects. A 56-year-old woman was given fludarabine 3 weeks earlier for multiple myeloma. (**a**) Axial fluid-attenuated inversion recovery (FLAIR) and (**b**) diffusion weighted imaging disclosed foci of hyperintense signal in the periventricular white matter. (**c**) Corresponding mild apparent diffusion coefficient (ADC) reduction was identified as hypointensity on the ADC map (arrows). (**d–f**) Follow-up magnetic resonance imaging (MRI) after 2 weeks showed more prominent findings, not only in the (**d**) FLAIR and (**e**) diffusion weighted images but also in (**f**) the areas of restricted diffusion in the ADC map (arrows).

disturbances. Cerebellar, extrapyramidal, and pyramidal syndromes can also occur. PRES and toxic lesions may ensue (the former is usually more common), and are usually associated with characteristic imaging features.[33]

Acute toxic lesions may present soon after the initiation of CSA. MRI findings are somewhat nonspecific and similar to those found in other toxic disorders. There is usually bilateral and symmetric hyperintensity involving the periventricular WM and corona radiata on T2-weighted and FLAIR images, associated with foci of restricted diffusion within these areas (▶ Fig. 9.15). Reversibility of

clinical symptoms and imaging features after CSA tapering confirms the diagnosis. Nonetheless, in some patients, residual FLAIR hyperintensity may persist, especially if initial FLAIR images showed severe brain involvement.[22] So far, the exact pathogenesis of CSA-neurotoxicity is not understood.

Metronidazole

Metronidazole is an antibiotic widely used to treat anaerobic and protozoal infections, hospital-acquired infections, *Helicobacter pylori*

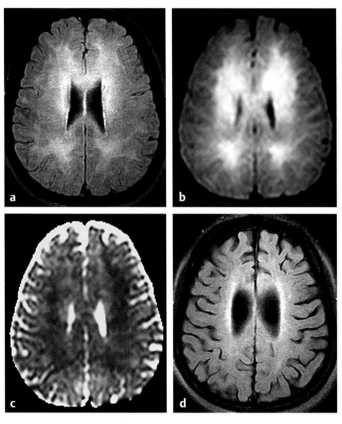

Fig. 9.14 Heroin toxicity, "chasing the dragon" syndrome. A 24-year-old woman inhaled heroin fumes and arrived at the emergency room quadriplegic and unresponsive. (**a-c**) The initial magnetic resonance imaging (MRI) showed signs of leukoencephalopathy, with symmetric hyperintense signal on (**a**) fluid-attenuated inversion recovery (FLAIR) from the periventricular to the subcortical white matter. Those areas demonstrated signs of restricted diffusion, hyperintensity on (**b**) diffusion weighted imaging, and hypointensity on (**c**) the apparent diffusion coefficient map. Symptoms had mostly resolved after 1 year, but follow-up MRI at that time showed (**d**) persistent white matter abnormalities on FLAIR associated with severe brain atrophy.

infections, and *Clostridium difficile* diarrhea. It also plays a role as a prophylactic agent after gastrointestinal surgery and to prevent recurrent bacterial infection, especially in Crohn's disease. Metronidazole is a safe and well tolerated drug at low doses, but it can be associated with encephalopathy, ototoxicity, and visual impairment when the dose exceeds 2 g/d or after prolonged administration.[34]

MRI typically shows bilateral symmetric hyperintense signal on T2-weighted and FLAIR sequences affecting the cerebellar dentate nuclei, superior olivary nuclei, dorsal pons and medulla, midbrain structures (tectum, red nucleus, tegmentum and in periaqueductal gray matter), and splenium of the corpus callosum, with variable involvement of the internal capsules, anterior commissure, and deep and subcortical WM.[34] More often there is restricted diffusion with low ADC values in the affected supratentorial WM (▶ Fig. 9.16), suggesting cytotoxic edema. However, increased diffusion in the cerebellar and brainstem nuclei has been

described, which perhaps corresponds to vasogenic edema in these locations.[34] The hyperintense T2 lesions and the DWI changes are thought to be almost entirely reversible after a few weeks of drug cessation, accompanied by progressive clinical improvement.[34]

Vigabatrin

Vigabatrin (VGB) is a drug used to treat infantile spasms, epilepsy associated with tuberous sclerosis, and complex partial seizures in children and adults. Although VGB is an effective antiepileptic drug, neurotoxic changes have been described with cumulative and high doses.[35]

Imaging findings include bilateral and symmetric hyperintensity on T2-weighted and FLAIR images in the basal ganglia, especially in the globi pallidi, thalami, dentate nuclei, and dorsal brainstem, with reduced diffusion in them (▶ Fig. 9.17).[35] MRI abnormalities may be reversible 12 to 16 weeks after drug discontinuation, but some patients show

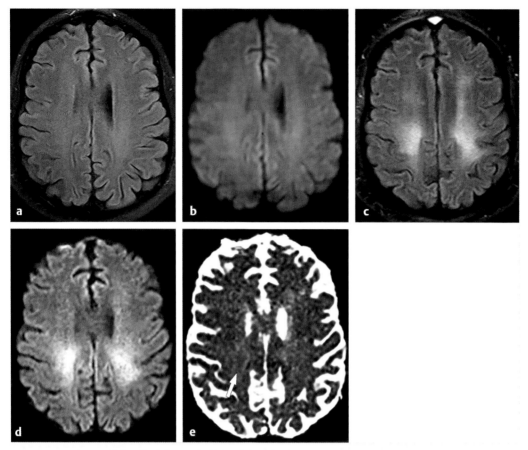

Fig. 9.15 Leukoencephalopathy following cyclosporine-A (CSA) treatment. CSA was given after bone marrow transplantation. Pretransplantation magnetic resonance imaging showed no significant abnormalities on (**a**) fluid-attenuated inversion recovery (FLAIR) and (**b**) diffusion weighted imaging (DWI). Nineteen days after CSA therapy hyperintensities on (**c**) FLAIR and (**d**) DWI appeared in the posterior cerebral periventricular white matter, associated with hypointense areas (arrow) in the (**e**) corresponding apparent diffusion coefficient map, thus confirming the presence of restricted diffusion.

improvement or resolution on MRI, even without cessation of VGB.[35] VGB-related MRI changes almost exclusively affect young infants, especially those diagnosed with infantile spasms.[35]

9.2.5 Environmental Toxins

Carbon Monoxide

Carbon monoxide (CO) is an odorless, colorless, and nonirritating gas produced by incomplete combustion of organic substances and carbon-containing fuel. CO has 210 times higher affinity to hemoglobin than oxygen; thus a small rise in its concentration can result in toxic levels of carboxyhemoglobin. Intoxication is often accidental.[36]

MRI shows marked ADC reduction with involvement of the basal ganglia and periventricular and subcortical WM (▶ Fig. 9.18), corpus callosum, and internal capsules. T2-weighted and FLAIR images show variable signal abnormalities dependent on the severity of the intoxication. WM abnormalities frequently reverse within 2 weeks to 10 months.[37] However, because of the higher metabolic activity in gray matter, the basal ganglia are more susceptible to permanent damage. In the chronic stages, it is not infrequent to find signs of striatal necrosis, especially in severe intoxications.[37]

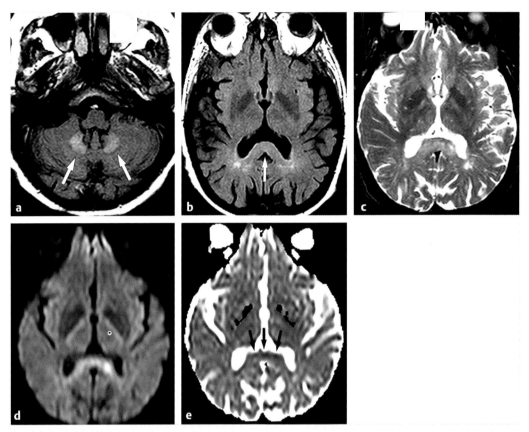

Fig. 9.16 Metronidazole encephalopathy. A 69-year-old woman was put on increasing doses of metronidazole over 2 months for recurrent vaginal infection. An initial magnetic resonance imaging (MRI) examination with fluid-attenuated inversion recovery images showed (**a**) bilateral and symmetric hyperintense signal involving the cerebellar dentate nuclei (arrows), which, in a less intense manner, could also be appreciated in (**b**) the splenium of the corpus callosum (arrow). (**c**) Follow-up MRI examination after 20 days demonstrated more severe signal changes in the splenium, in an axial T2-weighted image, with (**d**) hyperintensity on diffusion weighted imaging and (**e**) hypointense areas on the apparent diffusion coefficient map (arrows), confirming the presence of restricted diffusion.

Methanol

Methanol is a component of commercially available varnishes, solvents, antifreeze, and gasoline mixtures. Methanol intoxication may be accidental, intentional, or due to adulteration of alcoholic beverages. There is a latency period between ingestion of methanol and clinical onset of symptoms, probably because of the concomitant ingestion of ethanol. Early symptoms are nonspecific, including nausea, vomiting, and abdominal pain, followed by variable visual disturbances. Late manifestations are associated with acidosis and accumulation of formic and lactic acids. Methanol intoxication can be fatal within 6 to 36 hours after ingestion.[38]

The typical imaging features of methanol poisoning are bilateral lentiform nuclei necrosis with hyperintensity on T2-weighted, FLAIR images and DWI and reduced ADC. Hemorrhagic putaminal lesions can also occur.[21] Other affected areas included are corona radiata, centrum semiovale, and subcortical WM (▶ Fig. 9.19).[38]

9.2.6 Reversible Splenial Lesions

An important type of lesion that should be mentioned here are "reversible splenial lesions." These are found in a wide spectrum of clinical conditions that share common and typical MRI features of hyperintensity on T2-weighted and FLAIR images

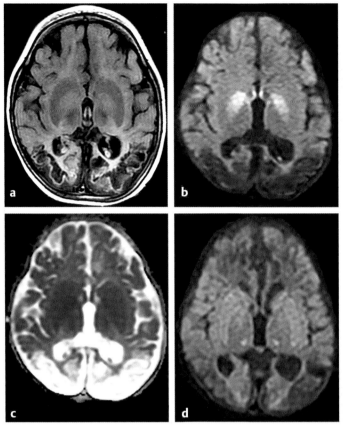

Fig. 9.17 Vigabatrin-related magnetic resonance imaging changes in an 8-month-old child, with chronic epilepsy secondary to neonatal hypoxia. (**a**) A few weeks after starting vigabatrin, there were slight bilateral and symmetric pallidal hyperintensities on a fluid-attenuated inversion recovery image, which also showed the residual posterior cerebral lesions secondary to the neonatal ischemic event. (**b**) Pallidal restricted diffusion was detected, seen as hyperintensity on diffusion weighted imaging and (**c**) hypointensity on the apparent diffusion coefficient map. (**d**) Five months after drug discontinuation, diffusion weighted imaging was unremarkable in the pallidal region.

and have reversible reduced diffusion within the posterior corpus callosum[39] (▸ Fig. 9.20). Because most lesions are transient and incidentally found on MRI, no therapy is warranted.

Countless disorders may be associated with reversible splenial lesions. Reported cases are often related to encephalitis/encephalopathy syndromes (usually secondary to viral infections), antiepileptic drug toxicity/withdrawal, and metabolic disorders (hypoglycemia and hypernatremia).[39,40] Several other conditions with transient splenial lesions, which can also involve other segments of the corpus callosum, include Marchiafava–Bignami disease, Wernicke encephalopathy, Kawasaki disease, hemolytic-uremic syndrome, traumatic brain injury, and high-altitude cerebral edema. Pharmacological agents associated with these reversible callosal lesions are methylbromide, cisplatinum, carboplatin, olanzapine, and citalopram.[26]

In patients with epilepsy, reversible splenial lesions may be attributed either to seizures or to their treatments. Almost every antiepileptic drug has been associated with this type of lesion, including carbamazepine, phenytoin, valproic acid, vigabatrin, lamotrigine, oxcarbazepine, topiramate, clonazepam, and others.[40]

The main DWI findings in toxic lesions are summarized in ▸ Table 9.1.

9.3 Summary

In demyelinating diseases, the findings on DWI reflect their neuropathological substrates, and thus are very heterogeneous. Occasionally, DWI can provide additional valuable information regarding lesion age and activity and also about the type of cellular damage. DTI can show abnormalities in the NAWM, confirming the findings reported using magnetization transfer and proton spectroscopy.

Toxic diseases affecting the CNS may affect specific structures, especially the WM in ATL, but overall the MRI findings are often nonspecific. In these disorders the lesions are usually bilateral and in the acute phase show restricted diffusion. Drug withdrawal results in improvement or resolution of the lesions in most patients.

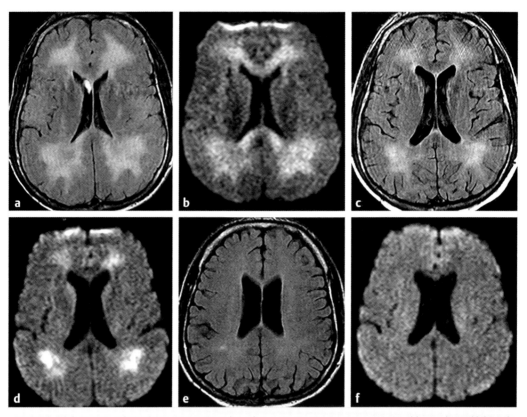

Fig. 9.18 Carbon monoxide (CO) intoxication. Five days after acute CO intoxication, a 33-year-old man showed bilateral and diffuse cerebral white matter hyperintensity on (**a**) fluid-attenuated inversion recovery (FLAIR) and (**b**) diffusion weighted images. After 2 months, corresponding (**c**) FLAIR and (**d**) DWI demonstrated improvement of the abnormalities, which mostly resolved at 9 months follow-up on (**e**) FLAIR and (**f**) DWI.

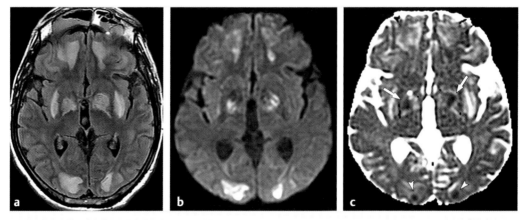

Fig. 9.19 Methanol intoxication. A 56-year-old man arrived in the emergency room with acute blindness, severe neurological impairment, and systemic symptoms. (**a**) Axial fluid-attenuated inversion recovery image revealed extensive symmetric damage to the cerebral white matter, more evident in the frontal and occipital lobes seen as areas of hyperintensity; there were also similar lesions in the basal ganglia, especially involving the lentiform nuclei. (**b**) Diffusion weighted imaging showed hyperintensity in these areas, and (**c**) corresponding apparent diffusion coefficient maps demonstrated restricted diffusion, more clearly depicted in the lentiform nuclei (arrows) and occipital white matter (arrowheads).

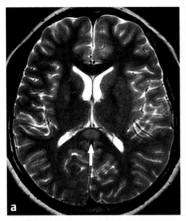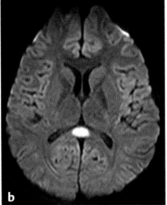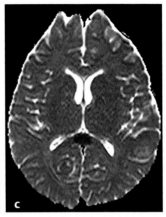

Fig. 9.20 Reversible splenial lesion in an 18-year-old woman with epilepsy. (a) Magnetic resonance imaging shows a focal splenial hyperintensity on (a) T2-weighted (arrow) and (b) diffusion weighted images. (c) The apparent diffusion coefficient map confirmed diffusion restriction in the affected area.

Table 9.1 Lesion location and main diffusion weighted imaging findings in toxic cerebral lesions

Agent	Lesion location[a]	DWI findings
Radiation subacute leukoencephalopathy	Periventricular WM	No abnormalities or slightly increased ADC
Fluorouracil	Cerebral WM, especially within the centrum semiovale and splenium of the corpus callosum	Restricted diffusion
Methotrexate	Periventricular WM, less likely affects cerebral and cerebellar cortex, subcortical WM, and thalamus	Restricted diffusion
Fludarabine	Periventricular WM	Restricted diffusion
Heroin (spongiform leukoencephalopathy)	Cerebral and cerebellar WM and posterior limb of internal capsules	Restricted diffusion
Cocaine (direct excitotoxic effect)	Cerebral white matter, globus pallidus, and splenium of the corpus callosum	Variable diffusion
Cyclosporine	Periventricular WM and corona radiata	Foci of restricted diffusion
Metronidazole	Cerebellar dentate nuclei, superior olivary nuclei, dorsal pons and medulla, midbrain, splenium of the corpus callosum, with variable involvement of the internal capsule, anterior commissure, deep and subcortical WM	Restricted diffusion in the supratentorial WM, increased diffusion in the cerebellar and brainstem nuclei
Vigabatrin	Basal ganglia, especially in the globi pallidi, thalami, dentate nuclei, and dorsal brainstem	Restricted diffusion
Carbon monoxide	Basal ganglia, periventricular and subcortical WM, corpus callosum, and internal capsule	Restricted diffusion
Methanol	Lentiform nuclei, usually hemorrhagic in putamen; WM lesions can occur	Restricted diffusion in lentiform nuclei

Abbreviations: ADC, apparent diffusion coefficient; DWI, diffusion weighted imaging; WM, white matter.
[a]Usually the lesions are bilateral.

References

[1] Koelblinger C, Fruehwald-Pallamar J, Kubin K, et al. Atypical idiopathic inflammatory demyelinating lesions (IIDL): conventional and diffusion weighted MR imaging (DWI) findings in 42 cases. Eur J Radiol 2013; 82(11): 1996–2004

[2] Karaarslan E, Arslan A. Diffusion weighted MR imaging in non-infarct lesions of the brain. Eur J Radiol 2008; 65(3): 402–416

[3] Inglese M, Salvi F, Iannucci G, Mancardi GL, Mascalchi M, Filippi M. Magnetization transfer and diffusion tensor MR imaging of acute disseminated encephalomyelitis. AJNR Am J Neuroradiol 2002; 23(2): 267–272

[4] Castriota Scanderbeg A, Tomaiuolo F, Sabatini U, Nocentini U, Grasso MG, Caltagirone C. Demyelinating plaques in relapsing-remitting and secondary-progressive multiple sclerosis: assessment with diffusion MR imaging. AJNR Am J Neuroradiol 2000; 21(5): 862–868

[5] Lerner A, Mogensen MA, Kim PE, Shiroishi MS, Hwang DH, Law M. Clinical Applications of Diffusion Tensor Imaging. World Neurosurg 2014; 82: 96–109

[6] Rimkus CM, Junqueira TF, Callegaro D, Otaduy MC, Leite CdaC. Segmented corpus callosum diffusivity correlates with the Expanded Disability Status Scale score in the early stages of relapsing-remitting multiple sclerosis. Clinics 2013; 68(8): 1115–1120

[7] Vrenken H, Pouwels PJ, Geurts JJ, et al. Altered diffusion tensor in multiple sclerosis normal-appearing brain tissue: cortical diffusion changes seem related to clinical deterioration. J Magn Reson Imaging 2006; 23(5): 628–636

[8] Yu CS, Zhu CZ, Li KC, et al. Relapsing neuromyelitis optica and relapsing-remitting multiple sclerosis: differentiation at diffusion tensor MR imaging of corpus callosum. Radiology 2007; 244(1): 249–256

[9] Huston JM, Field AS. Clinical applications of diffusion tensor imaging. Magn Reson Imaging Clin N Am 2013; 21(2): 279–298

[10] Werring DJ, Brassat D, Droogan AG, et al. The pathogenesis of lesions and normal-appearing white matter changes in multiple sclerosis: a serial diffusion MRI study. Brain 2000; 123(Pt 8): 1667–1676

[11] Young NP, Weinshenker BG, Lucchinetti CF. Acute disseminated encephalomyelitis: current understanding and controversies. Semin Neurol 2008; 28(1): 84–94

[12] Bernarding J, Braun J, Koennecke HC. Diffusion- and perfusion-weighted MR imaging in a patient with acute demyelinating encephalomyelitis (ADEM). J Magn Reson Imaging 2002; 15(1): 96–100

[13] Straus Farber R, Devilliers L, Miller A, et al. Differentiating multiple sclerosis from other causes of demyelination using diffusion weighted imaging of the corpus callosum. J Magn Reson Imaging 2009; 30(4): 732–736

[14] Wingerchuk DM, Lennon VA, Lucchinetti CF, Pittock SJ, Weinshenker BG. The spectrum of neuromyelitis optica. Lancet Neurol 2007; 6(9): 805–815

[15] Rueda Lopes FC, Doring T, Martins C, et al. The role of demyelination in neuromyelitis optica damage: diffusion tensor MR imaging study. Radiology 2012; 263(1): 235–242

[16] Enzinger C, Strasser-Fuchs S, Ropele S, Kapeller P, Kleinert R, Fazekas F. Tumefactive demyelinating lesions: conventional and advanced magnetic resonance imaging. Mult Scler 2005; 11(2): 135–139

[17] Toh CH, Wei KC, Ng SH, Wan YL, Castillo M, Lin CP. Differentiation of tumefactive demyelinating lesions from high-grade gliomas with the use of diffusion tensor imaging. AJNR Am J Neuroradiol 2012; 33(5): 846–851

[18] Martin RJ. Central pontine and extrapontine myelinolysis: the osmotic demyelination syndromes. J Neurol Neurosurg Psychiatry 2004; 75 Suppl 3: iii22–iii28

[19] Ruzek KA, Campeau NG, Miller GM. Early diagnosis of central pontine myelinolysis with diffusion weighted imaging. AJNR Am J Neuroradiol 2004; 25(2): 210–213

[20] Filley CM, Kleinschmidt-DeMasters BK. Toxic leukoencephalopathy. N Engl J Med 2001; 345(6): 425–432

[21] Rimkus CM, Andrade CS, Leite CC, McKinney AM, Lucato LT. Toxic leukoencephalopathies, including drug, medication, environmental, and radiation-induced encephalopathic syndromes. Semin Ultrasound CT MR 2014; 35(2): 97–117

[22] McKinney AM, Kieffer SA, Paylor RT, SantaCruz KS, Kendi A, Lucato LT. Acute toxic leukoencephalopathy: potential for reversibility clinically and on MRI with diffusion weighted and FLAIR imaging. AJR Am J Roentgenol 2009; 193(1): 192–206

[23] Soussain C, Ricard D, Fike JR, Mazeron JJ, Psimaras D, Delattre JY. CNS complications of radiotherapy and chemotherapy. Lancet 2009; 374(9701): 1639–1651

[24] Chawla S, Wang S, Kim S, et al. Radiation Injury to the Normal Brain Measured by 3D-Echo-Planar Spectroscopic Imaging and Diffusion Tensor Imaging: Initial Experience. J Neuroimaging 2013; 3: 9

[25] Deprez S, Amant F, Smeets A, et al. Longitudinal assessment of chemotherapy-induced structural changes in cerebral white matter and its correlation with impaired cognitive functioning. J Clin Oncol 2012; 30(3): 274–281

[26] Tha KK, Terae S, Sugiura M, et al. Diffusion weighted magnetic resonance imaging in early stage of 5-fluorouracil-induced leukoencephalopathy. Acta Neurol Scand 2002; 106 (6): 379–386

[27] Kim JY, Kim ST, Nam DH, Lee JI, Park K, Kong DS. Leukoencephalopathy and disseminated necrotizing leukoencephalopathy following intrathecal methotrexate chemotherapy and radiation therapy for central nerve system lymphoma or leukemia. J Korean Neurosurg Soc 2011; 50(4): 304–310

[28] Ziereisen F, Dan B, Azzi N, Ferster A, Damry N, Christophe C. Reversible acute methotrexate leukoencephalopathy: atypical brain MR imaging features. Pediatr Radiol 2006; 36(3): 205–212

[29] Antunes NL, Souweidane MM, Lis E, Rosenblum MK, Steinherz PG. Methotrexate leukoencephalopathy presenting as Klüver-Bucy syndrome and uncinate seizures. Pediatr Neurol 2002; 26(4): 305–308

[30] Lee MS, McKinney AM, Brace JR, Santacruz K. Clinical and imaging features of fludarabine neurotoxicity. J Neuroophthalmol 2010; 30(1): 37–41

[31] Cunha-Oliveira T, Rego AC, Oliveira CR. Cellular and molecular mechanisms involved in the neurotoxicity of opioid and psychostimulant drugs. Brain Res Brain Res Rev 2008; 58(1): 192–208

[32] Bartlett E, Mikulis DJ. Chasing "chasing the dragon" with MRI: leukoencephalopathy in drug abuse. Br J Radiol 2005; 78(935): 997–1004

[33] Gijtenbeek JM, van den Bent MJ, Vecht CJ. Cyclosporine neurotoxicity: a review. J Neurol 1999; 246(5): 339–346

[34] Heaney CJ, Campeau NG, Lindell EP. MR imaging and diffusion weighted imaging changes in metronidazole (Flagyl)-induced cerebellar toxicity. AJNR Am J Neuroradiol 2003; 24 (8): 1615–1617

[35] Dracopoulos A, Widjaja E, Raybaud C, Westall CA, Snead OC, III. Vigabatrin-associated reversible MRI signal changes in patients with infantile spasms. Epilepsia 2010; 51(7): 1297–1304

[36] Blumenthal I. Carbon monoxide poisoning. J R Soc Med 2001; 94(6): 270–272

[37] Prockop LD, Chichkova RI. Carbon monoxide intoxication: an updated review. J Neurol Sci 2007; 262(1–2): 122–130

[38] Takao H, Doi I, Watanabe T. Serial diffusion weighted magnetic resonance imaging in methanol intoxication. J Comput Assist Tomogr 2006; 30(5): 742–744

[39] Gallucci M, Limbucci N, Paonessa A, Caranci F. Reversible focal splenial lesions. Neuroradiology 2007; 49(7): 541–544

[40] Ruscheweyh R, Marziniak M, Evers S. Reversible focal splenial lesions in facial pain patients treated with antiepileptic drugs: case report and review of the literature. Cephalalgia 2009; 29(5): 587–590

10 Diffusion Weighted Imaging and Diffusion Tensor Imaging of White Matter Diseases In Children

Julie H. Harreld and Zoltan Patay

10.1 Physics

In diffusion imaging, directional diffusion gradients are applied to a T2-weighted (spin-echo) echo-planar imaging (EPI) sequence before and after a 180-degree refocusing pulse. Water protons moving freely through these gradients acquire random spins and are thus dephased, causing signal loss in voxels where water motion (diffusion) is significant. Conversely, stationary or slowly moving protons generate increased signal on diffusion weighted images (DWIs). The apparent diffusion coefficient (ADC) may be calculated from images acquired without and with a diffusion gradient and allows quantitation of the displacement of water molecules over time (mm^2/s) in a particular voxel.[1,2]

In tissues, water mobility may be restricted by cell membranes, macromolecules, or decreased extracellular spaces. In such cases, the signal on DWI is increased, and the ADC is decreased. For example, tissues with high cell density, such as small, round blue cell tumors like medulloblastoma and lymphoma, have decreased or "restricted" water diffusion and therefore appear bright on DWI. Hypercellularity due to a regional influx of cells, such as macrophages or glia, may also cause restricted diffusion (decreased ADC) and high signal on DWI. Cellular swelling due to cytotoxic edema, as in cerebral ischemia, also results in restricted diffusion due to resultant decreases in extracellular freely mobile water. Shift of water into the myelin sheath from the extracellular space, as occurs in intramyelinic edema or myelin vacuolation, may cause restricted diffusion in a similar or related fashion.[3] This is in contrast to vasogenic edema, in which there is an accumulation of extracellular water due to blood–brain barrier (BBB) breakdown or osmotic shifts, causing increased ADC.[4] Though all types of white matter edema may appear bright on T2-weighted imaging, ADC is increased in vasogenic edema (peritumoral edema, infection/inflammation), but decreased in cytotoxic edema (affecting oligodendrocytes and astrocytes) or intramyelinic edema, permitting differentiation. However, different types of edema may coexist (see "maple syrup urine disease" later in this chapter) and even shift during the course of disease. By providing insight into the dominant edema type, diffusion imaging may help characterize dynamic white matter disease processes.

Although diffusion is apparently equal in all directions (isotropic) in gray matter, in white matter it is greatest parallel to the fiber bundles ("tracts") and restricted perpendicular to the tracts, a property known as anisotropy. This is exploited in diffusion tensor imaging (DTI) and fiber tracking, and may be quantified as fractional anisotropy (FA), a measure of the propensity of water to diffuse in a single direction (e.g., along a white matter tract). An FA of 0 indicates isotropic diffusion, and the maximal FA of 1 indicates perfectly linear, anisotropic diffusion along the primary (longitudinal) eigenvector, which indicates axonal orientation. The mean of the second and third eigenvectors, which are perpendicular to the axon, is known as radial diffusivity and can provide further quantitation of myelin integrity. These metrics offer exciting, noninvasive, and reproducible approaches to qualitative and quantitative evaluation of white matter diseases.

10.2 Clinical Applications

In the central nervous system (CNS), the lamellar myelin sheath is formed by the wrapping of specialized oligodendrocyte membrane layers around intact axons, a process that is driven by neuronal electrical activity, coordinated activation of myelin protein genes, and growth and trophic factors produced by neurons and astrocytes. Disorders of any of these components may primarily or secondarily affect myelin to a variable degree. *Hypomyelination* describes early and permanent arrest in myelination (Pelizaeus–Merzbacher disease, trichothiodystrophy), as opposed to *delayed myelination*, in which myelin is quantitatively inappropriate for the age of the patient, typically infants. When myelination progresses but is abnormal due to defective, absent, or accumulated myelin components, it is termed *dysmyelination.*[5] *Demyelination*, the loss of qualitatively normal myelin, may be secondary (due to neuronal or axonal loss, as in trauma) or primary (due to abnormalities of myelin or oligodendrocytes). Primary demyelinating disorders may be heritable (metachromatic leukodystrophy, X-linked adrenoleukodystrophy), or acquired (infection, inflammation, immune disorders, toxins, ischemia).

Because these classic categories are descriptive rather than histopathologic, they may overlap and coexist. Dysmyelination predisposes to demyelination; hypomyelination often accompanies or may mimic delayed myelination. Similarly, though MRI-based patterns of pediatric white matter diseases may occasionally provide a high degree of diagnostic specificity,[6] conventional imaging abnormalities are not specific to underlying histopathologic processes. T1 hypointensity may occur due to rarefaction of myelin (and tissue matrix) or edema; T2 hyperintensity may be due to cytotoxic, intramyelinic, or vasogenic edema, or increased white matter water content due to decreased myelin. The precise pathomechanisms for many pediatric white matter disorders remain unknown, limited by the rarity of the disorders and limited availability of pathological material at various stages of disease. The ability of diffusion imaging to differentiate white matter pathologies contributes to our growing understanding of the pathological mechanisms underlying these disorders, and becomes stronger as more radiological–pathological–molecular biological correlation becomes available. Because patterns of diffusion abnormalities differ based on underlying mechanism, diffusion imaging may contribute to the imaging semiology and improve the specificity of traditional pattern-based diagnosis. Because many white matter diseases are characterized by diffusion abnormalities in their early stages, which subsequently progress to nonspecific increases in water diffusivity and decreased anisotropy due to demyelination and destruction of the white matter matrix, DWI/DTI may also be helpful in assessing the stage and rate of progression of these diseases, particularly in the early stages of disease.

The overall number of pediatric white matter disorders is already significant, and new entities are identified almost every year; the precise mechanisms of white matter damage and changes on brain magnetic resonance imaging (MRI) have yet to be elucidated in most. We therefore focus on disorders for which pathomechanisms and how they relate to diffusion imaging findings are understood (with a reasonable degree of confidence) to illustrate how DWI/DTI can contribute to pathological understanding and diagnosis in these and other pediatric white matter disorders.

10.2.1 Restricted Diffusion: Active Inflammatory Demyelination

Accumulation of microglia and myelin-laden macrophages (hypercellularity) and cytotoxic edema of oligodendrocytes due to proinflammatory cascades and/or metabolic stress results in restricted diffusion in areas of active demyelination.[7,8] Once most or all myelin is lost, these areas demonstrate increased diffusivity and decreased FA in the "burned-out" phase.[9]

Inherited: X-linked Adrenoleukodystrophy

In X-linked adrenoleukodystrophy (X-ALD), a single-enzyme defect in peroxisomal function results in accumulation of very long chain fatty acids (VLCFAs), which disrupt membranes and are toxic to oligodendrocytes and, to a lesser degree, astrocytes. Early demyelination becomes suddenly inflammatory in 90%, with rapid progression.[10] Progression is typically centrifugal and posterior to anterior.[11] Diffusion is relatively decreased in the inflammatory "leading edge" (▶ Fig. 10.1), which pathologically consists of perivascular inflammatory infiltrates, lipid-laden macrophages, and reactive astrocytes. In the central demyelinated zone, where myelinated axons and oligodendrocytes are essentially absent, diffusivity is increased and FA is decreased.[12]

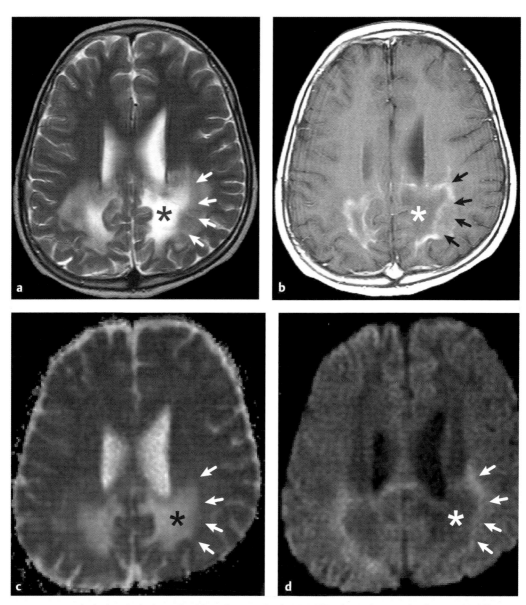

Fig. 10.1 X-Linked adrenoleukodystrophy. (a) Axial T2-weighted image, (b) enhanced T1-weighted image, (c) diffusion weighted image, and (d) apparent diffusion coefficient map. Diffusion is relatively decreased in the peripheral, enhancing inflammatory zone (arrows) surrounding the central demyelinated zone (*), in which water diffusivity is increased.

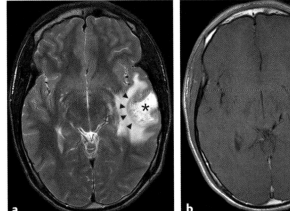
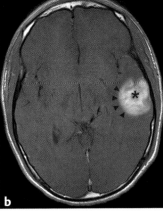
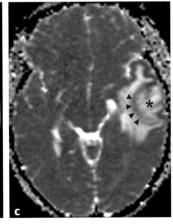

Fig. 10.2 Tumefactive demyelination. (**a**) Axial T2-weighted image, (**b**) enhanced T1-weighted image, and (**c**) apparent diffusion coefficient map show three distinct zones: an enhancing core with increased water diffusion (*) surrounded by a rim of enhancing restricted diffusion corresponding to active inflammation (arrowheads), and peripheral vasogenic edema. (Courtesy of Dr. W. K. Chong, Ormond Street Hospital for Children, NHS Trust, London, UK.)

Acquired: Multiple Sclerosis, Acute Disseminated Encephalomyelitis

Multiple sclerosis is a clinically and pathologically heterogeneous chronic inflammatory demyelinating disorder. Active inflammatory lesions show variable perivascular inflammation, T lymphocytes, and lipid-laden macrophages, whereas chronic lesions are hypocellular and show variable remyelination.[13] Though most white matter lesions demonstrate increased diffusion, restricted diffusion has been reported in ~ 30% of acute lesions, usually the tumefactive type, likely reflecting the heterogeneity of underlying pathological mechanisms.[7,8] Axons are relatively preserved. When present in the acute phase, restricted diffusion is most common at the periphery of the lesion, may precede T2 signal abnormality and enhancement, and correlates with attack severity.[9] FA is lower in enhancing than in nonenhancing lesions.[14]

Acute disseminated encephalomyelitis is characterized pathologically by perivenular demyelination and inflammation, occurring after viral illness or infection.[13] Monophasic white matter lesions tend to be large and bilaterally asymmetric, with increased diffusion in the core and variable, often decreased, ADC at the periphery in the acute phase (▶ Fig. 10.2).[15]

10.2.2 Restricted Diffusion: Diffuse Cytotoxic/Intramyelinic Edema with White Matter Cavitation

Inherited: Mitochondrial Respiratory Chain Deficiency

In mitochondrial disorders, the mitochondria are unable to meet the metabolic requirements of the cell (metabolic imbalance), resulting in cytotoxic edema in the acute phase.[16] Though most mitochondrial disorders involve deep gray matter with or without some white matter involvement, some selectively affect white matter. Isolated deficiencies of respiratory chain complexes may result in a characteristic cavitating leukoencephalopathy, with a distinct pattern of strikingly restricted diffusion throughout the white matter (including the corpus callosum) during the acute phase, with the leading edge apparently moving centrifugally, which may coexist with increased diffusivity and loss of FA in white matter cavitations in the central burned-out areas (▶ Fig. 10.3).[17]

Acquired: Global Neonatal Hypoxic Injury

In certain instances, severe perinatal hypoxia in term infants may result in acute global neonatal

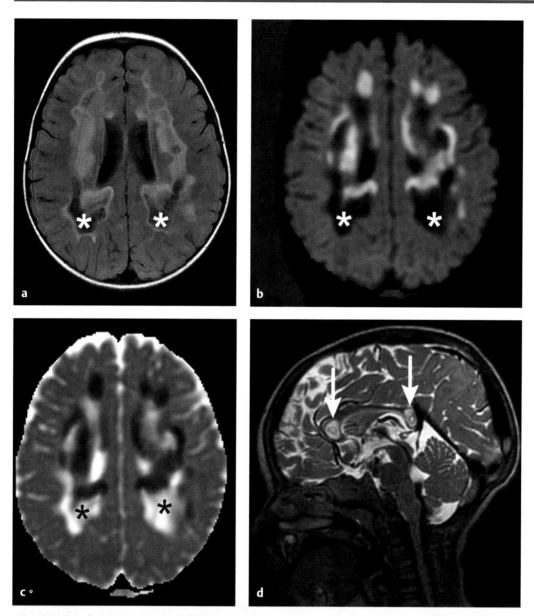

Fig. 10.3 Complex I (respiratory chain) deficiency in a 12-month-old infant with seizures and rapid neurological deterioration. (**a**) Axial fluid-attenuated inversion recovery images show extensive white matter abnormality with sparing of the subcortical white matter and presence of central cavitations (*). (**b**) Diffusion weighted image and (**c**) apparent diffusion coefficient map show strikingly restricted diffusion in affected white matter and increased diffusivity in cavitations. (**d**) Involvement of the corpus callosum (arrows) is evident on sagittal T2-weighted imaging. (Courtesy of Drs. Fred Laningham and Natalie Hauser, Children's Hospital of Central California, Madera, CA, USA.)

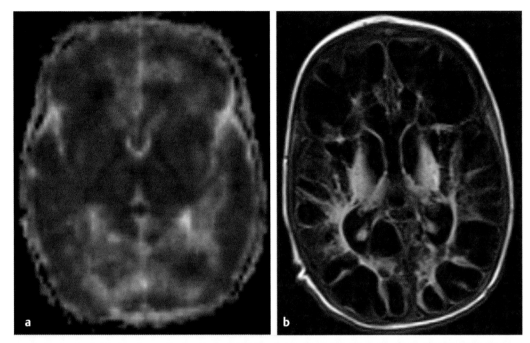

Fig. 10.4 Severe global hypoxic injury in a 4-day-old infant delivered at 38 weeks with vasa previa. (a) Diffusely abnormal diffusion on apparent diffusion coefficient map at 4 days, which (b) progressed to diffuse cerebral cavitation and atrophy on fluid-attenuated inversion recovery magnetic resonance imaging by 26 days of life.

ischemia with diffuse supratentorial cytotoxic edema due to cerebral energy depletion, with restricted diffusion predominantly involving subcortical white matter (▶ Fig. 10.4a), progressing to widespread cavitation (▶ Fig. 10.4b) with increased diffusivity. The brainstem and posterior fossa are generally spared.[6,18] Neonatal herpes infection and isolated sulfite oxidase deficiency are in the differential diagnosis for this appearance.[19]

10.2.3 Restricted Diffusion, Regional: Neurotoxicity

In these disorders, rapid extracellular-to-intracellular or intramyelinic fluid shift results in decreased free water diffusion.

Inherited: Maple Syrup Urine Disease (Classic Type)

In classic maple syrup urine disease, autosomal recessive deficiency in branched-chain ketoacid dehydrogenase (a mitochondrial enzyme complex)

results in accumulation of branched-chain amino acids (especially L-leucine) and their keto-acids (especially α-ketoisocaproic acid (αKIC). Overabundant leucine competitively inhibits uptake of other amino acids into cells, inhibiting protein synthesis; myelin synthesis is impaired leading to dysmyelination. At the same time, αKIC inhibits adenosine triphosphate (ATP) synthesis, disrupting sodium–potassium–ATP (NA/K ATPase) function. Because myelination in the newborn and young infant is extremely active, hence energy dependent, cytotoxic and intramyelinic edema (and restricted diffusion) develop exclusively in myelinated areas, superimposed on a background of diffuse vasogenic edema as a sign of global neurotoxicity (▶ Fig. 10.5).[20,21]

Acquired: Methotrexate Toxicity

Methotrexate (MTX) inhibits dihydrofolate reductase, resulting in adenosine release, which dilates cerebral blood vessels and slows presynaptic neurotransmitter release.[22] Because symptoms improve rapidly with aminophylline, a competitive adenosine antagonist, MTX neurotoxicity is

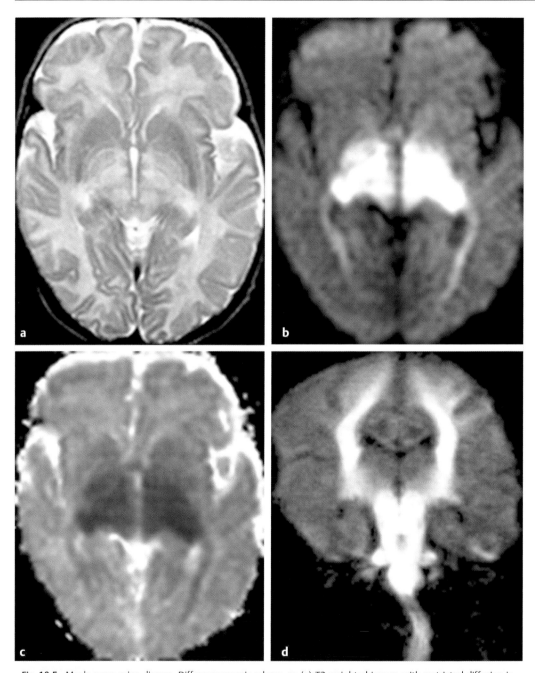

Fig. 10.5 Maple syrup urine disease. Diffuse vasogenic edema on (**a**) T2-weighted image, with restricted diffusion in myelinated white matter on (**b**) diffusion weighted image (DWI) and (**c**) apparent diffusion coefficient map. (**d**) Coronal DWI shows involvement of myelinated white matter not only intracranially, but also in the spinal cord.

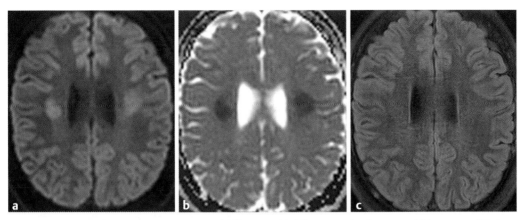

Fig. 10.6 Acute methotrexate toxicity. Restricted diffusion on (**a**) diffusion weighted image and (**b**) apparent diffusion coefficient map, unaccompanied by (**c**) fluid-attenuated inversion recovery (FLAIR) signal abnormality, consistent with cytotoxic/intramyelinic edema.

favored to be mediated by the actions of adenosine in the CNS via unknown mechanisms, potentially via oxidative stress.[22,23] Homocysteine may be increased or normal.[24] Ten to 14 days after MTX administration, and within hours after the appearance of clinical signs and symptoms, restricted diffusion develops in the centrum semiovale of affected patients (▶ Fig. 10.6a,b). This is unaccompanied by T2 or fluid-attenuated inversion recovery (FLAIR) evidence of vasogenic edema in the early stage (▶ Fig. 10.6c), consistent with a "pure" cytotoxic and/or intramyelinic edema. Therefore DWI is critical for early, confident diagnosis of MTX neurotoxicity. This restricted diffusion subsequently subsides, but in some cases may progress to loss of tissue matrix, with increased diffusivity and T2 signal in the primarily involved areas.[24]

10.2.4 Restricted Diffusion: Progressive Oligodendrocyte Toxicity and Metabolic Failure

Inherited: Krabbe Disease (Globoid Cell Leukodystrophy), Metachromatic Leukodystrophy

In Krabbe disease (globoid cell leukodystrophy), early myelin is normal, but autosomal recessive deficiency of lysosomal β-galactocerebrosidase causes accumulation of β-galactocerebroside (a major component of myelin) and its catabolic derivative psychosine, which is toxic to oligodendrocytes, as early myelination progresses.[25,26] Reduced diffusivity is possible early in the disease, which may correspond to cytotoxic and/or intramyelinic edema in the stage of rapid oligodendrocyte death and myelin breakdown, followed by progressive increases in diffusion and decreased anisotropy as demyelination progresses.[5,11,19,26] T2-weighted images may show a "tigroid" pattern of radiating lines.[5] ADC is lower than in primarily vacuolating disorders, due to influx of microglia and macrophages.[27]

In metachromatic leukodystrophy, an autosomal recessive deficiency of lysosomal arylsulfatase A causes accumulation of sulfatides and deficiency of cerebrosides, the main component of myelin, in the lysosomes of oligodendrocytes and Schwann cells. Though oligodendrocytes are initially able to compensate and maintain myelin membrane homeostasis, they eventually undergo metabolic failure.[26] Demyelination is the result of oligodendrocyte dysfunction/death and instability of abnormal myelin.[26,28] Diffuse white matter signal abnormality with a tigroid pattern of perivascular sparing (particularly in the juvenile form) may be accompanied by restricted diffusion in the early stage (▶ Fig. 10.7), suggesting relatively rapid extracellular to intracellular/intramyelinic water shifts; inflammation is not a characteristic feature. In the burned-out phase, ADC is increased (increased water diffusion) and FA is decreased, a

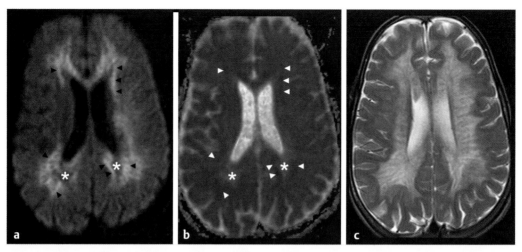

Fig. 10.7 Metachromatic leukodystrophy. (**a**) Axial diffusion weighted image and (**b**) apparent diffusion coefficient map show that water diffusion is relatively restricted in areas of active disease (arrowheads) and increased in demyelinated white matter (asterisks). (**c**) Both processes contribute to diffuse white matter hyperintensity on T2-weighted imaging.

nonspecific appearance common to demyelinated white matter.[11]

10.2.5 Diffusion Negative: Hypomyelination

In disorders characterized primarily by hypomyelination, axonal density is normal but myelination is permanently arrested. Myelin destruction is not a dominant feature. There is no cytotoxicity or influx of microglia/macrophages to cause restricted diffusion. Anisotropy is only slightly decreased because FA is not entirely dependent on myelin; normal axonal density may be sufficient to maintain FA.[27]

Inherited: Pelizaeus–Merzbacher Disease

In Pelizaeus–Merzbacher disease, X-linked recessive mutations in the *PLP1* gene result in abnormal proteolipid protein, a major myelin structural protein, resulting in diffuse hypomyelination in the CNS and increased water diffusion (▶ Fig. 10.8a–c). There is no pathological evidence of active demyelination, and peripheral nervous system (PNS) myelin is spared. There is relative sparing of the cortex, subcortical white matter, spinal cord, and brainstem. Atrophy is not a prominent feature. In

areas where myelin is rare or absent, oligodendrocytes are few and abnormal. Axonal integrity is preserved, which may be sufficient to maintain near-normal anisotropy because FA is only slightly decreased (▶ Fig. 10.8d,e).[27]

Imaging-based differential considerations for this appearance include other hypomyelinating disorders, such as trichothiodystrophy, 18q syndrome, and Salla disease.[29]

Acquired: Congenital Hypothyroidism, Severe Early Malnutrition

The generation of myelin by oligodendrocytes is dependent on coordinated upregulation of myelin protein genes by trophic factors, deficits in which may cause delayed or hypomyelination. In congenital hypothyroidism, absent or deficient thyroid hormone (T3) inhibits terminal differentiation of oligodendrocytes and reduced expression of myelin genes, resulting in hypomyelination.[30] This hypomyelination is reversible with early thyroxine therapy.[31] Insulin-like growth factor 1 (IGF-1), which promotes myelination and oligodendrocyte maturation, may be reduced in severe undernourishment. Permanent hypomyelination may occur if this undernourishment occurs during critical growth periods.[5]

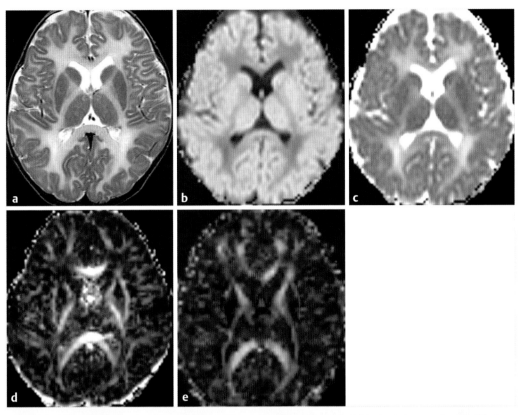

Fig. 10.8 Pelizaeus–Merzbacher disease. Diffuse white matter T2 hyperintensity (**a**) is due to increased water diffusion on diffusion weighted imaging (**b**) and apparent diffusion coefficient map (**c**) in the setting of hypomyelination. Fractional anisotropy (FA) is only mildly decreased on the FA map (**d**) and the directionally encoded color map (**e**). (Courtesy of Dr. Ata Siddiqui, Kings College Hospital, London, UK.)

10.2.6 Increased Diffusion: Abnormal Water Homeostasis with Myelin Vacuolation

Inherited: Megalencephalic Leukoencephalopathy with Subcortical Cysts

In addition to regulating myelin formation and neurogenesis, and supplying neurons with metabolic substrates, astrocytes play a key role in water and ion homeostasis in the CNS, including at the BBB via astrocyte endfeet. In the classic, most common form of megalencephalic leukoencephalopathy with subcortical cysts, autosomal-recessive mutations in the astrocyte-specific MLC1 gene

product disrupt brain ion and water homeostasis, leading to vacuolating myelin degeneration. Vacuoles form in the outer lamellae of the myelin sheath, and in the intracellular structures and endfeet of astrocytes.[32] Early diffuse cerebral white matter swelling, with increased ADC (▶ Fig. 10.9b, c) and decreased anisotropy, ultimately leads to atrophy by the adult years. Bilateral anterior temporal lobe (▶ Fig. 10.9a), and sometimes parietal and frontal lobes, subcortical cysts follow white matter rarefaction in infancy.[33]

In Canavan disease, autosomal recessive defects in oligodendrocyte aspartoacylase causes accumulation of *N*-acetyl aspartate (NAA) in the extracellular space and unavailability of acetate for myelin lipid synthesis. Altered osmotic-hydrostatic pressures due to accumulation of NAA in the

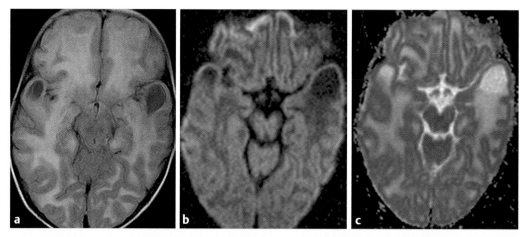

Fig. 10.9 Megalencephalic leukoencephalopathy with subcortical cysts. Generalized hyperintensity of white matter on (a) T2-weighted imaging is due to rarefaction and cystic degeneration of white matter and myelin vacuolation, resulting in increased water diffusion as evidenced by decreased signal on (b) diffusion weighted imaging and increased on (c) the apparent diffusion coefficient map.

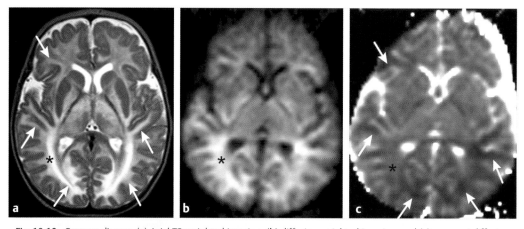

Fig. 10.10 Canavan disease. (a) Axial T2-weighted imaging, (b) diffusion weighted imaging, and (c) apparent diffusion coefficient (ADC) map. ADC differentiates T2 hyperintensity due to restricted water diffusion in the subcortical white matter (dark on ADC, arrows) from T2 hyperintensity due to white matter rarefaction and increased size of water spaces (asterisks). (Courtesy of Dr. Ata Siddiqui, Kings College Hospital, London, UK.)

extracellular space are the proposed cause for the extracellular and astrocytic edema and myelin vacuolation observed at pathological section.[34] Progression is centripetal, with early changes in the subcortical white matter accompanied by restricted diffusion (▶ Fig. 10.10), which persists over an extended period of time. This is likely due to restriction of the extracellular spaces due to early cellular swelling and myelin vacuolation. Ultimately, diffusion is increased in demyelinated white matter due to increased size of the extracellular spaces later in the disease.[5]

Acquired: Osmotic Demyelination Syndrome (Central Pontine And Extrapontine Myelinolysis)

Very high or low levels of sodium, or rapid correction of hyponatremia, which may occur in chronically ill or undernourished children,[35] cause osmotic cerebral stress, to which oligodendrocytes are particularly vulnerable. Signal abnormalities correspond to the distribution of oligodendrocytes associated with large neurons in the pons and in extrapontine sites, including the thalamus.

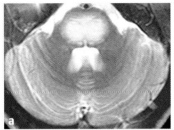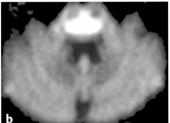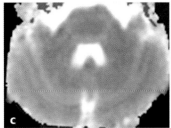

Fig. 10.11 Osmotic demyelination syndrome. Pontine signal abnormality on (**a**) T2-weighted image is predominantly due to intracellular and intramyelinic water shifts, as evidenced by restricted diffusion on (**b**) diffusion weighted image and (**c**) apparent diffusion coefficient map, with minimal surrounding vasogenic edema.

Restricted diffusion may be present in the early stages (▶ Fig. 10.11), likely secondary to characteristic cellular swelling and myelin vacuolation prior to myelin rupture. Inflammation is not a feature; lipid-laden macrophages appear later.[36] Findings on T2-weighted imaging may lag behind the diffusion abnormalities in both the acute and the recovery phases; normalization of ADC has been found to parallel clinical recovery.[36]

10.2.7 Increased Diffusion: Myelin Rarefaction and Cystic Degeneration

Inherited: Vanishing White Matter Disease (Myelin Rarefaction, Cystic Degeneration)

In vanishing white matter disease, also known as childhood ataxia with diffuse CNS hypomyelination (CACH), abnormal cellular stress responses due to autosomal recessive mutations in eukaryotic translation initiation factor 2B (eIF2B) result in abnormal astrocyte and oligodendrocyte proliferation. Recurrent episodes of ataxia, spasticity, and cognitive decline are characteristic, with rapid progression after minor head trauma or fright.[32] Diffuse, progressive white matter rarefaction with cystic degeneration results in increased water diffusion (ADC) and decreased FA.[27] Diffusion may be restricted early in the disease due to increased numbers of oligodendrocytes and their precursors (hypercellularity)

in regions where myelin is relatively spared, such as the subcortical U fibers (▶ Fig. 10.12), cerebellar white matter, and peduncles.[3]

Acquired: End-Stage Demyelination

In burned-out white matter disease, diffusion characteristics of white matter lesions are typically nonspecific, as are pathological findings, reflecting extensive severe devastation and resultant tissue matrix rarefaction. Increased diffusion and decreased FA reflect general pathological findings of hypocellularity, decreased myelin and oligodendrocytes, and an increase in white matter water to myelin ratio.[23]

10.3 Summary

Though identifiable patterns of pediatric WM diseases exist on T2-weighted imaging, many are nonspecific in appearance. Diffusion imaging permits distinction of mechanistically and histopathologically distinct areas within the affected white matter, enhancing understanding of underlying processes, and providing important clues to stage/activity of disease and underlying pathology. Relationships of diffusion imaging findings to underlying pathology in the examples covered in this chapter are summarized in ▶ Table 10.1. As new white matter diseases continue to be discovered, an understanding of these relationships will contribute to our growing understanding of these dynamic disease processes.

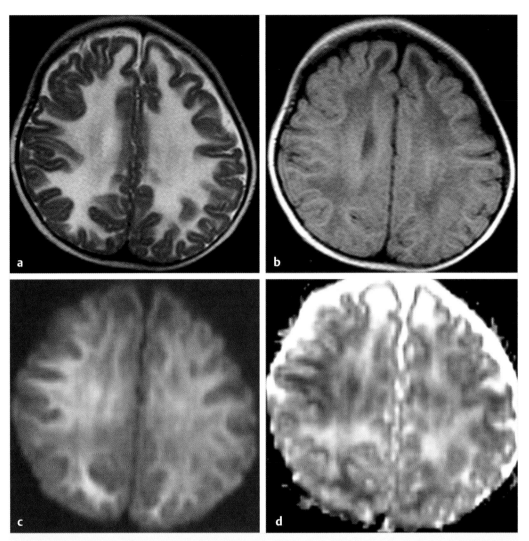

Fig. 10.12 Early vanishing white matter disease. Diffusely rarefied white matter appears hyperintense on (**a**) T2-weighted imaging and hypointense on (**b**) T1-weighted imaging. On (**c**) diffusion weighted imaging and (**d**) apparent diffusion coefficient map, diffusion is restricted in relatively spared subcortical white matter due to glial proliferation and relative hypercellularity. (Courtesy of Dr. Ata Siddiqui, Kings College Hospital, London, UK.)

Table 10.1 Diffusion characteristics and patterns of pediatric white matter disease by underlying pathology

Disorder	ADC	FA	Pattern
Restricted diffusion: active inflammatory demyelination			
X-linked adrenoleukodystrophy	↓ leading edge, acute; ↑ demyelinated zone, late	↑ in demyelinated WM	Centrifugal, posterior to anterior
Tumefactive multiple sclerosis	↓ possible at leading edge, acute; ↑ demyelinated zone, late	FA lower in enhancing than in nonenhancing lesions	Most frequently periventricular or subcortical, corpus callosum, progressive or relapsing-remitting
ADEM	↓ possible at leading edge, acute; ↑ demyelinated zone, late	May be decreased	Most frequently subcortical, periventricular, asymmetric, monophasic
Restricted diffusion: diffuse cytotoxic/intramyelinic edema with white matter cavitation			
Mitochondrial disorder: complex I deficiency	↓↓ in affected WM; ↑ in cavitations		Centrifugal, cavitations in central burned-out WM
Global neonatal hypoxic injury	↓		Variable
Restricted diffusion, regional: neurotoxicity			
Maple syrup urine disease (classic form)	↓ in prenatally myelinated WM; ↑ in nonmyelinated areas		Diffuse vasogenic edema; restricted diffusion in prenatally myelinated WM
Methotrexate toxicity	↓ early, acute; precedes FLAIR abnormality; normalizes after resolution	Unknown	Centrum semiovale
Restricted diffusion: progressive oligodendrocyte toxicity and metabolic failure			
Metachromatic leukodystrophy	May be ↓ in acute phase, ↑ late in demyelinated WM	↓ late in demyelinated WM	Centrifugal, posterior to anterior, with eventual diffuse WM involvement. "tigroid" perivenular sparing and sparing of subcortical U fibers.
Krabbe disease (globoid cell leukodystrophy)	↓ early along leading edge, then progressive ↑ ADC.	↓	Centrifugal, posterior to anterior, with eventual diffuse WM involvement. "tigroid" sparing.
Diffusion negative: hypomyelination, delayed myelination			
Pelizaeus–Merzbacher disease	Normal	Slightly ↓; near normal	Diffuse WM T2 hyperintensity
Congenital/perinatal hypothyroidism	Normal		Diffuse
Severe nutrient deficiency	Normal		Diffuse
Increased diffusion: abnormal water homeostasis with myelin vacuolation			
Megalencephalic leukoencephalopathy with subcortical cysts	↑	↓↓	Diffuse; early anterior temporal subcortical cysts
Canavan disease	Early: ↓/= in peripheral WM, globi pallidi, thalami, brainstem, dorsal pons, dentate nuclei Late: ↑		Centripetal WM progression; globi pallidi, thalami involved

Table 10.1 continued

Disorder	ADC	FA	Pattern
Osmotic demyelination syndrome (central pontine and extrapontine myelinolysis)	↓ early; normalization parallels recovery		Pons, thalamus, cortex, putamen
Increased diffusion: myelin rarefaction and cystic degeneration			
Vanishing white matter disease	↓ in preserved WM (subcortical U fibers, internal capsule); ↑ in rarified WM	↓	Diffuse, symmetric
End-stage demyelination	↑	↓	Depends on underlying cause

Abbreviations: ADC, apparent diffusion coefficient; ADEM, acute demyelinating encephalomyelitis; FA, fractional anisotropy; FLAIR, fluid-attenuated inversion recovery; WM, white matter.

References

[1] Mukherjee P, Berman JI, Chung SW, Hess CP, Henry RG. Diffusion tensor MR imaging and fiber tractography: theoretic underpinnings. AJNR Am J Neuroradiol 2008; 29(4): 632–641

[2] McRobbie DW. MRI from Picture to Proton. 2nd ed. New York, NY: Cambridge University Press; 2007

[3] van der Lei HD, Steenweg ME, Bugiani M, et al. Restricted diffusion in vanishing white matter. Arch Neurol 2012; 69 (6): 723–727

[4] Liang D, Bhatta S, Gerzanich V, Simard JM. Cytotoxic edema: mechanisms of pathological cell swelling. Neurosurg Focus 2007; 22(5): E2

[5] Knaap MSd, Valk J, Barkhof F, Knaap MSd. Magnetic Resonance of Myelination and Myelin Disorders. 3rd ed. New York, NY: Springer, 2005

[6] Schiffmann R, van der Knaap MS. Invited article: an MRI-based approach to the diagnosis of white matter disorders. Neurology 2009; 72(8): 750–759

[7] Hyland M, Bermel RA, Cohen JA. Restricted diffusion preceding gadolinium enhancement in large or tumefactive demyelinating lesions. Neurol Clin Pract 2013; 3(1): 15–21

[8] Popescu BF, Lucchinetti CF. Pathology of demyelinating diseases. Annu Rev Pathol 2012; 7: 185–217

[9] Abou Zeid N, Pirko I, Erickson B, et al. Diffusion weighted imaging characteristics of biopsy-proven demyelinating brain lesions. Neurology 2012; 78(21): 1655–1662

[10] Kemp S, Berger J, Aubourg P. X-linked adrenoleukodystrophy: clinical, metabolic, genetic and pathophysiological aspects. Biochim Biophys Acta 2012; 1822(9): 1465–1474

[11] Patay Z. Diffusion weighted MR imaging in leukodystrophies. Eur Radiol 2005; 15(11): 2284–2303

[12] van der Voorn JP, Pouwels PJ, Powers JM, et al. Correlating quantitative MR imaging with histopathology in X-linked adrenoleukodystrophy. AJNR Am J Neuroradiol 2011; 32(3): 481–489

[13] Wingerchuk DM, Lucchinetti CF. Comparative immunopathogenesis of acute disseminated encephalomyelitis, neuromyelitis optica, and multiple sclerosis. Curr Opin Neurol 2007; 20(3): 343–350

[14] Filippi M, Agosta F. Imaging biomarkers in multiple sclerosis. J Magn Reson Imaging 2010; 31(4): 770–788

[15] Bernarding J, Braun J, Koennecke HC. Diffusion- and perfusion-weighted MR imaging in a patient with acute demyelinating encephalomyelitis (ADEM). J Magn Reson Imaging 2002; 15(1): 96–100

[16] Sofou K, Steneryd K, Wiklund LM, Tulinius M, Darin N. MRI of the brain in childhood-onset mitochondrial disorders with central nervous system involvement. Mitochondrion 2013; 13(4): 364–371

[17] Biancheri R, Rossi D, Cassandrini D, Rossi A, Bruno C, Santorelli FM. Cavitating leukoencephalopathy in a child carrying the mitochondrial A8344G mutation. AJNR Am J Neuroradiol 2010; 31(9): E78–E79

[18] Weidenheim KM, Bodhireddy SR, Nuovo GJ, Nelson SJ, Dickson DW. Multicystic encephalopathy: review of eight cases with etiologic considerations. J Neuropathol Exp Neurol 1995; 54(2): 268–275

[19] Barkovich AJ. Pediatric Neuroimaging. 5th ed. Philadelphia, PA: Lippincott Williams & Wilkins; 2012

[20] Zinnanti WJ, Lazovic J, Griffin K, et al. Dual mechanism of brain injury and novel treatment strategy in maple syrup urine disease. Brain 2009; 132(Pt 4): 903–918

[21] Parmar H, Sitoh YY, Ho L. Maple syrup urine disease: diffusion weighted and diffusion tensor magnetic resonance imaging findings. J Comput Assist Tomogr 2004; 28(1): 93–97

[22] Bernini JC, Fort DW, Griener JC, Kane BJ, Chappell WB, Kamen BA. Aminophylline for methotrexate-induced neurotoxicity. Lancet 1995; 345(8949): 544–547

[23] Greenfield JG, Love S, Louis DN, Ellison D. Greenfield's Neuropathology. 8th ed. London: Hodder Arnold; 2008

[24] Brugnoletti F, Morris EB, Laningham FH, et al. Recurrent intrathecal methotrexate induced neurotoxicity in an adolescent with acute lymphoblastic leukemia: Serial clinical and radiologic findings. Pediatr Blood Cancer 2009; 52(2): 293–295

[25] Guo AC, Petrella JR, Kurtzberg J, Provenzale JM. Evaluation of white matter anisotropy in Krabbe disease with diffusion tensor MR imaging: initial experience. Radiology 2001; 218 (3): 809–815

[26] Scriver CR. The Metabolic and Molecular Bases of Inherited Disease. 8th ed. New York, NY: McGraw-Hill; 2001

[27] van der Voorn JP, Pouwels PJ, Hart AA, et al. Childhood white matter disorders: quantitative MR imaging and spectroscopy. Radiology 2006; 241(2): 510–517

[28] Patil SA, Maegawa GH. Developing therapeutic approaches for metachromatic leukodystrophy. Drug Des Devel Ther 2013; 7: 729–745

[29] Harreld JH, Smith EC, Prose NS, Puri PK, Barboriak DP. Trichothiodystrophy with dysmyelination and central osteosclerosis. AJNR Am J Neuroradiol 2010; 31(1): 129–130

[30] Mitew S, Hay CM, Peckham H, Xiao J, Koenning M, Emery B. Mechanisms regulating the development of oligodendrocytes and central nervous system myelin. Neuroscience 2014; 276: 29–47

[31] Jagannathan NR, Tandon N, Raghunathan P, Kochupillai N. Reversal of abnormalities of myelination by thyroxine therapy in congenital hypothyroidism: localized in vivo proton magnetic resonance spectroscopy (MRS) study. Brain Res Dev Brain Res 1998; 109(2): 179–186

[32] Lanciotti A, Brignone MS, Bertini E, Petrucci TC, Aloisi F, Ambrosini E. Astrocytes: emerging stars in leukodystrophy pathogenesis Transl Neurosci 2013; 4(2)

[33] van der Knaap MS, Boor I, Estévez R. Megalencephalic leukoencephalopathy with subcortical cysts: chronic white matter oedema due to a defect in brain ion and water homoeostasis. Lancet Neurol 2012; 11(11): 973–985

[34] Baslow MH, Guilfoyle DN. Are astrocytes the missing link between lack of brain aspartoacylase activity and the spongiform leukodystrophy in Canavan disease? Neurochem Res 2009; 34(9): 1523–1534

[35] Ranger AM, Chaudhary N, Avery M, Fraser D. Central pontine and extrapontine myelinolysis in children: a review of 76 patients. J Child Neurol 2012; 27(8): 1027–1037

[36] Ruzek KA, Campeau NG, Miller GM. Early diagnosis of central pontine myelinolysis with diffusion weighted imaging. AJNR Am J Neuroradiol 2004; 25(2): 210–213

11 Diffusion Imaging for the Assessment of Traumatic Brain Injury

Michael L. Lipton

11.1 Introduction

Diffusion sensitized MRI (dMRI) provides several useful metrics for the detection and characterization of traumatic brain injury (TBI).[1] This chapter discusses applications of directionally nonselective dMRI techniques, such as diffusion weighted MRI (DWI), as well as directionally sensitive approaches, such as diffusion tensor MRI (DTI), for detection of brain tissue injury in patients with TBI. The chapter emphasizes the unique contribution of DWI and DTI for detection of pathology that is not revealed by other imaging modalities.

11.2 Clinical Context and Diagnostic Criteria

TBI is a major cause of morbidity and mortality worldwide. Each year, in the United States alone, more than 2.5 million TBIs occur; over 55,000 individuals die, over 300,000 are hospitalized, and more than 2 million are treated and released from emergency departments.[2] An unknown but likely very large number of TBIs are unrecognized or dismissed.[3]

TBI is commonly classified as to its severity based on clinical examination at the time of injury. This classification, based largely on the Glasgow Coma Scale (GCS; scale range 3–15), delineates severe (GCS 3–8), moderate (GCS 9–12), and mild (GCS 13–15) TBI. This GCS-based classification is an excellent predictor of survival to hospital discharge, but does not effectively predict long-term outcome, especially with more mild degrees of injury.[4] Additional factors used for classification include the duration of unconsciousness, the duration of posttraumatic amnesia, and the presence of focal neurological deficits and imaging abnormalities.[5,6]

Mild TBI (mTBI, also termed concussion) is the most common form of TBI.[2] Patients with mTBI experience a disturbance of neurocognitive function following the injury, which may include confusion, disorientation, imbalance, and other features. Some, but by no means all, mTBI patients experience actual loss of consciousness.[7] Diagnostic criteria for mTBI include no more than 30 minutes of unconsciousness, no more than 24 hours of amnesia, and absence of focal neurological deficits.[8] mTBI is typically not associated with abnormalities on conventional computed tomography (CT) and magnetic resonance imaging (MRI).[1] Notwithstanding the relatively mild initial clinical features and absence of conventional imaging abnormalities, clinical manifestations of mTBI do arise from brain pathology, particularly traumatic axonal injury (TAI).[9]

Most patients with mTBI will recover, but a significant minority (15–30%,) will sustain long-term adverse consequences, including persistent postconcussive symptoms, cognitive impairment, and behavioral dysfunction.[7] Thus the consequences of "mild" TBI are by no means necessarily mild. High-profile coverage of sports and military-related mTBI and its long-term adverse effects, including delayed neurodegenerative disorders, such as chronic traumatic encephalopathy (CTE),[10] have driven increased awareness of mTBI. Patients with GCS scores in the mTBI range (13–15) who do have gross imaging abnormalities are often classified as mild-complicated TBI. These individuals may have worse prognosis for recovery.[11]

11.3 Pathology and Pathophysiology: Focal and Diffuse Injury

TBI pathology is commonly classified based on its gross pathological and imaging features as focal or diffuse injury.[9] Focal injury may be extra-axial (skull fracture and epidural, subdural, or subarachnoid hemorrhage) or intra-axial (contusion, laceration, and hematoma). Much TBI tissue pathology, however, is a diffuse (or, more properly, multifocal) microscopic injury to the white matter of the brain, caused by linear and rotational forces. This pathology is termed traumatic axonal injury (TAI). When widespread it is often referred to as diffuse axonal injury (DAI). Pathological evidence of TAI has been demonstrated in all degrees of TBI severity, including mTBI. Many types of focal TBI pathology, including hemorrhage and contusion, are readily detected using CT and conventional MRI techniques, particularly those sensitive to hemorrhage such as T1-weighted and T2*-weighted imaging. Although microhemorrhage, as detected with susceptibility-weighted MRI (SWI), may be detectable in patients with TAI, widespread TAI may go entirely undetected on conventional MRI scans.[1] This is because significant injury to axons occurs due to forces that do not rupture even the smallest blood vessels, which are at least 10 times the diameter of and more resilient than axons. Diffuse injury, TAI, is the major determinant of long-term symptoms, deficits, and disability in patients with TBI. Dysfunction arising from TBI is thought to be due to widespread brain network dysfunction, which can result from even microscopic axonal injury.[12,13]

In order to understand the nature of dMRI changes seen in the context of TBI, it is essential to understand the pathogenesis of brain tissue pathology underpinning the imaging changes. Moderate and severe TBI commonly entail frank physical trauma to the brain surface resulting in contusional injury. In all but the most severe TBI, however, frank disruption of deeper brain tissue does not result from the traumatic event. Rather, shear, stress and rotational force applied to white matter axons cause intra-axonal cytoskeletal alterations, such as microtubule damage and neurofilament misalignment, and set off a cascade of pathological cellular and molecular events.[14] Component mechanisms include membrane pump dysfunction, inflammation, apoptosis, impaired function of cell survival pathways, and, eventually, loss of myelin and axons. TAI pathology evolves over a period of time (▶ Fig. 11.1), and the underlying pathological processes are typically not detectable using conventional CT and MRI.[1,15] Tissue injury, particularly contusion as well as mass effect due to large hematomas, can lead to secondary ischemic injury or frank infarction, which may complicate the picture of focal TBI. Over the long term, loss of central nervous system (CNS) axons, due to processes including wallerian degeneration, ensues.[14] White matter fibers remote from the apparent site of injury as well as cortical regions connected by these fibers may subsequently exhibit volume loss.

11.4 Diffusion Weighted Imaging—Sensitive Detection of Traumatic Tissue Injury

11.4.1 Pathophysiology of Diffusion Weighted Imaging Abnormalities in TBI

As described elsewhere in this handbook, DWI has been known to be a sensitive means for detection of cytotoxic edema due to ischemic tissue injury since its clinical application to stroke became widespread in the 1990s.[16] Although the clinical utility and acceptance of DWI in stroke is well established, the cellular mechanisms underlying these diffusion changes remain controversial. Similar to stroke, restriction of isotropic diffusion is a manifestation of cytotoxic edema in patients with traumatic injury. As with stroke, the precise underlying cellular events remain unclear. Cytotoxic edema and its associated effect on diffusion most commonly occurs in traumatic cortical contusion, but may also be a feature of acute TAI and of intracranial hematoma.

Impact to the head, with or without consequent fracture, may cause contusion of the brain surface subjacent to the impact site, which is termed coup contusion. Subsequent acceleration of the brain and its impact against the skull opposite the site of the head impact leads to a secondary, typically more extensive, contusion. This secondary contusion is termed contrecoup contusion. Importantly, contusion also occurs in the absence of direct impact to the head. Acceleration of the head, as in a whiplash-type mechanism, can produce substantial acceleration of the brain, which subsequently impacts the skull, with potential for consequent cortical contusion.

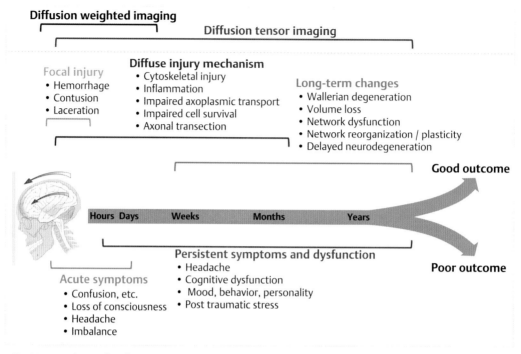

Fig. 11.1 Timeframe of evolving pathological, imaging, and clinical features after traumatic brain injury. Note that diffusion sensitized magnetic resonance imaging features overlap and that diffusion tensor imaging findings persist into the chronic phase.

Contusion initially results in cytotoxic edema, which characteristically affects a contiguous region of brain tissue, affecting both superficial cortical gray matter and subjacent white matter, a pattern similar to ischemic injury. Unlike infarct, however, contusional injury does not typically follow a vascular distribution (▸ Fig. 11.2). Concurrent vascular injury or ischemia secondary to mass effect, however, may complicate the imaging appearance of contusion on DWI.

Detection of DWI abnormalities in TBI

The earliest imaging manifestation of traumatic cortical contusion is restriction of isotropic diffusion. This appears as high signal on isotropic DWI and low apparent diffusion coefficient (ADC), seen on ADC images (see ▸ Fig. 11.2). Restricted diffusion in cortical contusion can be detected before CT or MRI reveal imaging evidence of tissue injury. However, DWI evidence of contusion is commonly

identified in conjunction with signs of extracranial as well as intracranial injury, including scalp hematoma, skull fracture, hemorrhage, and edema (▸ Fig. 11.3). In this regard, location of the diffusion abnormalities relative to other signs of injury is key to correct diagnosis. DWI findings of contusion follow the classical coup contrecoup distribution already provided. Typically, the extent of injury opposite the site of impact (contrecoup) is greater relative to that immediately subjacent to the site of impact (coup).

Differential Diagnosis of DWI Abnormalities in Trauma Patients

Restriction of isotropic diffusion is a nonspecific feature of many forms of brain tissue injury, including ischemia, infection, and inflammation (▸ Fig. 11.4). This lack of specificity, however, is typical of imaging findings in general and does not preclude the diagnostic utility of DWI in TBI. Additional features, when considered in conjunction

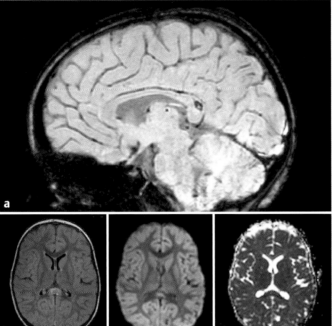

Fig. 11.2 Contusion and traumatic axonal injury (TAI) due to nonaccidental injury. This 2-year-old boy was brought to the emergency department with multiple injuries and lethargy. Computed tomography was entirely unremarkable. (**a**) Susceptibility-weighted magnetic resonance imaging (SWI) showed hemorrhage confined to the splenium. (**b**) Hyperintensity is present within the splenium on T2-weighted fluid-attenuated inversion recovery imaging. (**c**) More extensive high signal on diffusion weighted imaging co-located with (**d**) low apparent diffusion coefficient indicates cytotoxic edema due to acute TAI, later determined to be a result of severe shaking.

with the presence of low ADC, are useful in arriving at a correct diagnosis of traumatic injury. The spatial distribution of DWI abnormalities will occur in typical locations and follow expected patterns of contusion or TAI. Anterior and inferior frontal and temporal lobe location and a coup contrecoup distribution of diffusion restriction, association with findings of extracranial soft tissue injury, and skull fracture are typical findings in contusion. The absence of conformity to arterial vascular distributions provides further supporting evidence that cortical diffusion restriction is due to traumatic contusion. Clear conformance of diffusion restriction to an arterial vascular distribution, on the other hand, is typical of stroke.

Focal diffusion restriction involving the white matter may be a manifestation of acute TAI (▶ Fig. 11.5, ▶ Fig. 11.6). Other disorders, such as brain abscess and multiple sclerosis (MS), also manifest focal diffusion restriction. Predilection for involvement of the corpus callosum, especially the splenium, deep white matter structures, and the gray matter–white matter junction are typical features of TBI. Concurrent identification of additional imaging features is also helpful in narrowing the differential diagnosis. Useful features might include white matter hyperintensities typical of MS, other imaging features of abscess, or additional findings of TBI, such as hemorrhage and extracranial injury.

Clinical context is an essential factor in every differential diagnosis. History and other clinical evidence of TBI as well as the absence of known alternate diagnoses or their risk factors, including MS, cerebrovascular disease, or systemic infection, are necessary to support the correct attribution of DWI findings to TBI.

Differential diagnosis for intra-axial isotropic diffusion restriction

- Contusion and traumatic axonal injury
- Stroke
- Cerebritis and abscess
- Demyelination
- Radiation injury
- Surgery
- Hematoma
- Seizures and postictal changes

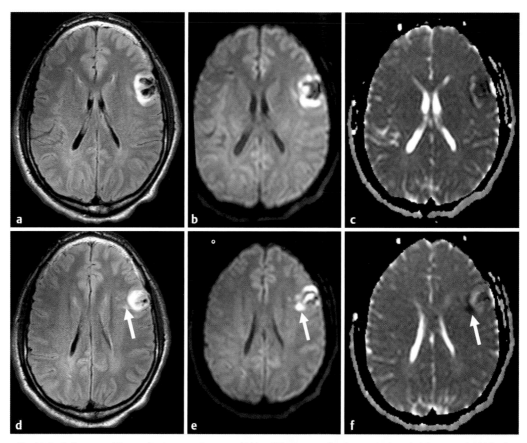

Fig. 11.3 Full extent of hemorrhagic contusion revealed by diffusion weighted imaging (DWI). (**a**) T2-weighted fluid attenuated inversion recovery, (**b**) diffusion weighted imaging and (**c**) apparent diffusion coefficient map shows heterogeneous signal due to hemorrhage, with areas of T2 shine-through (**c**) and diffusion restriction in the left frontal lobe. Note the additional area of diffusion restriction (white arrows; high signal on DWI (**e**) and (**f**) low apparent diffusion coefficient indicating tissue injury due to contusion beyond the area of hemorrhage. This area appeared relatively normal on computed tomography (not shown) and exhibited only minimal signal hyperintensity on (**d**) T2-weighted fluid attenuated inversion recovery.

11.5 Diffusion Tensor Imaging—Detection of Microstructural Traumatic Axonal Injury

11.5.1 Biophysical basis of DTI Abnormalities in TBI

DWI detects decline in the magnitude (ADC; direction-independent net spatial displacement) of water self-diffusion in tissue. Lower magnitude (high signal on DWI *and* low ADC; i.e., diffusion restriction) is a manifestation of cytotoxic edema (▶ Fig. 11.7). DTI, however, uniquely indexes diffusion direction. As explained in Chapter 1, DTI provides two directional characteristics of water

diffusion in tissue: the dominant direction of water diffusion (principle eigenvector) and the coherence (i.e., directional homogeneity, indexed by radial diffusivity [RD] and fractional anisotropy [FA]) of diffusion within the voxel. The normally high degree of anisotropic (directionally coherent) diffusion in normal white matter is conferred by its highly ordered microstructural environment, which includes multilayered parallel barriers to diffusion. These barriers include elements of the cytoskeleton, the axolemma and myelin sheath. As already described, one or more of these white matter constituents is affected and altered in TAI. The consequent loss of barriers to diffusion leads to less coherence of diffusion direction across the voxel, which manifests as lower FA. Higher RD may

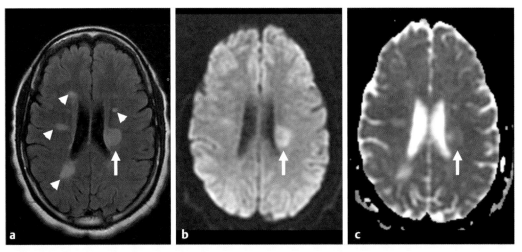

Fig. 11.4 Differentiating diffusion restriction in multiple sclerosis from traumatic axonal injury (TAI). Axial T2-weighted fluid attenuated inversion recovery -FLAIR (**a**), diffusion weighted imaging (**b**) and apparent coefficients map (**c**). Diffusion restriction involves the large lesion adjacent to the ventricle (arrows in **a**, **b** and **c**) that can be differentiated from TAI by its location and association with other findings of multiple sclerosis (arrowheads in **a**).

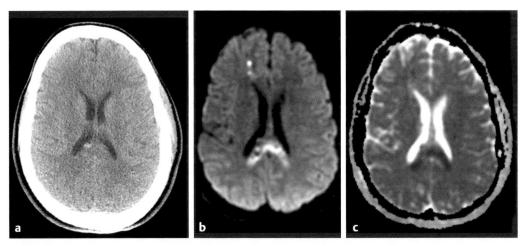

Fig. 11.5 (**a**) Computed tomography shows splenial hemorrhage typical of traumatic axonal injury (TAI) as well as diffuse edema, in a patient who was comatose following a high-speed motor vehicle accident. (**b**) Diffusion restriction due to TAI, however, is seen to involve the entire splenium, evidenced by high signal on diffusion weighted imaging and (**c**) low apparent diffusion coefficient. The additional area of diffusion restriction in the right frontal lobe represents cytotoxic edema due to surgical placement of an intracranial pressure monitor. (Images courtesy of: George Lantos, M. D., Jacobi Medical Center, Bronx, NY.)

be the predominant factor driving increases in FA and may be a better predictor of adverse functional consequences of TAI. Loss of barriers to diffusion also facilitates an increase in the overall magnitude of diffusion (mean diffusivity [MD]), which has been repeatedly reported as a feature of TAI. FA, however, is the most widely studied and applied DTI parameter.[17]

Newer dMRI methods, such as diffusion kurtosis imaging (DKI), high angular resolution diffusion imaging (HARDI), and others, provide more sophisticated and potentially more accurate characterization of directional diffusion. Although these techniques hold much promise for improving clinical assessment of TBI, they have been much less widely studied, compared to FA from

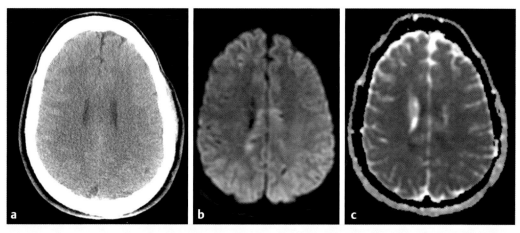

Fig. 11.6 In the same patient as in ▶ Fig. 11.4, **(a)** computed tomography at a more craniad level shows only diffuse edema. **(b)** High signal on diffusion weighted imaging and **(c)** low apparent diffusion coefficient delineate extensive traumatic axonal injury involving the corpus callosum and parasagittal gray–white junction bilaterally. (Images courtesy of: George Lantos, M.D., Jacobi Medical Center, Bronx, NY.)

DTI, and the incremental clinical benefit of these approaches remains to be demonstrated and quantified. The approaches for DTI image analysis described later in the chapter can be applied to any DTI metric as well as to DKI, HARDI, and other approaches. This chapter, however, focuses on the detection of low FA as a marker of TAI in TBI.

11.5.2 DTI Abnormalities in TBI

Lower FA has been repeatedly identified in multiple white matter locations when patients with TBI are compared to healthy controls. Moreover, this finding has held up across studies that differed significantly with regard to patient selection and imaging technique. Patients at all levels of TBI severity and at all stages of injury (acute, subacute, and chronic) have shown low FA in studies that performed DTI at a range of magnetic field strength, using a variety of technical parameters and applying different approaches to quantifying and analyzing the DTI data. This convergence of study findings despite methodological variance underscores the robustness of DTI as a means for detecting tissue abnormalities in TBI.[1,17]

Abnormally high FA has also been detected in TBI patients at various times following injury, though less frequently.[18] Abnormally high MD has also been identified in TBI patients.[19] Both changes in FA and MD have been associated with adverse clinical outcomes, including postconcussion symptoms and cognitive impairment, but it remains unclear how DTI findings near the time of TBI

might be able to *predict* future recovery and ultimate outcome. To date, relatively few studies have reported eigenvalue results in TBI.[17]

11.5.3 Detection of DTI Abnormalities in TBI

Detection of abnormally low FA as an indicator of TAI (▶ Table 11.1) can be accomplished by a number of approaches. Qualitative visual assessment of either grayscale or color-encoded directional FA images may, in some cases, reveal areas of abnormally low FA as dark areas within the white matter (▶ Fig. 11.8). This approach, however, is fraught with difficulty and may be unreliable, due to the normal variability of FA across white matter. The spatial variation in FA results from dispersion, turning, and crossing of fibers within the voxel. Thus, although normal white matter appears homogeneous on standard structural (e.g., T1- or T2-weighted) images, FA varies from voxel to voxel and from region to region to a much greater degree, conferring a "noisy" appearance. In the face of this normal variation, only very large reductions in FA, if any, will be visibly apparent and distinguishable from normal spatial variation. As a result, the visual assessment of FA images for TAI is very insensitive (highly significant abnormalities may be invisible) and may be unreliable (differences due to disease cannot be easily distinguished from differences due to normal variation).

Another qualitative approach to DTI interpretation entails the visual assessment of tractography

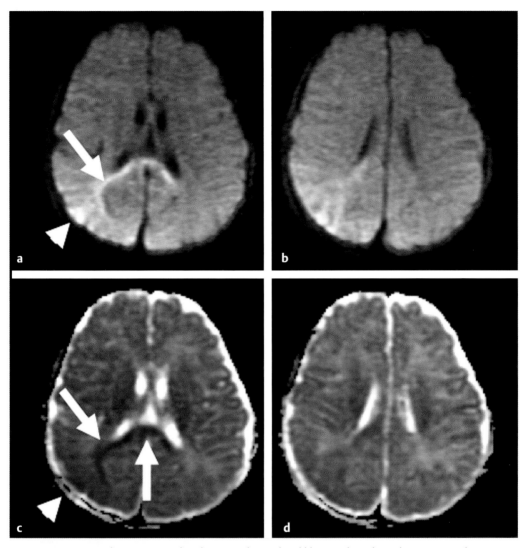

Fig. 11.7 Cytotoxic edema in nonaccidental trauma. This 90-day-old boy was brought to the emergency department with lethargy and fussiness. Computed tomography (not shown) revealed skull fractures and a thin right convexity subdural collection. Edema was suspected, but no parenchymal brain abnormality was evident. (**a, b**) High signal on diffusion weighted imaging with (**c, d**) co-located low apparent diffusion coefficient delineates extensive right parietooccipital contusion (arrowheads) as well as traumatic axonal injury involving the splenium and deep right parietal white matter (arrows). Note that the region of cortical contusion crosses the middle cerebral artery -posterior cerebral artery border zone.

(▶ Fig. 11.8, ▶ Fig. 11.9, ▶ Fig. 11.10, ▶ Fig. 11.11). Tracts are generated using image processing software and then assessed for completeness, volume, and branching. In cases of significant injury, changes related to injury can be visualized. However, tractography results are highly dependent on the parameters chosen by the user, including FA and turning thresholds for tract termination (▶ Fig. 11.12). It is thus essential to ensure that

abnormal appearances are not the result of technical factors.

FA images contain quantitative diagnostic information. Each pixel in the image contains a measurement, which can be analyzed to determine if it is abnormal. The assessment of a patient's FA images can thus be treated in much the same way as other laboratory tests. When the measurement is obtained in a group of healthy, normal

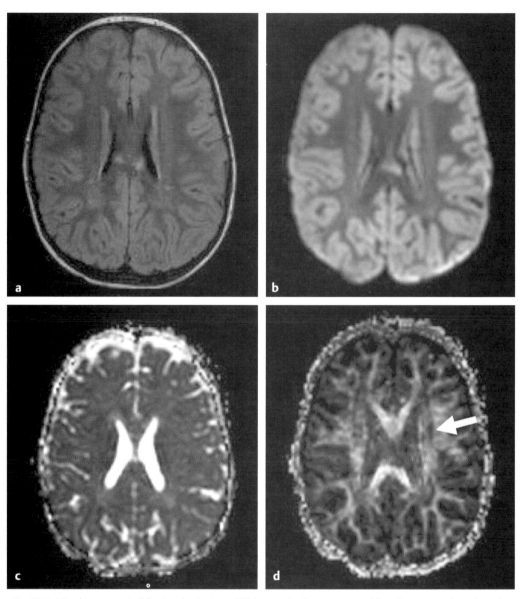

Fig. 11.8 Visual assessment of fractional anisotropy (FA) images. In the same nonaccidental trauma patient shown in ▶ Fig. 11.2, images at a more craniad level show additional signal abnormality on (**a**) T2-weighted fluid-attenuated inversion recovery images and (**b, c**) diffusion restriction, indicating traumatic axonal injury (TAI) within the body of the corpus callosum. (**d**) Areas of low FA, however, reveal additional foci of TAI (white arrow) not detected by other imaging modalities. Note that it is very difficult to discriminate these abnormalities from normal variation of FA.

individuals, the normal range of FA at a given brain location can be determined. Subsequently, a patient's FA can be compared to this normal range to determine if FA is normal or abnormal at that location in this particular patient. This same quantitative analysis process can be repeated for other areas. For the general approach just described, we

can identify two essential prerequisites to quantitative analysis of FA, which can be achieved through several possible analytic approaches. The requirements include the following:

1. **Measurement Standardization:** FA must be measured in the same way in the patient as in the individuals in whom the normal range is

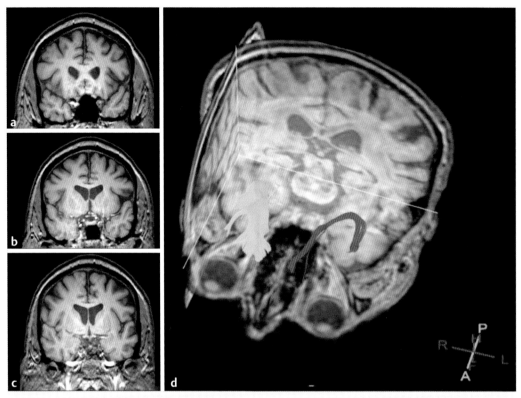

Fig. 11.9 Tract volume and traumatic axonal injury (TAI). In this man with persistent verbal memory dysfunction after traumatic brain injury, (**a-c**) T1-weighted magnetic resonance imaging shows volume loss of the left frontal and temporal lobes as asymmetric prominence of the sulci and sylvian fissure. In this right-handed individual, left language dominance is expected and, consequently, the left uncinate fasciculus should be larger. (**d**) Tractography, however, shows the left uncinate fasciculus is smaller than the right, consistent with TAI and the distribution of atrophy.

determined. This step is to avoid detecting differences between the patient and controls that are a result of technical factors and may lead to false-positive findings.

2. **Spatial Standardization:** The same brain location must be compared between the patient and the individuals in whom the normal range is determined. This step is important to avoid both false-negative and false-positive findings.

Measurement Standardization

Published studies suggest that FA is likely invariant, to a large degree, across MRI scanners and institutions performing DTI. This may hold true only when the parameters of the DTI acquisition (e.g., field strength, echo time (TE), b value, number and orientation of diffusion sensitizing directions) remain the same. The use of different acquisition parameters, however, may lead to differences in FA that are the result of technical factors, not disease. This requirement is similar to that of many widely used laboratory tests, which must be assessed in light of normative data generated using the same equipment and settings applied to test the patient. The quantitative nature of FA can then be leveraged when placed into the context of similarly acquired normative data. Comparison of absolute FA values between images obtained with different acquisition parameters *may* be a source of error, although the magnitude of this potential has not been demonstrated.

Another important measurement consideration is related to the individuals included in the group used to characterize the range of normal FA measurements. If, for example, we compare the FA measurements from a young, otherwise healthy TBI patient to a group of elderly individuals with cerebrovascular disease, who may have areas of low FA related to aging or stroke, the TBI patient may appear normal in comparison to this group, although this patient harbors true abnormalities

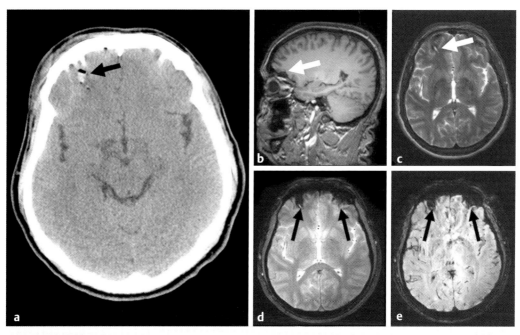

Fig. 11.10 This 23-year-old woman was injured in a boating accident. (**a**) Computed tomography performed on the day of the injury shows extracranial soft tissue injury in the right supraorbital region. Acute hemorrhage and air are present within the right orbitofrontal lobe (thick black arrow), due to laceration by a bone fragment from a fracture of the right orbital roof (not shown). (**b, c**) Magnetic resonance imaging performed 18 months later shows right orbitofrontal encephalomalacia on T1 and T2-weighted images (white arrows) and (**d**) bifrontal hemosiderin deposition on gradient echo and (**e**) susceptibility-weighted imaging (thin black arrows) due to hemorrhagic contusion. No other areas of brain injury were evident.

due to TAI. Conversely, when abnormally low FA is identified in an elderly patient with cerebrovascular disease, compared to a group of young, healthy individuals, these abnormalities might be due to TBI and/or stroke. To minimize the chance of false-negative and false-positive results, two approaches can be taken. One approach is to employ comparison subjects who are as similar to the patient as possible, such as all being of the same gender and age. Although at first glance this might seem an ideal approach, its limitation is that, each time a patient is assessed, a different comparison group will be required. An alternate approach is to employ methods for adjusting for the effects of potential confounding factors, most commonly for age and gender.

Spatial Standardization

The FA images constitute a three-dimensional (3-D) brain volume. To determine whether the patient's brain is abnormal, specific brain regions must be chosen for assessment. This can be performed either by delineating, a priori, regions of interest (ROIs) for analysis, or by assessing each voxel in the entire brain volume to identify all areas of abnormality. Each of these approaches has limitations and advantages, which will be discussed here.

ROI can be specified as discrete volumes of interest (e.g., ellipse, box, etc.), typically hand drawn, by an experienced radiologist or technician, on the patient's brain images using the ROI drawing tools available on most basic clinical image processing workstations and MRI scanner operator consoles. FA is then averaged across each ROI. Measurements are obtained from the patient and from a group of normal control subjects, which are then compared. The comparison can be quantified using various statistics. Computing the Z-score is one common approach. Once the Z-score is computed, a threshold for abnormality must be applied to determine if the area tested is abnormal, typically at least $Z \leq -2$. For the ROI approach to be valid, the location of the ROI within the brain of the patient must be identical to its location in

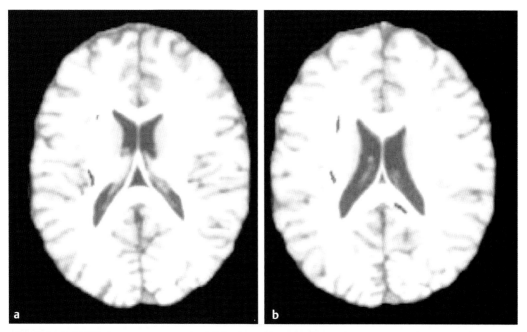

Fig. 11.11 (a,b) Diffusion tensor imaging (DTI) delineates additional widespread traumatic axonal injury (TAI). Voxelwise analysis of fractional anisotropy (FA) images from DTI in the patient presented in ▶ Fig. 11.8 reveals multiple areas of abnormally low FA (red), indicating areas of TAI not detectable on prior computed tomographic and magnetic resonance imaging studies.

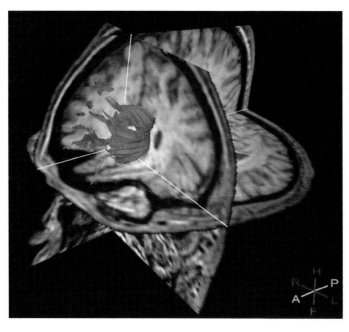

Fig. 11.12 Tractography delineates axonal degeneration secondary to gross white matter injury: Truncation of fibers (long arrow) projecting to the region of brain laceration in the right frontal lobe, compared to normal branching fibers (short arrows).

each normal control subject. Because each individual has a unique head shape and size and the position and orientation of slices may not be identical across individuals, this is a challenging process. Moreover, it is advantageous for ROIs to be drawn on a non-FA image, such as the $b = 0$ or T1-weighted image. This ensures that visual impressions of the FA images cannot bias the ROI placement. Best practice is to quantify the reliability of ROI placement by conducting a formal reliability study. ROIs are drawn on the same subject's brain multiple times by the same radiologist or technician. This procedure is then repeated for additional subjects. The variability of the resultant average FA across the ROI in each subject is quantified, typically using the intraclass correlation coefficient. Without such quality assurance measures, differences between a patient and the normal control subjects may be attributable to observer bias.

ROIs can also be defined using tractography. In this approach, a tract of interest is delineated and the average FA across the entire tract is assessed by comparing it to FA averaged across the same tract in each normal control. Because tracts are delineated by manual placement of seed and target ROI, definition of tracts as ROIs entails the same limitations and considerations already described. In particular, quality assurance procedures are essential to ensuring reliable and reproducible tract delineation across individuals.

To entirely avoid the difficulties and risk of error arising from manual delineation of ROIs for analysis, whole brain approaches can be employed to quantitatively assess FA. Histograms displaying FA across all brain (or all white matter) voxels can be computed using image-processing software. This approach is free from the risk of observer bias because no manual delineation of ROIs is required when the entire brain volume is assessed as one. Although this approach has shown differences between patients and normal individuals, it has inherently limited sensitivity.[20] TBI is a multifocal disease in which most brain voxels are normal. Averaging these few abnormal voxels with myriad unaffected voxels limits detection of true abnormalities.

Another whole brain approach to the assessment of FA is the brainwide voxelwise approach.[18, 19,21] Prior to the actual assessment of FA, a series of image processing steps are applied to coregister the brain volumes of the patient and each of the normal control subjects. This process transforms the size and shape of each brain to match that of a "template" brain. As a result, any individual voxel in the 3-D brain volume will represent the same brain location in each individual. Next, FA from each voxel in the patient's brain is compared to FA from the same voxel in the group of normal control subjects, employing a statistical threshold to classify each voxel as normal or abnormal. Because the typical FA brain volume will contain hundreds of thousands of voxels, this procedure entails hundreds of thousands of comparisons between the patient and the normal control subjects. In addition to the need for high-performance computing to complete this analysis, whenever many simultaneous comparisons are made, the potential increases that significant differences will occur due to chance alone. Thus such voxelwise analyses must employ steps to account and minimize this risk. Two basic approaches are employed. First, a more stringent statistical threshold is either chosen a priori or computed, such as using the false discovery rate method.[22] Whereas, for example, $Z < -2$ might be an acceptable significance level in a single comparison, $Z < -3$ or even stricter thresholds might be employed in voxelwise analyses. Second, spatial clustering is employed to reduce the chance of false-positive findings. In this latter approach, individual voxels are not recorded as abnormalities, even though they meet a strict criterion for abnormality. Only where multiple contiguous voxels, each meeting the threshold for abnormality, constitute a minimum volume of tissue is an abnormality recorded. This approach dramatically reduces the chance that a false-positive finding will be reported as a real abnormality. In any of the quantitative approaches described, the choice of threshold is always a balance between sensitivity (risk of false-negative findings) and specificity (risk of false-positive findings).[18]

11.5.4 Differential Diagnosis of DTI Abnormalities in Patients with TBI

The foregoing procedures and approaches allow for the detection and delineation of brain regions (ROIs, tracts or clusters of voxels) that differ significantly from the same locations in a group of normal control subjects. Building on the extensive literature identifying low FA as manifestation of TAI,[1,17] low FA detected in a TBI patient can thus be attributed to TAI (▶ Fig. 11.12, ▶ Fig. 11.13, ▶ Fig. 11.14, ▶ Fig. 11.15, ▶ Fig. 11.16, ▶ Fig. 11.17, ▶ Fig. 11.18). As with all imaging findings,

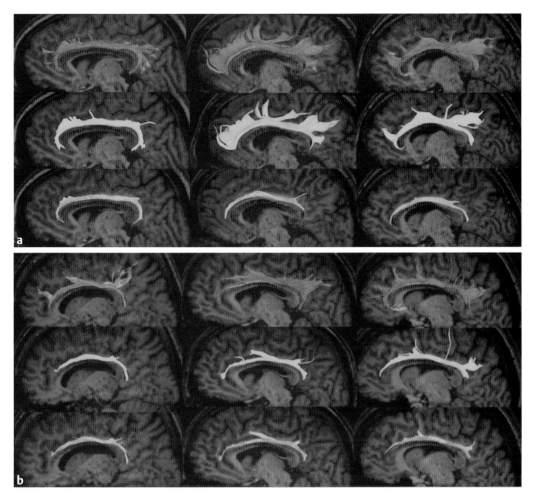

Fig. 11.13 Impact of tractography parameters on visual appearance of tracts and their volume. The cingulum has been delineated in three normal individuals in (**a**) (top, columns 1–3) and in three patients with traumatic brain injury (TBI) (**b**) (bottom, columns 1–3). Three different tracts were generated for each individual (blue, green, lavender) by using three different fractional anisotropy termination thresholds (0.15–0.30). Note the overall lesser volume of each tract in the TBI patients as well as the loss of peripheral branching of the tracts. (Republished from Kurki T. Diffusion tensor tractography-based analysis of the cingulum: clinical utility and findings in traumatic brain injury with chronic sequels. Neuroradiology 2014;56:833–841. With kind permission from Springer Science and Business Media.)

however, a differential diagnosis must consider other potential causes for the low FA findings.

The use of an appropriate normal control group addresses concerns regarding demographic factors, such as age and gender, which may impact FA. Assuming that other potentially confounding conditions have been excluded from the normal control subjects, such as medical and psychiatric disease, the primary source of potential confounding factors is the patients themselves. That is, does the patient harbor a brain disorder that could reasonably manifest the type of abnormal FA detected? To address this question, several factors must be considered. First, what other disorders have been shown to result in reductions in FA to the degree seen in TBI? Second, which of these potential differential diagnoses are relevant in the patient under assessment?

Multiple sclerosis, stroke, and brain tumors are examples of disorders that have been shown to reduce FA to a degree that is distinguishable, at least in some patients, from normal control

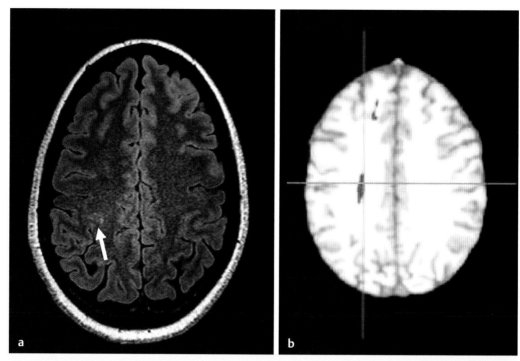

Fig. 11.14 Diffusion tensor imaging reveals more extensive traumatic axonal injury than conventional magnetic resonance imaging (MRI). (**a**) A small cluster of hyperintensities (white arrow) is shown on T2-weighted fluid-attenuated inversion recovery (FLAIR) MRI. (**b**) Areas of abnormally low fractional anisotropy (red) are more extensive than those shown on T2-weighted FLAIR.

subjects. Changes in FA have also been associated with other disorders, such as depression, autism, schizophrenia, and substance abuse. In these research studies, which compare groups of patients to groups of normal control subjects, significant differences can be, and have been, reported despite substantial overlap in the distribution of measurements from the two groups.[23] In light of these results, however, it is not possible to ascribe the FA changes in a specific individual to the disease in question. Multiple studies of TBI, on the other hand, have shown that FA exceeding a threshold such as $Z \leq -2.5$, especially when found at multiple white matter locations, is detectable in TBI patients, but only rarely, if at all, in normal control subjects.[24] Thus FA exceeding a validated threshold can be attributed to TBI, with the understanding that not all patients with TBI will evince changes of this magnitude. Ultimately, such an approach sacrifices some degree of sensitivity in exchange for greater diagnostic certainty.

11.6 Summary

dMRI, including DWI as well as DTI and its variants, is an important addition to the imaging toolbox for the clinical assessment of TBI. As with all imaging methods, dMRI results must be interpreted in context with the results of other imaging and nonimaging clinical information to reliably attribute dMRI findings to TBI or other potential etiologies. DWI abnormalities in acute TBI, including contusion and TAI, may be detected by visual assessment, though this approach remains insensitive to microstructural injury. The major advantage of dMRI is its ability to detect abnormalities where standard images appear normal. To realize this diagnostic improvement and maximize sensitivity and specificity, quantitative analysis techniques must be employed. Quantitative analysis of dMRI, however, is quite technically demanding. Improved availability of turnkey solutions for the postprocessing of dMRI are thus needed to facilitate wider use by clinical radiologists and greater benefit to patients.

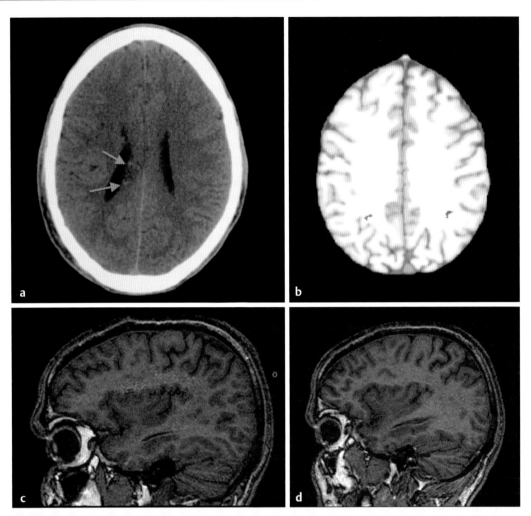

Fig. 11.15 Wallerian degeneration following traumatic axonal injury (TAI). This previously healthy 22-year-old laborer fell head first from a height of 15 feet, impacting his head at the vertex. He was unconscious for several minutes and had prolonged confusion and amnesia. (**a**) Computed tomography (CT) on the day of injury showed two punctate hemorrhages in the body of the corpus callosum (arrow), typical of TAI and unchanged on follow-up CT 24 hours later (not shown). The patient suffered persistent cognitive impairment, especially slowed processing speed. (**b**) Areas of abnormally low fractional anisotropy (red), consistent with TAI, were identified in the corpus callosum (not shown) and in the biparietal deep white matter. These findings indicate wallerian degeneration of axons traversing the corpus callosum, projecting to the parietal cortex and thus explaining the localized biparietal atrophy. (**c,d**) T1-weighted magnetic resonance imaging was performed 7 years later to investigate persistent cognitive impairment and showed biparietal atrophy. No additional areas of hemorrhage were identified.

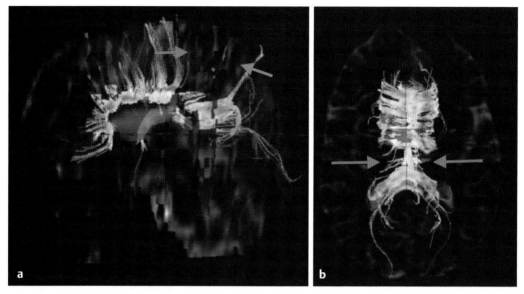

Fig. 11.16 (a) Lateral and (b) superior views of diffusion tensor imaging tractography performed in the same patient shown in ▶ Fig. 11.11. Tractography was performed using a seed region of interest encompassing the corpus callosum. Paucity and frank absence of fibers are evident traversing the location of prior hemorrhage in the body of the corpus callosum (arrows) and projecting to the regions of biparietal atrophy.

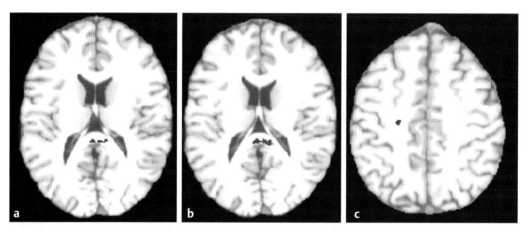

Fig. 11.17 A 45-year-old man was struck by a large metal component that fell from an adjacent truck, crashed through his car window, and struck him in the head. He was taken by ambulance to the emergency department, where a computed tomographic scan was normal. Standard magnetic resonance imaging performed 6 days after the injury, when the patient was suffering from severe postconcussion symptoms, showed no abnormality. Voxelwise analysis of fractional anisotropy (FA) images shows extensive abnormally low FA in the splenium and an additional area of low FA (red areas) in the right centrum semiovale.

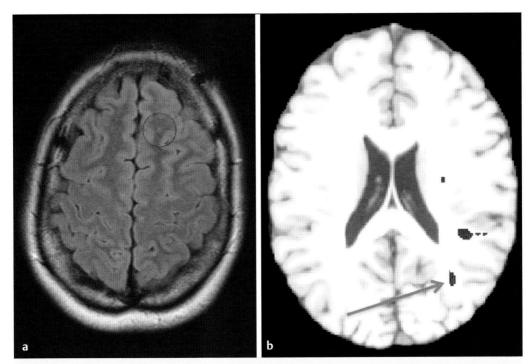

Fig. 11.18 A 27-year-old, previously healthy woman suffered mild traumatic brain injury with loss of consciousness when the car she was driving was struck on the rear driver's side. Computed tomographic scan was normal. (**a**) Magnetic resonance imaging performed 11 months later due to persistent symptoms and impaired cognitive function showed only small peripheral white matter hyperintensities on T2-weighted fluid-attenuated inversion recovery images (red circle). (**b**) Voxelwise analysis of fractional anisotropy (FA) images identified multiple areas of abnormally low FA (red areas), consistent with traumatic axonal injury, in the cerebral white matter subjacent to the left posterior location of impact (green arrow), which occurred in the motor vehicle accident.

References

[1] Shenton ME, Hamoda HM, Schneiderman JS, et al. A review of magnetic resonance imaging and diffusion tensor imaging findings in mild traumatic brain injury. Brain Imaging Behav 2012; 6(2): 137–192

[2] Faul M, Xu L, Coronado VG. Traumatic brain injury in the United States: emergency department visits, hospitalizations and deaths 2002–2006. Atlanta, GA, Centers for Disease Control and Prevention: 2010

[3] Centers for Disease Control and Prevention. Report to Congress on mild traumatic brain injury in the United States: steps to prevent a serious public health problem. Atlanta, GA: Centers for Disease Control and Prevention; 2003

[4] McCullagh S, Oucherlony D, Protzner A, Blair N, Feinstein A. Prediction of neuropsychiatric outcome following mild trauma brain injury: an examination of the Glasgow Coma Scale. Brain Inj 2001; 15(6): 489–497

[5] Saatman KE, Duhaime AC, Bullock R, Maas AI, Valadka A, Manley GT Workshop Scientific Team and Advisory Panel Members. Classification of traumatic brain injury for targeted therapies. J Neurotrauma 2008; 25(7): 719–738

[6] Mataró M, Poca MA, Sahuquillo J, et al. Neuropsychological outcome in relation to the traumatic coma data bank classification of computed tomography imaging. J Neurotrauma 2001; 18(9): 869–879

[7] Sterr A, Herron KA, Hayward C, Montaldi D. Are mild head injuries as mild as we think? Neurobehavioral concomitants of chronic post-concussion syndrome. BMC Neurol 2006; 6: 7

[8] American Congress of Rehabilitation Medicines. Definition of mild traumatic brain injury. J Head Trauma Rehabil 1993; 8: 86–87

[9] Bigler ED, Maxwell WL. Neuropathology of mild traumatic brain injury: relationship to neuroimaging findings. Brain Imaging Behav 2012; 6(2): 108–136

[10] McKee AC, Cantu RC, Nowinski CJ, et al. Chronic traumatic encephalopathy in athletes: progressive tauopathy after repetitive head injury. J Neuropathol Exp Neurol 2009; 68 (7): 709–735

[11] McMahon P, Hricik A, Yue JK, et al. TRACK-TBI Investigators. Symptomatology and functional outcome in mild traumatic brain injury: results from the prospective TRACK-TBI study. J Neurotrauma 201 4; 31(1): 26–33

[12] Messé A, Caplain S, Pélégrini-Issac M, et al. Specific and evolving resting-state network alterations in post-concussion syndrome following mild traumatic brain injury. PLoS ONE 2013; 8(6): e65470

[13] Sharp DJ, Scott G, Leech R. Network dysfunction after traumatic brain injury. Nat Rev Neurol 2014; 10(3): 156–166

[14] Povlishock JT, Katz DI. Update of neuropathology and neurological recovery after traumatic brain injury. J Head Trauma Rehabil 2005; 20(1): 76–94

[15] Povlishock JT. The window of risk in repeated head injury. J Neurotrauma 2013; 30(1): 1

[16] Provenzale JM, Sorensen AG. Diffusion weighted MR imaging in acute stroke: theoretic considerations and clinical applications. AJR Am J Roentgenol 1999; 173(6): 1459–1467

[17] Hulkower MB, Poliak DB, Rosenbaum SB, Zimmerman ME, Lipton ML. A decade of DTI in traumatic brain injury: 10 years and 100 articles later. AJNR Am J Neuroradiol 2013; 34 (11): 2064–2074

[18] Lipton ML, Kim N, Park YK, et al. Robust detection of traumatic axonal injury in individual mild traumatic brain injury patients: intersubject variation, change over time and bidirectional changes in anisotropy. Brain Imaging Behav 2012; 6(2): 329–342

[19] Lipton ML, Gulko E, Zimmerman ME, et al. Diffusion tensor imaging implicates prefrontal axonal injury in executive function impairment following very mild traumatic brain injury. Radiology 2009; 252(3): 816–824

[20] Benson RR, Meda SA, Vasudevan S, et al. Global white matter analysis of diffusion tensor images is predictive of injury severity in traumatic brain injury. J Neurotrauma 2007; 24 (3): 446–459

[21] Lipton ML, Gellella E, Lo C, et al. Multifocal white matter ultrastructural abnormalities in mild traumatic brain injury with cognitive disability: a voxel-wise analysis of diffusion tensor imaging. J Neurotrauma 2008; 25(11): 1335–1342

[22] Benjamini Y, Hochberg Y. Controlling the False Discovery Rate: a Practical and Powerful Approach to Multiple Testing. JRStatistSocB 1995; 57: 289–300

[23] White T, Nelson M, Lim KO. Diffusion tensor imaging in psychiatric disorders. Top Magn Reson Imaging 2008; 19(2): 97–109

[24] Mac Donald CL, Johnson AM, Cooper D, et al. Detection of blast-related traumatic brain injury in U.S. military personnel. N Engl J Med 2011; 364(22): 2091–2100

12 Diffusion Weighted Imaging in Hemorrhage

Joana Ramalho and Mauricio Castillo

Key Points

- The pattern of evolving hematomas on conventional magnetic resonance imaging (MRI) is well documented but remains somewhat complex, and its interpretation is further complicated by diffusion weighted imaging (DWI).
- T2 shine-through, T2 blackout effects, and susceptibility artifacts from blood products contribute to the appearance of hemorrhage on DWI and influence the apparent diffusion coefficient (ADC) measurements. Therefore, DWI of hemorrhage should be interpreted cautiously and in conjunction with T2- and T2*-weighted MRI.
- According to recent studies, DWI is accurate in detection, characterization, and staging of intraparenchymal hematomas; however, it should not be interpreted alone but in conjunction with other sequences. It is also accurate for detection of hemorrhagic venous infarcts or hemorrhagic transformation of arterial infarcts and subdural and epidural hematomas.
- Conversely, DWI has low diagnostic accuracy in microbleeds and acute subarachnoid hemorrhage and should not be used in the latter.

12.1 Introduction

Intracranial hemorrhage diagnosis and characterization depend on imaging studies because clinical signs and symptoms are usually nonspecific. Hemorrhage can be classified based on its location as (1) intra-axial, including parenchymal and intraventricular hemorrhages; and (2) extra-axial, including epidural, subdural, and subarachnoid hemorrhage, which may occur in isolation or in different combinations depending on the underlying etiology.

Computed tomography (CT) is commonly the first imaging modality used for suspected intracranial hemorrhage evaluation. Acute blood is markedly hyperdense compared to brain parenchyma, making its easy to diagnose. However, after the acute phase, CT provides little information regarding the precise stage of the hemorrhage, and because subacute hemorrhage becomes progressively less dense in a few days, CT's utility is confined to the acute period.

Conversely, magnetic resonance imaging (MRI) has excellent capabilities to determine the presence of blood, its underlying etiology, and the age of the hemorrhage. The MRI appearance of intracranial hemorrhage primarily depends on the oxygenation of hemoglobin, the chemical state of its iron-containing moieties, the integrity of the red blood cells (RBCs), and the MRI sequences and/or parameters used (▶ Table 12.1). Other factors that

Table 12.1 Signal intensities on different magnetic resonance sequences of intraparenchymal hematomas according to the various stages

Stage of the hematoma	Time (days)	Hemoglobin	T1-WI	T2-WI	GRE	DWI
Hyperacute	< 1	Oxyhemoglobin (intracellular)	Iso/Hypo	Hyper	Iso/Hyper	Hyper (core) Hypo (rim)
Acute	1–3	Deoxyhemoglobin (intracellular)	Iso/Hypo	Hypo	Hypo	Hypo
Early subacute	3–7	Methemoglobin (intracellular)	Hyper	Hypo	Hypo	Hypo
Late subacute	> 7	Methemoglobin (extracellular)	Hyper	Hyper	Hyper	Hyper
Chronic	> 14	Ferritin and hemosiderin (extracellular)	Iso/Hypo	Hyper/Iso Hypo (rim)	Iso/Hyper Hypo (rim)	Iso/Hypo Hypo (rim)

Abbreviations: DWI, diffusion weighted imaging; Iso, isointense; GRE, gradient-recalled echo imaging; Hyper, hyperintense; Hypo, hypointense; T1-WI, T1-weighted image; T2-WI, T2-weighted image.

influence the MRI appearance of blood are the hemorrhage location, the local partial pressure of oxygen, the local pH, the hematocrit, the local glucose concentration, the hemoglobin concentration, the integrity of the blood–brain barrier, and the patient's temperature.[1]

The characteristic MRI intensity patterns observed during the evolution of the hematomas are well known. Hyperacute hematomas show low to isointense signal on T1-weighted images and hyperintense signal on conventional T2-weighted images with a peripheral thin and irregular hypointense rim.[2] This pattern represents oxyhemoglobin forming the bulk of the hematoma with early deoxyhemoglobin at the periphery, and because oxyhemoglobin produces no paramagnetic effects it is a reflection of the water contained in blood.[2] Acute hematomas are seen as hypointense lesions on T2-weighted images[3] with isointense signal on T1-weighted images.[4] Although multifactorial, it has been generally accepted that the basis of this signal loss on T2-weighted images is mainly related to the intrinsic heterogeneity of magnetic field gradients due to compartmentalized paramagnetic deoxygenated blood.[3,5,6,7] Similarly, "early subacute" hematomas are hyperintense on T1-weighted images and markedly hypointense on T2-weighted images, due to the presence of methemoglobin within intact RBCs.[3] Over several days to weeks, the energy status of the RBCs declines, causing a loss of cellular integrity, and cellular lyses. In this late subacute phase, hematomas show an increased T1 and T2 signal intensity caused by the extracellular methemoglobin. Over months, the hematoma enters the chronic phase. The center of the hematoma may evolve into a fluid-filled cavity with signal intensity identical to that of cerebrospinal fluid (CSF). The walls of the cavity show low signal on T1- and T2-weighted images, related to extracellular hemosiderin and ferritin outside and within macrophages, and may collapse, leaving behind a thin, fluid-filled slit.

Despite the frequent use of conventional MRI to evaluate the extent, location, and underlying mechanism of intracranial hemorrhages, diffusion weighted imaging (DWI) has also been studied and used in this setting. DWI is not the best sequence for evaluation of intracranial hemorrhage; however, it is helpful to recognize blood's signal intensity changes over time to reduce the risk of misdiagnosis. Furthermore, the primary assessment of patients with early stroke is moving toward MRI, and DWI may play a crucial role in the emergent evaluation of these patients.[8,9,10] In this context, understanding the appearance of intracerebral hemorrhage on DWI is critical to instituting appropriate stroke management because hemorrhage is a contraindication for thrombolytic therapy.

On DWI, restricted diffusion shows hyperintensity, whereas fast diffusion shows hypointensity. However, because there is a contribution from the T2 echo-planar spin-echo baseline image to DWI signal intensity, not all areas of high signal intensity represent restricted diffusion, an effect termed T2 shine-through, and also not all areas with low signal represent fast diffusion, an effect known as T2 blackout effect.[4] These concepts are particularly important when interpreting the appearance of hemorrhage on DWI, and they influence the measurements of its apparent diffusion coefficient (ADC) values.

12.2 Clinical Applications

12.2.1 Intracerebral Hematomas

Hyperacute Hematomas

On DWI, hyperacute hematomas show a heterogeneous hyperintense core with focal areas of hypointensity surrounded by a peripherally hypointense incomplete rim[11,12,13] (▶ Fig. 12.1 and ▶ Fig. 12.2). The central hyperintensity probably represents intracellular oxyhemoglobin because it is also isointense on T1-weighted images, heterogeneously hyperintense on T2 and fluid-attenuated inversion recovery (FLAIR) images, with a variable appearance on gradient-echo images, but usually heterogeneously hyperintense. The hypointense incomplete rim has been reported to occur within the first few hours after a hemorrhage[8,11,14,15] and is thought to represent early intracellular deoxyhemoglobin at the periphery of the hematoma because it is also hypointense on T2-weighted images and is particularly obvious on gradient-echo images, which have a stronger susceptibility effect. However, some focal areas of low signal intensity on DWI, seen in different locations within the hematoma, show high signal on T2-weighted and gradient-echo images and may represent unclotted blood separate from the retracted clot (▶ Fig. 12.2).[2,16,17] These hypointense areas are consistently seen in patients with hyperacute intracranial hematomas and may represent an important imaging feature for differentiating hemorrhage from infarction.

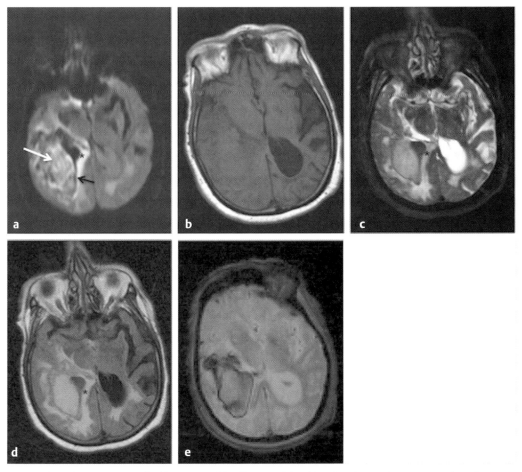

Fig. 12.1 Hyperacute intracerebral hematoma. (a) Diffusion weighted imaging shows a heterogeneous hyperintense core (white arrow) with focal areas of hypointensity surrounded by a peripherally hypointense irregular and incomplete rim (black arrow). Note the hyperintense area around the hematoma (*) that represents edema. (b) T1-weighted image shows an isointense hematoma, whereas (c) the T2-weighted image, (d) fluid-attenuated inversion recovery, and (e) gradient-echo image show a hyperintense hematoma with a well-defined hypointense rim. The surrounding edema is well depicted in all sequences.

Acute and Early Subacute Hematomas

Acute and early subacute hematomas appear markedly hypointense on DWI, T2-weighted, FLAIR, and gradient-echo images (▶ Fig. 12.3 and ▶ Fig. 12.4). As stated earlier, on T1-weighted images acute hematomas are heterogeneously isointense or of low intensity, whereas early subacute hematomas are markedly hyperintense. This lower signal intensity on DWI has been attributed to magnetic field inhomogeneity caused by paramagnetic intracellular deoxyhemoglobin in acute hematomas[14] and paramagnetic intracellular methemoglobin in early subacute hematomas,[18] which represent the T2 blackout effect.

In the hyperacute, acute, and early subacute stages, a bright rim of variable thickness and completeness at the periphery of a hematoma is seen on DWI.[11,12] This bright rim is hyperintense on T2-weighted images but is usually not seen on gradient-echo images. It probably is not caused by susceptibility artifacts but may represent the T2 shine-through effect caused by vasogenic edema.[11,19]

Late Subacute Hematomas

Late subacute hematomas are hyperintense on DWI, T1-weighted, T2-weighted, and FLAIR images

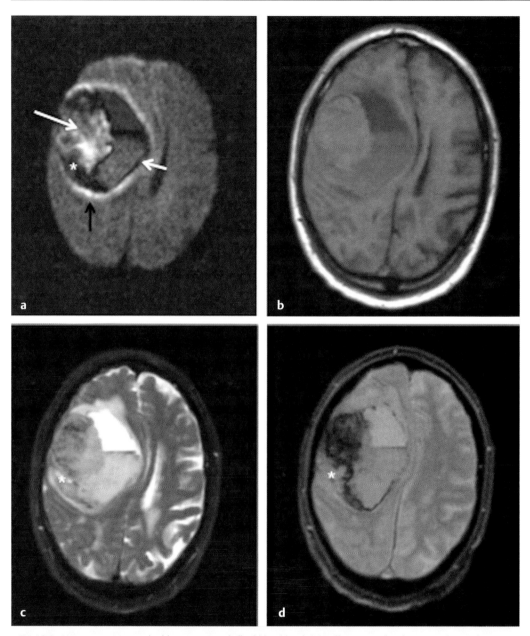

Fig. 12.2 Hyperacute intracerebral hematoma with fluid-blood level. (a) Diffusion weighted imaging (DWI) shows a heterogeneous hyperintense hematoma (white arrow) with focal areas of hypointensity, surrounded by a well-defined hypointense rim (small white arrow). The hematoma is isointense on (b) T1-weighted image, hyperintense on (c) T2-weighted image, and shows greater signal loss on (d) gradient-echo image. The fluid-blood level is well depicted in all sequences. It is seen as a horizontal interface between hypodense bloody serum layered above hyperdense settled blood. Note the thin area of edema well seen on DWI (black arrow) as a hyperintense rim surrounding the hematoma. Some of the areas of low signal intensity on DWI described above (*) show high signal on T2-weighted and gradient-echo images and may represent unclotted blood separated from the retracted clot.

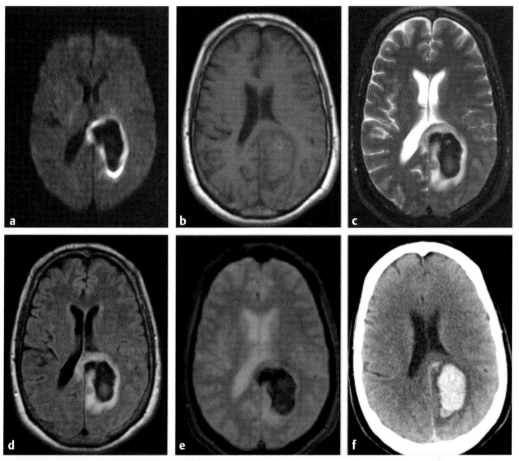

Fig. 12.3 Acute intracerebral hematoma. (a) Diffusion weighted imaging shows a markedly hypointense hematoma surrounded by a continuous rim of bright signal intensity that corresponds to edema. (b) T1-weighted image shows an isointense hematoma, whereas (c) T2-weighted image, (d) fluid-attenuated inversion recovery, and (e) gradient-echo image show a markedly hypointense hematoma with a well-defined hyperintensity area of edema. (f) Axial computed tomography shows a hyperdense hematoma surrounded by hypodense edema.

and heterogeneously hyperintense on gradient-echo images (▶ Fig. 12.5).

Chronic Stage

In the chronic stage, paramagnetic ferritin and hemosiderin are seen on DWI, T2-weighted images, and gradient-echo imaging as a dark rim at the periphery of the hematoma. The diffusion increases as the lesion becomes cystic, and for that reason the core of a chronic hematoma appears isointense in the early chronic stage and hypointense in the late chronic stage (▶ Fig. 12.6).

Apparent Diffusion Coefficient of Hematomas

The restriction of diffusion (reduced ADC values) of the intracranial hematomas varies over time according to different authors. Different postprocessing methods can strongly influence ADC measurements.[14]

Atlas et al[14] suggested that restricted diffusion (reduced ADC values) is seen within hematomas containing RBCs with membranes as follows: hyperacute (intracellular oxyhemoglobin), acute (intracellular deoxyhemoglobin), and early

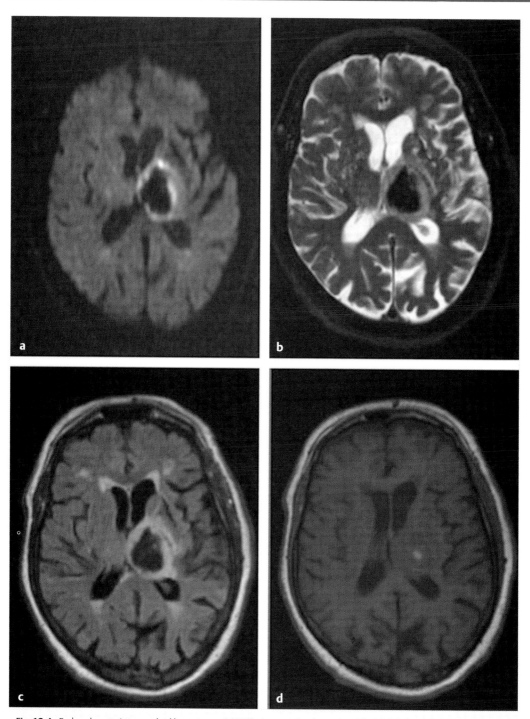

Fig. 12.4 Early subacute intracerebral hematoma. (**a**) Diffusion weighted imaging, (**b**) T2-weighted image, and (**c**) fluid-attenuated inversion recovery show a markedly hypointense hematoma surrounded by a rim of hyperintense edema. (**d**) T1-weighted image shows an isointense hematoma with a central area of hyperintensity that represents intracellular methemoglobin.

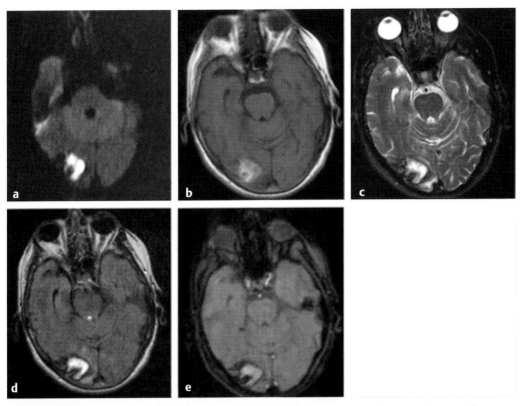

Fig. 12.5 Late subacute intracerebral hematoma. (**a**) Diffusion weighted imaging, (**b**) T1-weighted image, (**c**) T2-weighted image, (**d**) fluid-attenuated inversion recovery, and (**e**) gradient-echo image show a hyperintense hematoma with a small area of surrounding edema.

subacute (intracellular methemoglobin), and increased diffusion is seen after RBC lysis. However, Kang et al[11] found that ADC values of hematomas were reduced compared with normal brain tissues during hyperacute, acute, early, and late subacute phases, suggesting that diffusion is restricted in them before and after cell lysis. In the late subacute phase, cell organelles are found in the extracellular space, causing high viscosity. Other biological changes at this stage include high cellularity resulting from the infiltration of inflammatory cells and macrophages. All these changes may affect the molecular diffusion and the ADC values of a hematoma. Khedr et al[12] and Silvera et al[8] also found restricted diffusion in early stages of intracranial hematomas. Additional explanations for these findings include (1) shrinkage of the extracellular space with clot retraction; (2) change in the osmotic environment once blood becomes extravascular, which alters the shape of the RBCs (a phenomenon related to formation of the fibrin network associated with clots); (3)

conformational changes in the hemoglobin macromolecule within the RBC; and (4) the less likely possibility of contraction of intact RBCs (thereby decreasing intracellular space). All of these processes may alter the potential mobility of intracellular water protons and thus affect their diffusion properties.[4,12,20,21]

Maldjian et al[4] showed that T2- dark hematomas (with intact red cell membranes and intracellular blood products) have diffusion rates comparable with those of the brain (despite their low signal on DWI). The authors argued that obtaining accurate diffusion measurements in regions in which the T2 signal is low could be problematic because an individual pixel value may be dominated by the thermal and electronic noise of the imaging system. Wintermark et al[22] also found increased ADC values in hyperacute hematomas, although lower than the ADC values of CSF.

Does et al[23] and Schaefer et al[18] reported that magnetic susceptibility effects caused a drop in ADC, and suggested that an accurate ADC value for

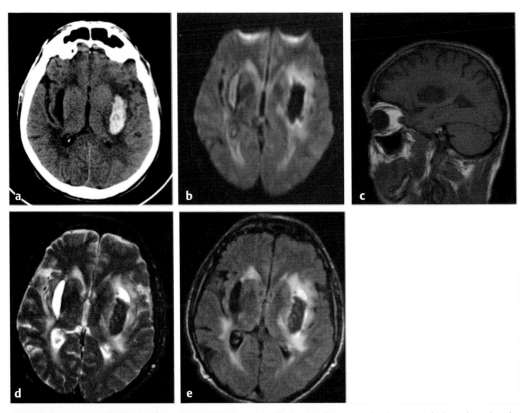

Fig. 12.6 Chronic and acute basal ganglia hematomas. **(a)** Axial computed tomography shows a right hypodense basal ganglia lesion suggestive of chronic hematoma. On the left, there is a basal ganglia hyperdense acute hematoma with surrounding edema. **(b)** Diffusion weighted imaging (DWI) shows the chronic hematoma as a hyperintense lesion with a hypointense rim. **(c)** Sagittal T1-weighted image, **(d)** axial T2-weighted image (T2-WI), and **(e)** fluid-attenuated inversion recovery (FLAIR) show the chronic hematoma as a cavity with signal intensity similar to cerebrospinal fluid. **(d)** A hypointense rim is also seen on T2-weighted image. The acute hematoma is seen as a markedly hypointense left basal ganglia lesion on **(b)** DWI, **(d)** T2-WI, and **(e)** FLAIR.

acute and early subacute hematomas could not be reliably calculated.

Importantly, the reduction in ADC values observed among different studies did not significantly differ between the different stages of the hematomas. Such a steady decrease in ADC values would be expected to produce DWI hyperintensity, which should remain stable throughout the time course of hematoma. The clear variations seen in DWI signal intensity according to the stage of the hematoma imply that factors other than ADC values influence their signal intensity on DWI.[8]

DWI is not a simple map of diffusion but is a composite of contributions from diffusion and paramagnetic effects on T1- and T2-weighted sequences, and the T2 shine-through effect of hyperacute hematomas and the T2 blackout effect of acute and

early subacute hematomas is an important component of their signal intensity on DWI. The T1 effect is probably not a main component of their DWI appearance given that DWI and T1-weighted sequences show different signal intensities during hyperacute and early subacute stages. In the hyperacute phase, the hematoma is mainly isointense on T1-weighted images and hyperintense on DWI, and during the early subacute phase high signal intensity is usually observed on T1-weighted images, whereas low signal is observed on DWI.[8] Because of these effects, DWI should not be interpreted alone but in conjunction with other sequences. Regarding the ADC values of a chronic hematoma, it is accepted that the ADC value increases as the lesion approaches a cystic state.

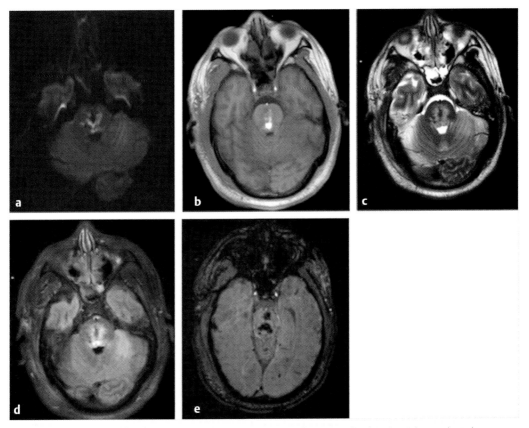

Fig. 12.7 Small intracranial hemorrhage: Duret hemorrhage. (**a**) Diffusion weighted imaging shows a hypodense midline midbrain lesion, surrounded by hyperdense edema suggestive of a Duret hemorrhage. (**b**) A T1-weighted image shows a hyperintense lesion, whereas (**c**) T2-weighted and (**d**) fluid-attenuated inversion recovery images show a hypointense small hematoma, surrounded by edema. (**e**) The lesion is also markedly hypointense on a susceptibility-weighted image (SWI). Note also other small lesions on SWI.

12.2.2 Small Intracranial Hemorrhages

DWI can detect relatively small amounts of hemorrhage (▶ Fig. 12.7), as reported by Chung et al[13] However, it has been reported that DWI is not able to detect microhemorrhages.[24] In fact, acute medium to large hematomas show the typical MRI appearance of mixed signal intensity surrounded by edema, but small hemorrhages usually show minimal surrounding edema and may have similar appearance to calcifications, microinfarcts, and intravascular thrombus.

Hyperacute and late subacute microhemorrhages, which show high signal on DWI, may go unnoticed on gradient echo sequences (due to insufficient T2 shortening and/or lack of paramagnetic properties) and cannot be differentiated from acute microinfarctions.

12.2.3 Hemorrhagic Infarctions

According to several studies, DWI can differentiate hemorrhage from pure infarction in hemorrhagic arterial (▶ Fig. 12.8) or venous (▶ Fig. 12.9) infarcts by showing areas of low signal intensity within areas of restricted diffusion. The signal intensity of these hemorrhagic lesions corresponds to acute or early subacute hematomas, but the clinical relevance of these findings is unclear.[8,12,13,25]

The thrombus inside a venous sinus can also be depicted on DWI images (▶ Fig. 12.10).

12.2.4 Extra-axial Hematomas

The evolution of the MRI signal in extra-axial hematomas is less predictable than the signal changes occurring in intraparenchymal hematomas. Like parenchymal hemorrhage, subdural hematomas

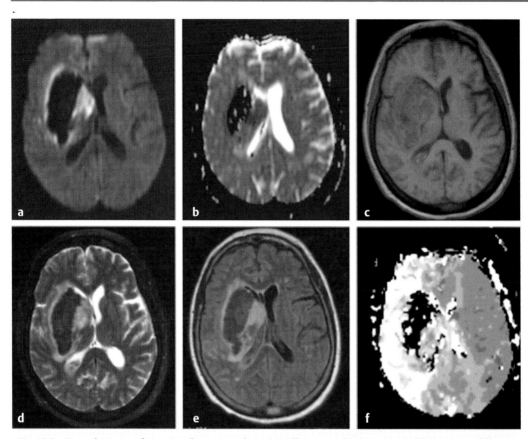

Fig. 12.8 Hemorrhagic transformation of an acute infarct. (**a**) Diffusion weighted imaging and (**b**) apparent diffusion coefficient map show restricted diffusion around an acute hemorrhagic lesion. (**c**) A T1-weighted image shows an iso-/hypointense hematoma. (**d**) T2-weighted and (**e**) fluid-attenuated inversion recovery images show a well-demarcated hypointense hematoma surrounded by a hyperintense area of cytotoxic and vasogenic edema. (**f**) Mean transit time magnetic resonance perfusion shows a delayed transit time in the right middle cerebral artery vascular territory.

(SDHs) have five distinct stages of evolution. However, because the dura is well vascularized and oxygen tension is high, progression from one stage to another is slower. Additionally, recurrent bleeding occurs frequently, further complicating the expected MRI signal intensity. Subdural hematomas usually show heterogeneous low signal on DWI (▶ Fig. 12.11) that may be explained by the mixed nature of these lesions, which usually contain acute, early, and late subacute blood products and CSF. Hypointensity is probably caused by paramagnetic intracellular deoxyhemoglobin and paramagnetic intracellular methemoglobin.[12] Epidural hematomas (EDHs) evolve in a manner similar to that of SDHs. EDHs are differentiated from SDHs on the basis of their classic biconvexity versus medial concavity and on the basis of the intensity of the fibrous dura mater (▶ Fig. 12.12).

12.2.5 Subarachnoid Hemorrhage

In the evaluation of acute subarachnoid hemorrhage (SAH) DWI is probably not clinically relevant because these patients usually undergo CT, which is over 90% sensitive for its detection. Conventional MRI, particularly FLAIR, is also very sensitive for SAH detection, leaving little if any use for DWI in this setting. Furthermore, several studies have concluded that DWI is not accurate in the detection of SAH.[12,20,21,26] However, Busch et at[9] detected DWI changes during acute SAH in an animal model.

12.3 Summary

The appearance of intracerebral hematomas on DWI is influenced not only by restriction of diffusion but also by magnetic susceptibility and T2

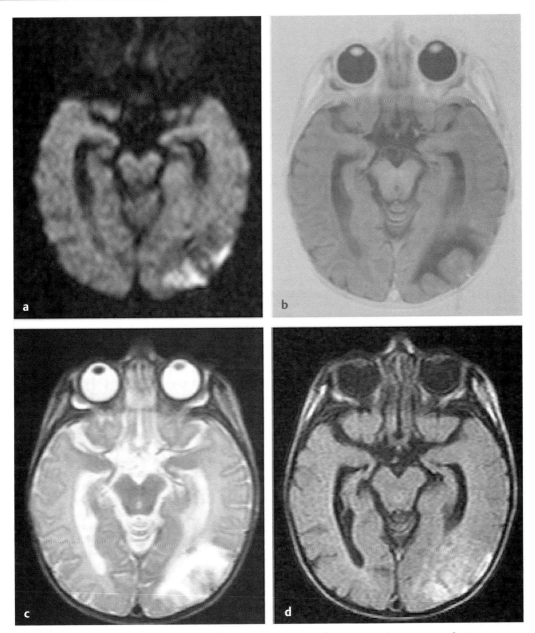

Fig. 12.9 Venous hemorrhagic infarct. (**a**) Diffusion weighted imaging shows a hemorrhagic venous infarct seen as an area of restricted diffusion with a small hemorrhagic central hypointense lesion. (**b**) On T1 inversion recovery, (**c**) T2-weighted, and (**d**) fluid-attenuated inversion recovery images the hemorrhagic area is difficult to depict.

signal intensity. T2 shine-through effects may contribute to the hyperintensity of hematomas on DWI, whereas T2 blackout effects may be responsible for the hypointense signal in hematomas. Further research is required to confirm the pathophysiological and biochemical basis underlying the imaging findings and ADC values of intracerebral hemorrhages. However, the findings here described reinforce the well-known principle that DWI signal intensity changes should be interpreted in light of T2 signal intensity changes, especially during the early period. DWI is also accurate for detection of hemorrhagic venous or arterial infarctions and subdural hematomas but has low

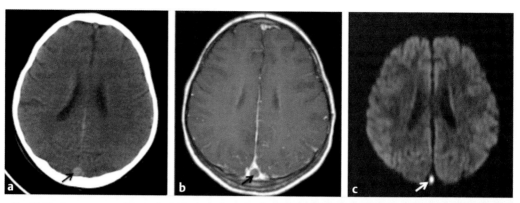

Fig. 12.10 Superior sagittal sinus thrombosis. (**a**) Axial computed tomography shows the hyperdense thrombus inside the superior sagittal sinus (arrow). (**b**) Postcontrast T1-weighted imaging shows filling defect caused by the thrombus (delta sign) (arrow). (**c**) Diffusion weighted imaging shows the hyperintense thrombus (arrow), probably in the hyperacute stage.

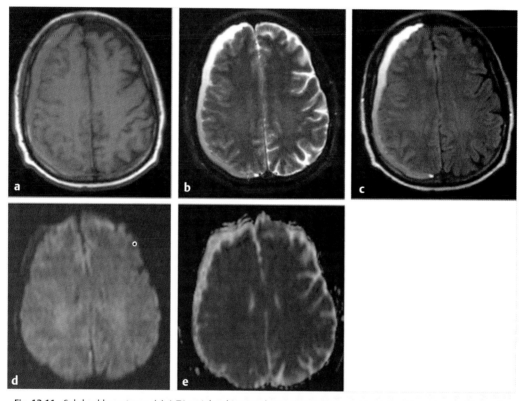

Fig. 12.11 Subdural hematoma. (**a**) A T1-weighted image shows an isointense right subdural hematoma with small areas of high signal intensity. (**b**) On T2-weighted and (**c**) fluid-attenuated inversion recovery images the hematoma is seen as a hyperintense subdural collection with an ill-defined blood-fluid level. (**d**) Diffusion weighted imaging shows a heterogeneous hypointense hematoma with hyperintensity on (**e**) the apparent diffusion coefficient map.

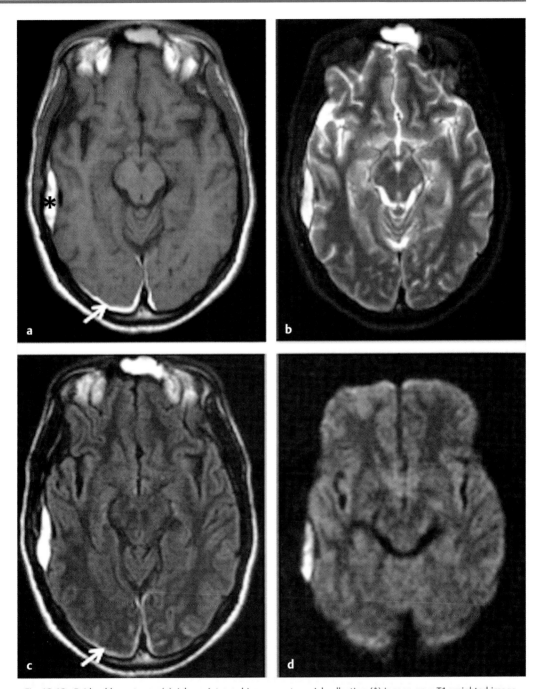

Fig. 12.12 Epidural hematoma. (a) A hyperintense biconvex extra-axial collection (*) is seen on a T1-weighted image, (b) T2-weighted image, (c) fluid-attenuated inversion recovery (FLAIR), and (d) diffusion weighted imaging. Note the subdural hematoma (arrow) well depicted on (a) T1-weighted and (c) FLAIR images.

diagnostic accuracy in small parenchymal hemorrhage and SAH.

References

[1] Bradley WG. Hemorrhage and brain iron. In: Stark DD, Bradley WG. Eds. Magnetic Resonance Imaging. 2nd ed. St Louis, MO: Mosby; 1992

[2] Atlas SW, Thulborn KR. MR detection of hyperacute parenchymal hemorrhage of the brain. AJNR Am J Neuroradiol 1998; 19(8): 1471–1477

[3] Gomori JM, Grossman RI, Goldberg HI, Zimmerman RA, Bilaniuk LT. Intracranial hematomas: imaging by high-field MR. Radiology 1985; 157(1): 87–93

[4] Maldjian JA, Listerud J, Moonis G, Siddiqi F. Computing diffusion rates in T2-dark hematomas and areas of low T2 signal. AJNR Am J Neuroradiol 2001; 22(1): 112–118

[5] Thulborn KR, Waterton JC, Matthews PM, Radda GK. Oxygenation dependence of the transverse relaxation time of water protons in whole blood at high field. Biochim Biophys Acta 1982; 714(2): 265–270

[6] Bryant RG, Marill K, Blackmore C, Francis C. Magnetic relaxation in blood and blood clots. Magn Reson Med 1990; 13 (1): 133–144

[7] Clark RA, Watanabe AT, Bradley WG, Jr, Roberts JD. Acute hematomas: effects of deoxygenation, hematocrit, and fibrin-clot formation and retraction on T2 shortening. Radiology 1990; 175(1): 201–206

[8] Silvera S, Oppenheim C, Touzé E, et al. Spontaneous intracerebral hematoma on diffusion weighted images: influence of T2-shine-through and T2-blackout effects. AJNR Am J Neuroradiol 2005; 26(2): 236–241

[9] Busch E, Beaulieu C, de Crespigny A, Moseley ME. Diffusion MR imaging during acute subarachnoid hemorrhage in rats. Stroke 1998; 29(10): 2155–2161

[10] Shoamanesh A, Catanese L, Sakai O, Pikula A, Kase CS. Diffusion weighted imaging hyperintensities in intracerebral hemorrhage: microinfarcts or microbleeds? Ann Neurol 2013; 73(6): 795–796

[11] Kang BK, Na DG, Ryoo JW, Byun HS, Roh HG, Pyeun YS. Diffusion weighted MR imaging of intracerebral hemorrhage. Korean J Radiol 2001; 2(4): 183–191

[12] Khedr SA, Kassem HM, Hazzou AM, et al. MRI diffusion weighted imaging in intracranial hemorrhage (ICH). Egypt J Radiol Nucl Med 2013; 44: 625–634

[13] Chung SP, Ha YR, Kim SW, Yoo IS. Diffusion weighted MRI of intracerebral hemorrhage clinically undifferentiated from ischemic stroke. Am J Emerg Med 2003; 21(3): 236–240

[14] Atlas SW, DuBois P, Singer MB, Lu D. Diffusion measurements in intracranial hematomas: implications for MR imaging of acute stroke. AJNR Am J Neuroradiol 2000; 21 (7): 1190–1194

[15] Linfante I, Llinas RH, Caplan LR, Warach S. MRI features of intracerebral hemorrhage within 2 hours from symptom onset. Stroke 1999; 30(11): 2263–2267

[16] González RG, Schaefer PW, Buonanno FS, et al. Diffusion weighted MR imaging: diagnostic accuracy in patients imaged within 6 hours of stroke symptom onset. Radiology 1999; 210(1): 155–162

[17] Schellinger PD, Jansen O, Fiebach JB, Hacke W, Sartor K. A standardized MRI stroke protocol: comparison with CT in hyperacute intracerebral hemorrhage. Stroke 1999; 30(4): 765–768

[18] Schaefer PW, Grant PE, Gonzalez RG. Diffusion weighted MR imaging of the brain. Radiology 2000; 217(2): 331–345

[19] Wiesmann M, Mayer TE, Yousry I, Hamann GF, Brückmann H. Detection of hyperacute parenchymal hemorrhage of the brain using echo-planar T2*-weighted and diffusion weighted MRI. Eur Radiol 2001; 11(5): 849–853

[20] Mitchell P, Wilkinson ID, Hoggard N, et al. Detection of subarachnoid haemorrhage with magnetic resonance imaging. J Neurol Neurosurg Psychiatry 2001; 70(2): 205–211

[21] Rajeshkannan R, Moorthy S, Sreekumar KP, et al. Clinical applications of diffusion weighted MR imaging: a review. Indian J Radiol Imaging 2006; 16: 705–710

[22] Wintermark M, Maeder P, Reichhart M, Schnyder P, Bogousslavsky J, Meuli R. MR pattern of hyperacute cerebral hemorrhage. J Magn Reson Imaging 2002; 15(6): 705–709

[23] Does MD, Zhong J, Gore JC. In vivo measurement of ADC change due to intravascular susceptibility variation. Magn Reson Med 1999; 41(2): 236–240

[24] Lin DD, Filippi CG, Steever AB, Zimmerman RD. Detection of intracranial hemorrhage: comparison between gradient-echo images and b(0) images obtained from diffusion weighted echo-planar sequences. AJNR Am J Neuroradiol 2001; 22(7): 1275–1281

[25] Packard AS, Kase CS, Aly AS, Barest GD. "Computed tomography-negative" intracerebral hemorrhage: case report and implications for management. Arch Neurol 2003; 60(8): 1156–1159

[26] Wiesmann M, Mayer TE, Yousry I, Medele R, Hamann GF, Brückmann H. Detection of hyperacute subarachnoid hemorrhage of the brain by using magnetic resonance imaging. J Neurosurg 2002; 96(4): 684–689

13 Diffusion Weighted Imaging and Diffusion Tensor Imaging in Spine and Spinal Cord Diseases

Majda M. Thurnher

Key Points

- Diffusion weighted imaging (DWI) is the method of choice for the detection of spinal cord infarction.
- Diffusion tensor imaging (DTI) can be helpful for differentiating ependymoma from astrocytoma in adults.
- DTI is a promising technique for evaluating patients with spinal cord injury (detecting the injury epicenter, differentiating injured from normal spinal cord in the absence of T2-signal changes).
- DWI is a useful tool for differentiating benign from malignant vertebral body fractures (when used with conventional sequences).
- DWI can be a helpful tool for differentiating Modic I changes from acute spondylodiskitis.

13.1 Introduction

13.1.1 Technical Considerations

The role of diffusion weighted magnetic resonance imaging (DWI) in the evaluation of brain diseases was established shortly after its introduction. DWI became an irreplaceable part of the routine brain imaging protocol. Further developments with diffusion tensor magnetic resonance imaging (DTI) and fiber tractography (FT) have catapulted brain imaging to an even higher level.

Since the first published report on the usefulness of DWI in the differentiation between osteoporotic and malignant vertebral body fractures in 1998,[1] physicists and clinicians continue to grapple with constructing clinically applicable and reproducible DWI and DTI sequences for the spine and spinal cord. Nevertheless, obtaining spinal cord DWI and DTI remains a challenge due to numerous technical difficulties. The size of the spinal cord, the macroscopic motion related to the surrounding cerebrospinal fluid (CSF) pulsations, breathing and swallowing movement artifacts, and local field inhomogeneities are the major technical issues. Technical solutions are needed to optimize both image acquisition and image processing. Studies published on DWI and DTI of the spine are limited and have mainly been restricted to the cervical spine.

Recently, fairly good technical solutions have been developed, such as multishot echo-planar imaging (EPI), diffusion weighted periodically rotated overlapping parallel lines with enhanced reconstruction (PROPELLER), spin-echo navigator spiral DTI, and parallel imaging. The acquisition times have been reduced, allowing implementation of DWI/DTI in routine clinical protocols. Through spatially selective excitation, zoomed DWI allows for acquisition of high-resolution images, with a reduced scan time, due to a reduced field-of-view (rFOV) in the phase-encoding direction.[2] rFOV sequences[3,4] have shown promise in producing high-quality, *in vivo* human spinal cord DTI. In one larger study of 223 patients, performed on a 1.5 T clinical scanner, an rFOV DWI sequence added clinical utility in 33% of cases where pathology was done.[4] The rFOV DWI sequence was found to be helpful in the evaluation of acute infarction, demyelination, infection, neoplasm, and intradural and epidural collections.[4] In another study, the diagnostic value of DWI and the measurement of the apparent diffusion coefficient (ADC) were evaluated in 33 patients who presented with a spinal cord syndrome due to a noncompressive myelopathy.[5] ADC values measured in that study were significantly lower in spinal cord infarct (mean ADC 0.81×10^{-3} mm^2/s) when compared with inflammatory spinal cord lesions (mean ADC 1.37×10^{-3} mm^2/s) and with those measured in healthy control spinal cord (mean ADC 0.93×10^{-3} mm^2/s).[5]

The usefulness of DWI and DTI of the spine has also been reported in children. In one study, five controls and five children with cervical spinal cord injury (SCI) were imaged by using a single-shot, echo-planar, diffusion weighted sequence. Children with SCI showed reduced fractional anisotropy (FA) and increased diffusion (D) values compared with controls. The study has shown that the differences in diffusion metrics between non-injured and injured spinal cords can be demonstrated in the pediatric population.[6]

13.2 Clinical Applications for DWI and DTI of the Spinal Cord

13.2.1 Spinal Cord Ischemia

Acute spinal cord ischemia is an uncommon condition that accounts for 5 to 8% of acute myelopathies. It is associated with severe functional neurological loss, and paraplegia in up to 33% of the cases.[7] Aortic dissection, open thoracoabdominal aortic surgery (5–21% risk), mechanical trauma, and systemic hypotension are the most common causes of acute spinal cord ischemia.[7] Rarely, a fibrocartilaginous embolism (FCE) with a progressive onset (over several hours) could be the cause.[8] Linear T2-hyperintensity on sagittal magnetic resonance imaging (MRI) scans, and the appearance of "snake-eyes" on axial T2-weighted MRI in the cord, are typical MRI findings. The spinal cord will be swollen, and contrast enhancement will be present in the subacute stage. Although MRI is the method of choice in the detection of spinal cord ischemia, in a large number of cases, initial MRI will not show any abnormality.[7]

There have been only smaller series published that describe DWI findings in acute spinal cord ischemia.[9,10,11,12,13,14] The ADC measured in one published series of spinal cord infarction ranged between 0.23 and 0.86×10^{-3} mm^2/s.[14] The shortest time reported in the literature between the onset of clinical symptoms and abnormalities shown on DWI was 3 hours after the onset of symptoms (▶ Fig. 13.1). In one small series of four children with anterior spinal artery infarction after minor trauma, DWI confirmed the clinical diagnosis in all cases[15] and showed the feasibility of DWI in spinal cord ischemia in a pediatric population.

Clinical rationale for DWI/DTI in spinal cord ischemia:

- Early detection of spinal cord infarction when conventional sequences are unremarkable
- Detection of spinal cord infarction due to FCE in young athletes

13.2.2 Spinal Cord Tumors

The most common intramedullary tumors in adults are ependymomas, followed by astrocytomas, other gliomas, hemangioblastomas, and metastases. In the pediatric population, astrocytomas are diagnosed in a higher percentage of cases. Diagnostic challenges are the differentiation of ependymoma and astrocytoma, and the differentiation of resectable from nonresectable spinal cord tumors based on MRI findings. Ependymomas and hemangioblastomas are considered resectable, whereas astrocytomas, due to their infiltrative nature, are considered nonresectable. Therefore, the determination of resectability is essential. The value of DWI and DTI in predicting the resectability of intramedullary tumors has been shown in a recent study.[16] Patients were classified according to the fiber course with respect to the lesion. The results were compared with the surgical findings (existence or absence of cleavage plane). Despite the low number of patients in that study (14 patients), the results showed good interrater reliability for DTI and intraoperative findings, and the presence or absence of a cleavage plane.[16] Caution is necessary when DTI is used in the pediatric population. The pilocytic astrocytomas, that are common intramedullary neoplasms in children, show histological and structural differences from the infiltrating astrocytomas seen in adults. In one published series of 10 children with intramedullary neoplasms, preoperative DTI was performed to characterize the margins of tumors for surgical planning.[17] In all pilocytic astrocytomas (seven cases) (▶ Fig. 13.2) and one ependymoma (▶ Fig. 13.3), splaying of fibers was found. The ganglioglioma and high-grade glioma showed evidence of infiltration of fibers.[17] In another small series, displacement of the fibers was seen in three cases of ependymoma.[18]

Ducreaux et al described DTI findings in five cases of spinal cord astrocytoma (▶ Fig. 13.4).[18,19] The data suggest that FT can be used for visualization of warped and destroyed fibers in cases of solid astrocytomas, but showed some limitations in cystic astrocytomas. Furthermore, when using DTI metrics, astrocytomas, ependymomas, and metastases showed similar FA values.[18] The lowest FA values were measured in metastases and the highest in hemangioblastomas. Metastatic infiltration of nerve roots can also be detected by DTI (▶ Fig. 13.5).

It is imperative to identify drop metastases in children with brain tumors. The presence of drop metastases is associated with a poor prognosis, so early detection is crucial to allow modification of the treatment. Recently, a case of drop metastasis was reported in which readout-segmented echoplanar imaging (EPI) was used to identify hypercellular metastases in a child with a primary CNS tumor.[20]

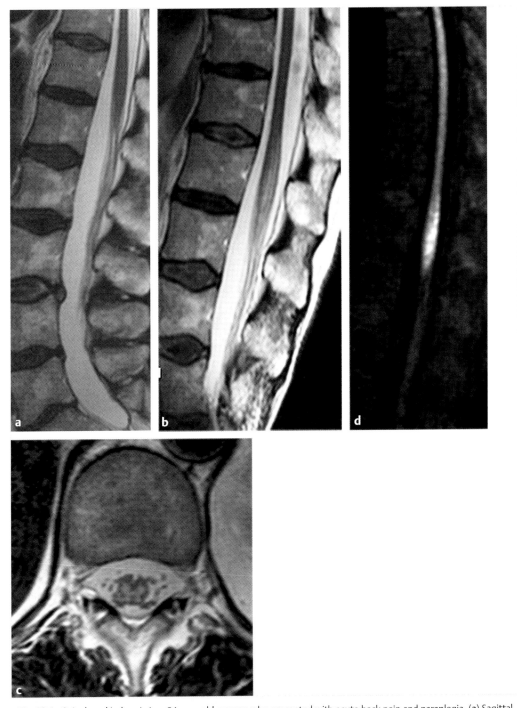

Fig. 13.1 Spinal cord ischemia in a 64-year-old woman who presented with acute back pain and paraplegia. (**a**) Sagittal T2-weighted image of the lumbar spine performed 4 hours after the onset of symptoms shows no abnormality. (**b**) Sagittal T2-weighted image 48 hours later demonstrates hyperintensity and swelling of the conus medullaris. (**c**) On the T2-weighted image, there is swelling of the anterior gray matter. (**d**) Diffusion weighted imaging shows high signal intensity as the result of restricted diffusion in the conus medullaris (with low apparent diffusion coefficient, not shown).

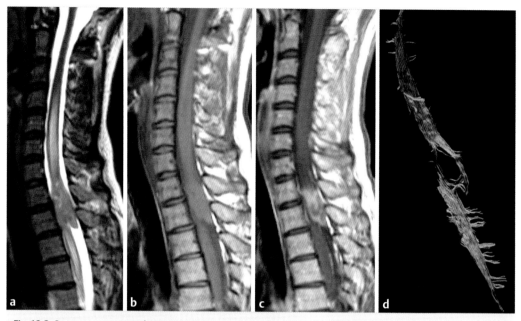

Fig. 13.2 Surgery-proven ependymoma in a 39-year-old female patient (**a**) On the sagittal T2WI image of the cervical spine, a bulky mass is noted in the spinal cord at the Th1–2 level, with cord hyperintensity above and below the mass, representing edema. (**b**) The mass is T1-isointense to the spinal cord. (**c**) On the post-contrast T1WI image, strong enhancement is shown of the solid tumor part. (**d**) DT-FT Diffusion tensor-Fiber tractograpy shows centrally located mass with displacement of the fibers.

The differentiation between an intramedullary tumor and tumorlike lesions (TLLs) in the cervicomedullary junction region and cervical spinal cord can sometimes be challenging. A recently published series evaluated DTI and perfusion-weighted imaging (PWI) in 12 patients with intramedullary tumors and 13 with TLL in the cervicomedullary junction and cervical spinal cord. The mean FA value of tumors was found to be significantly lower when compared with TLL, and the mean trace ADC and peak height values of tumors were significantly higher.[21]

Clinical Rationale for DWI/DTI in Spinal Cord Tumors

- Differentiation of ependymoma and astrocytoma in adults (not in children!) (splayed and destroyed fibers in ependymoma, diffuse involvement of fibers in astrocytoma)
- Determination of resectability of spinal cord tumors
- Identification of hypercellular drop metastases in children with central nervous system (CNS) neoplasms

- Differentiation between intramedullary tumor and tumefactive demyelinating lesions in the cervicomedullary junction or cervical spinal cord (high perfusion and low FA in tumors)

13.2.3 Multiple Sclerosis

Multiple sclerosis (MS) is an inflammatory demyelinating disorder of the brain and spinal cord, with cord lesions found in up to 99% of autopsy cases.[22,23]

Increased diffusivity has been found in focal MS lesions in the cord, with a significantly higher isotropic diffusion coefficient, when compared to healthy controls.[24] Valsasina et al have shown, in their study of 44 patients with MS and 17 healthy controls, that the average cervical cord FA was significantly lower in MS patients compared to controls.[25]

Early studies that performed DTI measurements in patients without T2-visible cord signal abnormalities have revealed significantly lower FA values in the lateral, dorsal, and central parts of the normal-appearing white matter (NAWM) in MS patients.[26] Several studies confirmed that significant changes in DTI metrics are present in the

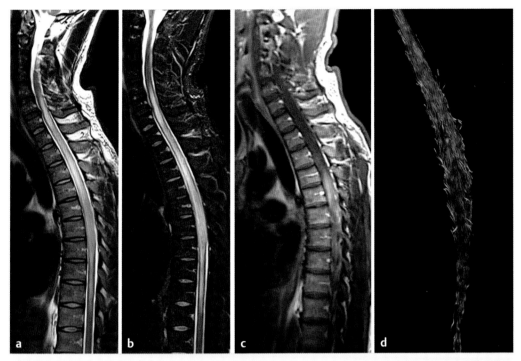

Fig. 13.3 Histology-proven the spinal cord astrocytoma (grade III) in a 38-year-old male patient who presented with pain in the thoracic region, sensory disturbances in the left lower extremity followed by left hemiparesis, and gait disorder. On spinal sagittal T2-weighted image (**a**) and Short tau inversion recovery (STIR) (**b**) hyperintensity and enlargement of the cord is detected from the C6 to the T10 level. (**c**) On enhanced T1-weighted image, an ill-defined enhancement is shown at the T3–6 level. (**d**) Fiber tractography shows diffuse infiltration of the fibers with no displacement.

cervical spinal cord of MS patients, in the absence of spinal cord signal abnormality at conventional MRI examination.[26,27,28] Diffusional kurtosis imaging of the spinal cord, used recently in one study, has demonstrated not only white but also gray matter damage in patients with MS.[29]

Furthermore, DTI metrics of the spinal cord in MS patients has been compared with electrophysiological studies. On DTI acquired in 28 healthy volunteers and 41 MS patients, FA and ADC were evaluated in NAWM at the cervical level and correlated with motor-evoked potentials ($n = 34$).[30] Asymmetric anatomical changes in spinal cord NAWM were found in DTI, which corresponded to asymmetric electrophysiological deficits for both arms and legs. Overall, DTI studies of the spinal cord in MS patients have demonstrated and confirmed the spinal cord damage and opened the pathway for further clinical studies.

13.2.4 Neuromyelitis Optica

The identification, in 2004, of a disease-specific autoantibody, neuromyelitis optica immunoglobulin G (NMO-IgG), in the serum of patients with NMO ended the debate about whether NMO is a variant of MS or a distinct disease.[31] NMO-IgG binds selectively to aquaporin-4 (AQP-4), a water channel that is densely expressed in astrocytic foot processes at the blood-brain barrier (BBB). NMO is currently defined as an autoimmune antibody-mediated disease, induced by a specific serum autoantibody, the NMO-IgG, directed against AQP-4. Unilateral or bilateral severe optic neuritis (ON) usually precedes longitudinally extensive transverse myelitis (LETM). Extensive signal abnormalities that extend to multiple segments (>three segments), with cavitations, and patchy enhancement are typical imaging findings. Reported brain abnormalities range from 20 to 89% of cases, depending on geographical area.[32]

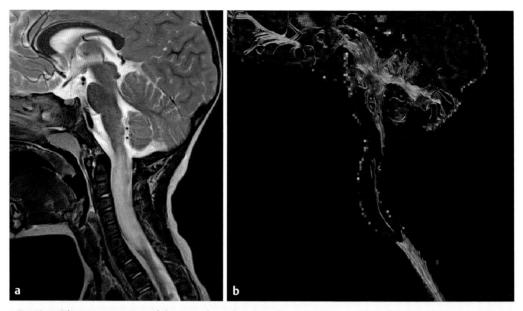

Fig. 13.4 Pilocytic astrocytoma of the cervical spinal cord in a five-year-old boy. (**a**) Sagittal T2-weighted image shows high signal intensity mass in the cervical spinal cord extending from C2 to the T1 levels, with cord enlargement. The mass did not show enhancement (not shown). (**b**) Fiber tractography nicely demonstrates splaying of the fibers.

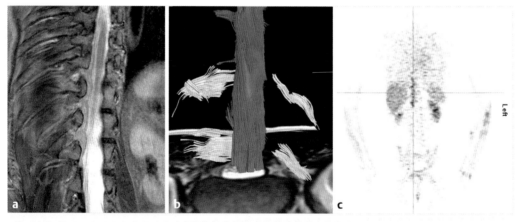

Fig. 13.5 Biopsy-proven metastatic neuropathy in a 44-year-old woman with breast carcinoma who presented with lumbar pain irradiating to the right side. (**a**) Thoracic spine coronal short tau inversion recovery (STIR) shows low signal linear abnormalities following the spinal roots over multiple segments. (**b**) Diffusion tensor imaging demonstrates asymmetry of the nerve roots with multiple thickened nerve roots on the right side. (**c**) Positron emission tomography/computed tomography confirmed metastatic disease affecting multiple thoracic nerve roots.

The crucial point is the differentiation from MS, because some MS treatments can exacerbate NMO. DTI of the cervical spinal cord was used in one study to assess cord damage in NMO.[33] Ten NMO patients showed reduced FA and increased MD, compared with 12 healthy controls. In another study, decreased FA was found in patients with NMO when compared with patients with relapsing-remitting MS.[34] The study demonstrated extensive normal-appearing spinal cord damage in NMO patients, including peripheral areas of the cervical spinal cord.

13.2.5 Transverse Myelitis

Transverse myelitis (TM) is an acute inflammatory disease of the spinal cord with a heterogeneous pathogenesis. MRI findings include central T2-hyperintensity usually extending over more than two segments, and involving more than two-thirds of the cross-sectional area of the cord, with or without enhancement.[35]

In one study, a pulse-triggered DTI sequence with an rFOV technique and coronal acquisition was used for the assessment of the cervical spinal cord in patients with myelitis.[36] Qualitative assessment of the spinal cord damage was evaluated in 12 healthy volunteers and 40 consecutive patients with myelitis (25 MS, 11 neuromyelitis optica, 1 sarcoidosis, 1 Gougerot–Sjögren syndrome, and 2 cases of idiopathic myelitis). FA and MD measurements clearly demonstrated a significant FA increase and an MD decrease in active lesions. In the absence of active lesions, and regardless of the pathology, FA decreased and MD increased significantly.[36]

Clinical Rationale for DWI/DTI in MS, NMO, and TM

- Not yet part of the routine protocols
- May be useful in the future for therapy monitoring
- Differentiation between demyelinating/inflammatory disorders and spinal cord ischemia

13.2.6 Spinal Cord Trauma

Knowing the limitations of conventional MRI techniques in estimation of the extent of Spinal cord injury (SCI), there is a need for the evaluation of new techniques. DWI has been first evaluated in animal studies showing promising results.[37] The comparison of conventional T2-weighted images and DWI in acute SCI showed comparable detection rates for spinal cord damage in 18 patients within 24 hours postinjury.[38] The detection rates of high signals on T2-weighted and DWI did not show significant differences, being 94 and 72%, respectively.[38] In another study, conventional MRI and multishot, navigator-corrected DWI were performed in 20 patients with acute spinal cord trauma using 1.5 T MRI within 72 h after the onset of trauma.[39] In that study 20 cases were classified

into four types: edema type (10 cases), mixed type (6 cases), hemorrhage type (2 cases), and compressed type (2 cases). DWI hyperintensity was detected in edema cases, most probably representing cytotoxic edema, as well as in two patients with cord compression. Inhomogeneous signals were seen in patients with mixed-type injury. An important limitation of the study is the lack of axial DWI images, lack of normal controls, and low b values (400 and 500 s/mm^2) used.[39]

Clinical Rationale for DWI/DTI in Traumatic Spinal Cord Injury

- Not yet part of the routine protocols
- Promising technique for evaluation of injury epicenter, differentiation of injured and normal spinal cord in the absence of T2-signal changes

13.3 Clinical Applications for DWI and DTI of the Vertebral Bodies

13.3.1 Vertebral Body Fracture

The normal bone marrow in an adult consists of approximately 50% fat and 50% water.

Osteoporotic fractured vertebra contains fat and edema. In malignant vertebral fractures, the tumor cells usually have replaced the bone marrow. The reliable imaging differentiation of benign and malignant vertebral body fractures remains a diagnostic challenge. In the first published study, all benign osteoporotic fractures were hypointense or isointense on steady-state free procession (SSFP)-based DWI, whereas malignant fractures showed hyperintensity.[1] Malignant fractures show restricted diffusion due to dense tumor-cell packing (▶ Fig. 13.6). Acute osteoporotic fractures demonstrate increased diffusion caused by increased water proton mobility in the bone marrow edema (▶ Fig. 13.7). Important exceptions to that rule are sclerotic metastases and treated metastases, which will be hypointense (false-negative results).[40] Reported ADC values of benign osteoporotic and benign traumatic fractures vary from 0.32 to 2.23×10^{-3} mm^2/s, whereas the range in malignant fractures or metastases is 0.19 to 1.04×10^{-3} mm^2/s.[41] The calculated diffusion coefficients will

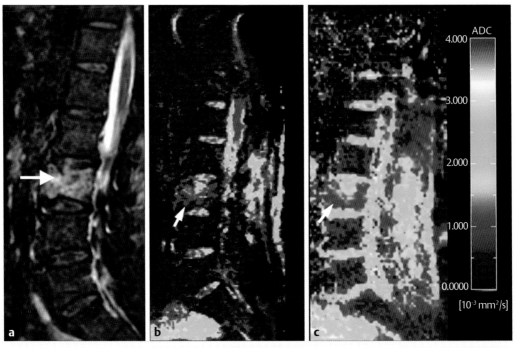

Fig. 13.6 Metastatic vertebral body fracture in a 71-year-old patient with a history of adenocarcinoma. (**a**) Sagittal short tau inversion recovery magnetic resonance imaging (STIR) shows high signal in the L3 vertebral body. Apparent diffusion coefficient (ADC) maps calculated from (**b**) diffusion weighted echo-planar imaging (DW-EPI) and (**c**) half-Fourier acquisition single-shot turbo-spin-echo diffusion weighted MR (DW-HASTE) images show average ADC values of 0.9×10^{-4} mm^2/s (DW-EPI) and 1.38×10^{-4} mm^2/s (DW-HASTE) (arrows). (Courtesy of Andrea Baur-Melnyk. From Magnetic Resonance Imaging of the Bone Marrow, 2013. With kind permission from Springer Science and Business Media.)

depend on the technique applied and also on fat saturation. The diffusion weighted reversed fast imaging with steady state free precession (DW-PSIF) sequence (delta = 3 ms) was reported in a recent study to have the highest accuracy in differentiating benign from malignant vertebral fractures. Qualitatively assessed opposed-phase, DW-EPI, and DW single-shot turbo spin echo (TSE) sequences and ADCs (DW-EPI) cannot be used to accurately differentiate benign from malignant vertebral fractures.[41]

In another recently published study, DWI (*b* values: 0, 800, and 1,400 s/mm^2) were analyzed in 62 patients with acute compression fractures.[42] At qualitative analysis, hyperintensity was seen in 87% of malignant compression fractures, but only in 22% of acute osteoporotic compression fractures. The median ADCs of malignant fractures were significantly lower than those of benign

fractures. When readers used a combination of conventional sequences and DWI, increased sensitivity, specificity, and accuracy were observed (97–100%).[42]

Clinical Rationale for DWI in Vertebral Body Fractures

- Differentiation between benign and malignant fractures (when used with conventional sequences)

13.3.2 Degenerative Changes and Spondylodiskitis

Degenerative end plate changes, such as Modic type I and spondylodiskitis, may both present with similar clinical symptoms and imaging findings.

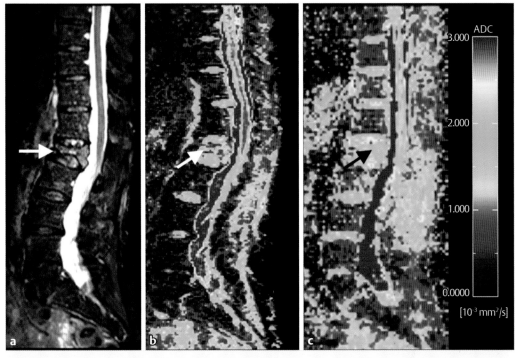

Fig. 13.7 Osteoporotic vertebral body fracture in a 70-year-old patient. **(a)** Sagittal short tau inversion recovery image shows hyperintense signal in the L2 vertebral body (arrow). Apparent diffusion coefficient (ADC) maps from L2 vertebral body (arrow in **b** and **c**) calculated from **(b)** diffusion weighted echo-planar imaging (DW-EPI) and **(c)** half-Fourier acquisition single-shot turbo-spin-echo diffusion weighted MR (DW-HASTE) images show higher average ADC values of 1.25×10^{-4} mm^2/s (DW-EPI) and 1.73×10^{-4} mm^2/s (DW-HASTE) (arrows). (Courtesy of Andrea Baur-Melnyk. From Magnetic Resonance Imaging of the Bone Marrow, 2013. With kind permission from Springer Science and Business Media.)

Moreover, a postcontrast MRI study will show enhancement in both diseases. In one study, 27 patients with erosive intervertebral osteochondrosis Modic type I, and 18 patients with spondylodiskitis were examined with conventional and DWI sequences.[43] All patients with spondylodiskitis showed DWI hyperintensity of the vertebral end plates (▶ Fig. 13.8), whereas in patients with Modic I changes, hypointensity was observed (▶ Fig. 13.9).[43]

In another study, a "claw sign" was described as highly suggestive of degeneration, and its absence is strongly indicative of diskitis/osteomyelitis.[44] Seventy-three patients with imaging features that suggested Modic type 1 changes were classified clinically into three groups: true degenerative Modic type 1 changes ($n = 33$); confirmed diskitis/osteomyelitis ($n = 20$); and suspected infection

($n = 20$). These patients were examined with DWI.[44] When a definite claw was seen, patients were proved to be infection-free. Conversely, in cases of absence of claw sign (diffuse DWI pattern), there was proved infection in 17 of 17 cases (100%) and 13 of 14 cases (93%).[44]

Clinical Rationale for DWI in Degenerative Spine Diseases

- Differentiation of Modic I changes and spondylodiskitis

13.4 Conclusion

Considering the absence of a true "gold standard," the variety of sequences used in published studies,

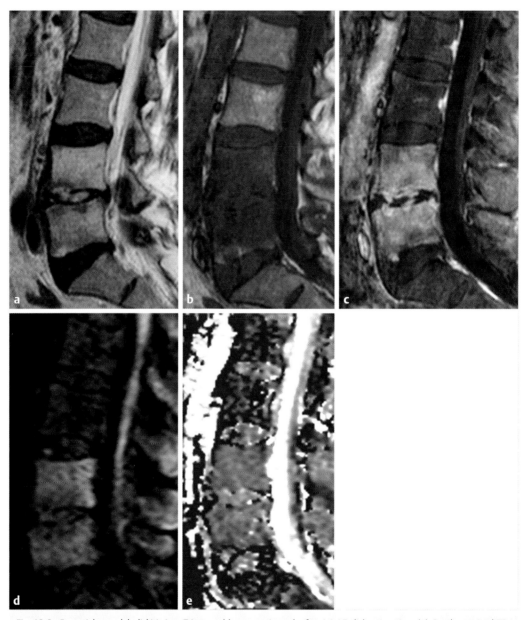

Fig. 13.8 Bacterial spondylodiskitis in a 74-year-old woman 1 week after L4–L5 disk extraction. (**a**) On the sagittal T2-weighted image, high signal is observed in the L4 and L5 vertebral bodies, as well as in the disk space. (**b**) Low signal is demonstrated on the sagittal T1-weighted image. (**c**) On the enhanced T1-weighted image, there is marked enhancement of the affected vertebral bodies. On (**d**) Diffusion weighted imaging and (**e**) the apparent diffusion coefficient map, homogeneous high signal is present in the L4 and L5 vertebral bodies.

and especially the small number of patients in published series, DTI and DT-FT of the spine and spinal cord have not been fully validated.

However, the results demonstrating the accuracy and utility of DWI and DTI in different spinal cord diseases and emerging technical solutions will help to increase confidence in these techniques.

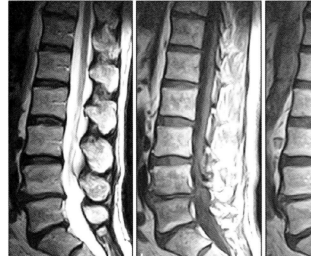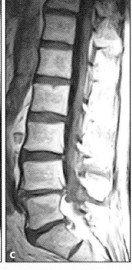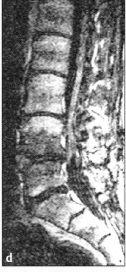

Fig. 13.9 Modic I changes. (**a**) On sagittal T2-weighted imaging, no signal change is seen. (**b**) Bandlike low signal is demonstrated on the sagittal T1-weighted image in the L4 and L5 vertebral bodies. (**c**) On the postcontrast T1-weighted image, enhancement of the affected vertebral bodies is shown. (**d**) On diffusion weighted imaging, low signal is present in the L4 and L5 vertebral bodies, suggestive of elevated diffusion. (Courtesy of Cem Calli.)

References

[1] Baur A, Stäbler A, Brüning R, et al. Diffusion weighted MR imaging of bone marrow: differentiation of benign versus pathologic compression fractures. Radiology 1998; 207(2): 349–356

[2] Seeger A, Klose U, Bischof F, Strobel J, Ernemann U, Hauser TK. Zoomed EPI DWI of acute spinal ischemia using a parallel transmission system. Clin Neuroradiol 2014

[3] Xu J, Shimony JS, Klawiter EC, et al. Improved in vivo diffusion tensor imaging of human cervical spinal cord. Neuroimage 2013; 67: 64–76

[4] Andre JB, Zaharchuk G, Saritas E, et al. Clinical evaluation of reduced field-of-view diffusion weighted imaging of the cervical and thoracic spine and spinal cord. AJNR Am J Neuroradiol 2012; 33(10): 1860–1866

[5] Marcel C, Kremer S, Jeantroux J, Blanc F, Dietemann JL, De Sèze J. Diffusion weighted imaging in noncompressive myelopathies: a 33-patient prospective study. J Neurol 2010; 257(9): 1438–1445

[6] Mohamed FB, Hunter LN, Barakat N, et al. Diffusion tensor imaging of the pediatric spinal cord at 1.5T: preliminary results. AJNR Am J Neuroradiol 2011; 32(2): 339–345

[7] Nedeltchev K, Loher TJ, Stepper F, et al. Long-term outcome of acute spinal cord ischemia syndrome. Stroke 2004; 35(2): 560–565

[8] Cuello JP, Ortega-Gutierrez S, Linares G, et al. Acute cervical myelopathy due to presumed fibrocartilaginous embolism: a case report and systematic review of the literature. J Spinal Disord Tech 2014; 27(8): E276–E281

[9] Loher TJ, Bassetti CL, Lövblad KO, et al. Diffusion weighted MRI in acute spinal cord ischaemia. Neuroradiology 2003; 45(8): 557–561

[10] Küker W, Weller M, Klose U, Krapf H, Dichgans J, Nägele T. Diffusion weighted MRI of spinal cord infarction—high

resolution imaging and time course of diffusion abnormality. J Neurol 2004; 251(7): 818–824

[11] Zhang JS, Huan Y, Sun LJ, Ge YL, Zhang XX, Chang YJ. Temporal evolution of spinal cord infarction in an in vivo experimental study of canine models characterized by diffusion weighted imaging. J Magn Reson Imaging 2007; 26(4): 848–854

[12] Fujikawa A, Tsuchiya K, Takeuchi S, Hachiya J. Diffusion weighted MR imaging in acute spinal cord ischemia. Eur Radiol 2004; 14(11): 2076–2078

[13] Stepper F, Lövblad KO. Anterior spinal artery stroke demonstrated by echo-planar DWI. Eur Radiol 2001; 11(12): 2607–2610

[14] Thurnher MM, Bammer R. Diffusion weighted magnetic resonance imaging of the spine and spinal cord. Semin Roentgenol 2006; 41(4): 294–311

[15] Beslow LA, Ichord RN, Zimmerman RA, Smith SE, Licht DJ. Role of diffusion MRI in diagnosis of spinal cord infarction in children. Neuropediatrics 2008; 39(3): 188–191

[16] Setzer M, Murtagh RD, Murtagh FR, et al. Diffusion tensor imaging tractography in patients with intramedullary tumors: comparison with intraoperative findings and value for prediction of tumor resectability. J Neurosurg Spine 2010; 13(3): 371–380

[17] Choudhri AF, Whitehead MT, Klimo P, Jr, Montgomery BK, Boop FA. Diffusion tensor imaging to guide surgical planning in intramedullary spinal cord tumors in children. Neuroradiology 2014; 56(2): 169–174

[18] Vargas MI, Delavelle J, Jlassi H, et al. Clinical applications of diffusion tensor tractography of the spinal cord. Neuroradiology 2008; 50(1): 25–29

[19] Ducreux D, Lepeintre J-F, Fillard P, Loureiro C, Tadié M, Lasjaunias P. MR diffusion tensor imaging and fiber tracking in 5 spinal cord astrocytomas. AJNR Am J Neuroradiol 2006; 27(1): 214–216

[20] Hayes LL, Jones RA, Palasis S, Aguilera D, Porter DA. Drop metastases to the pediatric spine revealed with diffusion weighted MR imaging. Pediatr Radiol 2012; 42(8): 1009–1013

[21] Liu X, Tian W, Kolar B, et al. Advanced MR diffusion tensor imaging and perfusion weighted imaging of intramedullary tumors and tumor like lesions in the cervicomedullary junction region and the cervical spinal cord. J Neurooncol 2014; 116(3): 559–566

[22] Ikuta F, Zimmerman HM. Distribution of plaques in seventy autopsy cases of multiple sclerosis in the United States. Neurology 1976; 26(6 PT 2): 26–28

[23] Toussaint D, Périer O, Verstappen A, Bervoets S. Clinicopathological study of the visual pathways, eyes, and cerebral hemispheres in 32 cases of disseminated sclerosis. J Clin Neuroophthalmol 1983; 3(3): 211–220

[24] Clark CA, Werring DJ, Miller DH. Diffusion imaging of the spinal cord in vivo: estimation of the principal diffusivities and application to multiple sclerosis. Magn Reson Med 2000; 43(1): 133–138

[25] Valsasina P, Rocca MA, Agosta F, et al. Mean diffusivity and fractional anisotropy histogram analysis of the cervical cord in MS patients. Neuroimage 2005; 26(3): 822–828

[26] Hesseltine SM, Law M, Babb J, et al. Diffusion tensor imaging in multiple sclerosis: assessment of regional differences in the axial plane within normal-appearing cervical spinal cord. AJNR Am J Neuroradiol 2006; 27(6): 1189–1193

[27] van Hecke W, Nagels G, Emonds G, et al. A diffusion tensor imaging group study of the spinal cord in multiple sclerosis patients with and without T2 spinal cord lesions. J Magn Reson Imaging 2009; 30(1): 25–34

[28] Miraldi F, Lopes FC, Costa JV, Alves-Leon SV, Gasparetto EL. Diffusion tensor magnetic resonance imaging may show abnormalities in the normal-appearing cervical spinal cord from patients with multiple sclerosis. Arq Neuropsiquiatr 2013; 71 9A: 580–583

[29] Raz E, Bester M, Sigmund EE, et al. A better characterization of spinal cord damage in multiple sclerosis: a diffusional kurtosis imaging study. AJNR Am J Neuroradiol 2013; 34(9): 1846–1852

[30] von Meyenburg J, Wilm BJ, Weck A, et al. Spinal cord diffusion tensor imaging and motor-evoked potentials in multiple sclerosis patients: microstructural and functional asymmetry. Radiology 2013; 267(3): 869–879

[31] Lennon VA, Kryzer TJ, Pittock SJ, Verkman AS, Hinson SR. IgG marker of optic-spinal multiple sclerosis binds to the aquaporin-4 water channel. J Exp Med 2005; 202(4): 473–477

[32] Kim W, Kim SH, Huh SY, Kim HJ. Brain abnormalities in neuromyelitis optica spectrum disorder. Mult Scler Int 2012; 2012: 735486

[33] Qian W, Chan Q, Mak H, et al. Quantitative assessment of the cervical spinal cord damage in neuromyelitis optica using diffusion tensor imaging at 3 Tesla. J Magn Reson Imaging 2011; 33(6): 1312–1320

[34] Pessôa FM, Lopes FC, Costa JV, Leon SV, Domingues RC, Gasparetto EL. The cervical spinal cord in neuromyelitis optica patients: a comparative study with multiple sclerosis using diffusion tensor imaging. Eur J Radiol 2012; 81(10): 2697–2701

[35] Goh C, Desmond PM, Phal PM. MRI in transverse myelitis. J Magn Reson Imaging 2014; 40(6): 1267–1279

[36] Hodel J, Besson P, Outteryck O, et al. Pulse-triggered DTI sequence with reduced FOV and coronal acquisition at 3 T for the assessment of the cervical spinal cord in patients with myelitis. AJNR Am J Neuroradiol 2013; 34(3): 676–682

[37] Schwartz ED, Chin CL, Shumsky JS, et al. Apparent diffusion coefficients in spinal cord transplants and surrounding white matter correlate with degree of axonal dieback after injury in rats. AJNR Am J Neuroradiol 2005; 26(1): 7–18

[38] Pouw MH, van der Vliet AM, van Kampen A, Thurnher MM, van de Meent H, Hosman AJ. Diffusion weighted MR imaging within 24 h post-injury after traumatic spinal cord injury: a qualitative meta-analysis between T2-weighted imaging and diffusion weighted MR imaging in 18 patients. Spinal Cord 2012; 50(6): 426–431

[39] Zhang JS, Huan Y. Multishot diffusion weighted MR imaging features in acute trauma of spinal cord. Eur Radiol 2014; 24 (3): 685–692

[40] Castillo M, Arbelaez A, Smith JK, Fisher LL. Diffusion weighted MR imaging offers no advantage over routine non-contrast MR imaging in the detection of vertebral metastases. AJNR Am J Neuroradiol 2000; 21(5): 948–953

[41] Geith T, Schmidt G, Biffar A, et al. Quantitative evaluation of benign and malignant vertebral fractures with diffusion weighted MRI: what is the optimum combination of b values for ADC-based lesion differentiation with the single-shot turbo spin-echo sequence? AJR Am J Roentgenol 2014; 203 (3): 582–588

[42] Sung JK, Jee WH, Jung JY, et al. Differentiation of acute osteoporotic and malignant compression fractures of the spine: use of additive qualitative and quantitative axial diffusion weighted MR imaging to conventional MR imaging at 3.0 T. Radiology 2014; 271(2): 488–498

[43] Oztekin O, Calli C, Kitis O, et al. Reliability of diffusion weighted MR imaging in differentiating degenerative and infectious end plate changes. Radiol Oncol 2010; 44(2): 97–102

[44] Patel KB, Poplawski MM, Pawha PS, Naidich TP, Tanenbaum LN. Diffusion weighted MRI "claw sign" improves differentiation of infectious from degenerative modic type 1 signal changes of the spine. AJNR Am J Neuroradiol 2014; 35(8): 1647–1652

14 Diffusion Weighted Imaging and Diffusion Tensor Imaging in Head and Neck Diseases

Eloisa M Santiago Gebrim, Regina Lucia Elia Gomes, Flavia K. Issa Cevasco, and Marcio Ricardo Taveira Garcia

Key Points

Diffusion Weighted Imaging in the Head and Neck

- **Diffusion weighted imaging (DWI)** helps differentiate solid from cystic lesions and benign from malignant head and neck lesions.
- The DWI imaging findings should always be correlated with the morphological anatomical images, and interpreting the findings requires experience and knowledge.
- Some of the indications for DWI are tissue characterization for primary tumors and nodal metastases, prediction and monitoring of treatment response, differentiation of recurrent tumor from posttherapeutic changes, evaluation of inflammatory and infectious lesions, and study of salivary and thyroid glands.
- Generally, malignant tumors show greater restriction of diffusion and a lower apparent diffusion coefficient (ADC) compared to normal tissues and benign tumors.
- Lymphomas tend to have some of the lowest ADCs of all tumors in the head and neck.
- Exceptions occur, such as nasopharyngeal adenoid hypertrophy, which has greater restriction of diffusion and a lower ADC, similar to malignant tumors, probably due to the high cellularity.
- Other exceptions are classic chordomas and low-grade chondrosarcomas, which show high ADC values.
- One of the most important indications for DWI in the head and neck is the evaluation of cholesteatomas, especially in their postoperative follow-up; they are hyperintense on DWI.

14.1 Introduction

The addition of diffusion weighted imaging (DWI) to magnetic resonance imaging (MRI) protocols in the evaluation of head and neck malignancies increases lesion detection and helps with differentiating solid from cystic lesions and benign from malignant lesions. Both the DWI and apparent diffusion coefficient (ADC) maps are valuable for assessing various head and neck pathological conditions; however, the DWI findings should always be correlated with the anatomical images, and good collaboration between radiologists, physicists, and clinicians is a prerequisite for optimal patient management.[1] The recent studies of diffusion in the head and neck suffer from small samples, susceptibility artifacts associated with single-shot echo-planar image (EPI) sequences, and low resolution of diffusion images and ADC maps. Because of these issues, DWI characteristics and ADC values should not be used in isolation because there may be overlap between different tumor types.[2] Correct interpretation of DWI requires experience and knowledge.[3]

Optimization and standardization of DWI technical parameters, comparison of DWI with morphological images, and increasing experience are prerequisites for successful application of this challenging technique to head and neck lesions. For this anatomical region, indications for DWI include, but are not limited to, tissue characterization for primary tumors and nodal metastases, prediction and monitoring of treatment response, differentiation of recurrent tumor from posttherapeutic changes, evaluation of inflammatory and infectious lesions, and study of salivary and thyroid glands.[1]

In general, malignant tumors tend to show greater restriction of diffusion and, hence, a lower ADC when compared with normal tissues and benign tumors. Lymphomas tend to have some of the lowest ADCs of all tumors in the head and neck. Furthermore, cancers that show only small changes (increase or decrease) in ADC during treatment or in the early posttreatment phase are more likely to fail treatment. For tumors in general, variations in ADC may arise from heterogeneity in cell size and density, as well as microscopic hemorrhage or calcification.

Future improvement of methods to analyze ADC maps, including histogram analysis and functional

Table 14.1 Head and neck lesions with most common apparent diffusion coefficient (ADC) characteristics for low and high ADC

Lesions of the head and neck with low ADC	Lesions of the head and neck with high ADC
Lymphoma	Pleomorphic adenoma
Squamous cell carcinoma	Inflammatory process
Soft tissue sarcoma	Chordoma
Metastatic lymph node	Low-grade chondrosarcoma
Warthin tumor	Low-grade glioma (optic)
Rhabdomyosarcoma	Vascular lesion
Primitive neuroectodermal tumor	Hemangioma
Eosinophilic granuloma	Cholesterol granuloma
Inflammatory process	
Fungal lesions	
Abscess	
Hemorrhage following recent surgery	
Cerumen in the external ear canal	
Meningioma	
Fibrous histiocytoma	
Cholesteatoma	
Dermoid cyst	
Nasopharyngeal adenoid hypertrophy	

maps, should advance the applications of DWI in the head and neck, especially for treatment monitoring. Recently, several attempts have been made to determine perfusion and diffusion parameters separately by using intravoxel incoherent motion MRI (IVIM-MRI). Perfusion is an important marker of many physiological and pathological processes and can be used as a predictive indicator for effectiveness of chemoradiation and radiotherapy. Therefore, analyzing DWI and perfusion may be helpful in the preoperative tumor evaluation. A simplified IVIM-MRI technique based on the IVIM model has been used to assess perfusion-related parameters (PPs) and molecular diffusion (D) of head and neck tumors, which can be determined with three or four b values (0, 500 and 1,000 s/mm^2; or 0, 200, 400 and 800 s/mm^2). This technique is both fast and easy to apply compared with

IVIM-MRI using multiple b values (e.g., 0, 10, 20, 30, 50, 80, 100, 200, 300, 400, and 800 s/mm^2). The time–signal intensity curve (TIC) profiles obtained after dynamic contrast-enhanced (DCE) MRI represent tumor tissue perfusion properties. Therefore, the use of any single technique may not be effective in the differentiation of head and neck tumors. IVIM-MRI is a technique with the potential for simultaneously assessing both tissue perfusion and diffusion. This multiparametric approach using a TIC and IVIM criteria can help in the differentiation between benign and malignant head and neck tumors and between different histological tumor types with high levels of accuracy.[4]

This chapter emphasizes the main indications for DWI in the differentiation of tumors and inflammatory processes (▶ Table 14.1). The chapter closes with some comments about diffusion

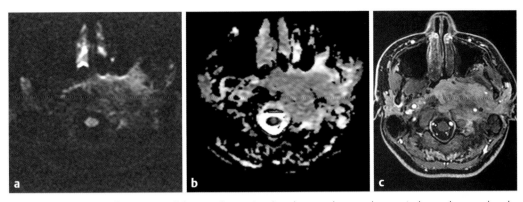

Fig. 14.1 Squamous cell carcinoma of the nasopharynx invading the retropharyngeal, paraspinal, parapharyngeal, and masticator left spaces. The lesion shows (**a**) heterogeneous signal on the *b* 1,000 diffusion weighted imaging, (**b**) middle intensity signal on the apparent diffusion coefficient map, and (**c**) diffuse gadolinium enhancement.

tensor imaging (DTI) applications in the head and neck.

14.2 Tumors

14.2.1 Squamous Cell Carcinoma

Squamous cell carcinoma (SCC) is the most prevalent tumor of the head and neck region, and MRI has aided in lesion detection and characterization, particularly for areas that are difficult to access during physical examination, such as the skull base, nasopharynx, palatine and lingual tonsils, laryngeal cartilages, and hypopharynx. When a patient presents with a clinical suspicion of a malignancy in the head and neck, the first step is to confirm the diagnosis with imaging. If the diagnosis is confirmed, the second step is to assess the disease extent, regional spread, and metastases. The third step is to supply specific information about the tumor nature, trying to identify which tumors will be more responsive to conventional chemoradiation. This step is important to select which cancers will need other therapies, such as surgery or different radiation types. DWI is the most important and established technique for the third step.[2]

Beyond the structural images, DWI is a functional technique used mostly for detection and characterization of head and neck tumors. Restriction of water diffusion is observed in malignant tumors that present low ADC values, due to high cellularity, dense cellular populations, and/or a high nucleocytoplasmic ratio. Necrosis and nonmalignant changes, such as fibrosis and inflammation, have less cellularity compared to viable tumor and hence show high ADC values[3] (▶ Fig. 14.1).

There are several studies emphasizing the importance of DWI in the evaluation and differentiation of tumors in the head and neck.[5,6,7] Wang et al[6] and Maeda et al[7] reported that it is possible to differentiate tumors applying the mean ADC value, showing that benign lesions have higher ADC values, lymphomas have lower values, and carcinomas had intermediate values. Wang et al determined a threshold ADC value of 1.22×10^{-3} mm^2/s, with high accuracy (86%), sensitivity (84%), and specificity (91%) to predict malignancy.[6] Other authors have presented different ADC values for malignant tumors of the head and neck, with lesser values for lymphomas, intermediate values for SCC, and greater ADC values for malignant salivary gland tumors.[2] Other capacity attributed to DWI is to distinguish between well-differentiated and poorly differentiated SCCs by virtue of their ADC values. The most differentiated tumors have higher ADC values, whereas poorly differentiated tumors have lower ADC values.[2,6,8] This difference is due to the higher concentration of cytoplasmic macromolecules, the higher nucleus–cytoplasm relationship, increased cellularity, and the presence of necrotic foci in undifferentiated neoplastic tissues.

On the other hand, a recent retrospective study by Surov et al found that the ADC values of nasopharyngeal adenoid hypertrophy (NAH) were as low those previously reported in carcinomas of

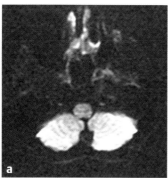 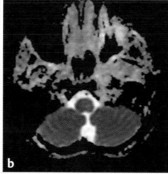 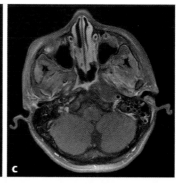

Fig. 14.2 The same patient as in ▶ Fig. 14.1, with nasopharynx squamous cell carcinoma after 6 months of chemoradiation, presented (**a**) a reduction in the size of the lesion and signal reduction on the *b* 1,000 diffusion weighted imaging, (**b**) absence of reduced apparent diffusion coefficient, and (**c**) no gadolinium enhancement. The findings suggest treatment response with significant reduction in cellularity of the lesion.

the head and neck region, both in children and adults, a finding that was attributed to the NAH high cellularity. Because of this behavior, NAH can be misinterpreted as carcinoma or malignant lymphoma, especially in patients over 40 years of age.[9]

A recent review of the literature on DWI in the head and neck demonstrates that it shows no added value in the detection of primary epidermoid carcinoma, but it may show potential value in nodal staging and discrimination of recurrence from posttreatment changes.[10]

MRI has good diagnostic performance in the overall pretreatment evaluation of node staging in patients with SCC. A limited number of small studies suggest that DWI has a higher accuracy as compared with turbo spin-echo (TSE) MRI for the detection of nodal metastases. DWI can be complementary to conventional MRI because size-related and morphological criteria lack sufficient reliability for the identification of small nodal metastases in patients with SCC. Malignant lymph nodes have a lower ADC than benign lymph nodes, and DWI is most beneficial in the detection of subcentimeter metastatic lymph nodes.[11,12]

Oral inspection, laryngoscopy under general anesthesia, conventional image analysis of computed tomography (CT) and MRI can also be impaired by actinic changes, such as local edema, inflammation, necrosis, fibrosis, mucosal thickening, and diffuse contrast enhancement, limiting the identification of residual or recurrent tumors or suggesting false-positive diagnoses, which may

result in unnecessary procedures. Moreover, some residual or recurrent tumors may not show increased contrast enhancement, further hindering the identification of disease.[13]

The need for early diagnosis of cancer recurrence is essential, so MRI techniques have been developed to increase the sensitivity and specificity for its detection. Diffusion imaging sequences have also been used to distinguish recurrent tumor from postoperative and postradition changes.[14] The *b* = 0 signal intensity is lower in malignant lesions than in benign tissues with postradiation changes. The *b* = 1,000 signal intensity is higher in malignancy than in nonneoplastic tissues. Consequently, ADC values are significantly lower in cancer. These characteristics hold for before, during, or after the chemoradiation therapy between inflammatory, fibrotic, and persistent tumor.[14] Some authors demonstrated that cellular death and vascular changes by therapy could be detected by DWI before a reduction of lesion diameter became apparent by conventional images. DWI allows monitoring of tumor response during radiotherapy because loss of tumor cells and increased free water in tissues result in increased ADC values[14] (▶ Fig. 14.2).

DWI helps to distinguish responders from nonresponders, as well as early identification of nonresponding tumors. Radio resistance and poor outcomes during treatment are determined by lower cellularity and necrosis mediated by hypoxia. Radio sensitivity is determined by solid and

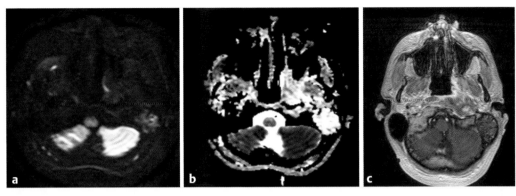

Fig. 14.3 The same patient as in ▶ Fig. 14.1 and ▶ Fig. 14.2 with nasopharynx squamous cell carcinoma after 42 months of chemoradiation shows (**a**) significant reduction in the dimensions of the tumor and signal normalization on *b* 1,000 diffusion weighted imaging, (**b**) high signal on the apparent diffusion coefficient map, and (**c**) faint gadolinium enhancement. The results suggest complete response after treatment, with fibrous scarring at the site of the primary lesion.

hypercellular tissues with low pretreatment ADC values.[14] Early studies show that changes in ADC values may occur before morphological changes, such as tumor dimension, volume or contrast enhancement, mainly in the first 3 months posttreatment. An increase in ADC during treatment is associated with higher survival rates[15] (▶ Fig. 14.3 and ▶ Fig. 14.4). DWI can detect nonresponders and can lead to stopping ineffective treatments and avoiding delays in the administration of other, potentially more effective, treatment alternatives. Thus DWI has increased sensitivity and accuracy to detect recurrence and in the differential diagnosis in the posttreatment setting, providing better results than CT and fludeoxyglucose positron emission tomography (FDG-PET), including fewer false-positive results in persistent primary sites and in metastatic lymph nodes.[15]

One technical advantage of DWI is the ability to acquire reproducible images in a short time period. One disadvantage is its magnetic susceptibility, especially that due to dental fillings. One potential solution to reduce susceptibility artifacts is acquisition time parallel imaging. The overlapping ADC values may be caused by partial volume effects in tiny structures and lowered ADC (false-positive) in fibrosis and higher ADC in necrotic parts of recurrent tumor (false-negative).[13]

Diffusion sequences should be used routinely in standard MRI studies as an adjunct to evaluated response of cancers to nonsurgical treatment.[14]

14.2.2 Lymphomas

Lymphomas are tumors with high cellularity and scarce stroma. The usual imaging analysis based on the characterization of lymph node morphology, size, and shape is not reliable to differentiate benign from malignant nodes. Molecular imaging is a noninvasive modality that has the potential of tissue characterization based on the results of DWI, spectroscopy, single-photon emission computed tomography (SPECT), and PET-CT.[16] Even though ADC varies with *b* value, field strength, lesion size, and presence of necrosis, Maeda et al found that the mean ADC for lymphoma is consistent in $0.65 + - 0.09 \times 10^{-3}$ mm^2/s[7] range. According to these authors an ADC of 0.76×10^{-3} mm^2/s may be used to distinguish between SCC and lymphoma with an accuracy of 98%.[7] Sumi et al found differences in ADC values in lymph nodes and benign lymphadenopathy; the latter had higher values, whereas lymphomas had the lowest values (▶ Fig. 14.5), and metastatic lymph nodes had values that were slightly higher than those in lymphomas.[8]

Compared to PET-CT, which is considered the gold standard in the detection and monitoring of lymphoma, DWI has sensitivity and specificity of 90% and 94%, respectively, for this purpose.[16] IVIM-MRI may improve the use of DWI and allow differentiation of benign from malignant head and neck tumors. According to Sumi et al the ADC

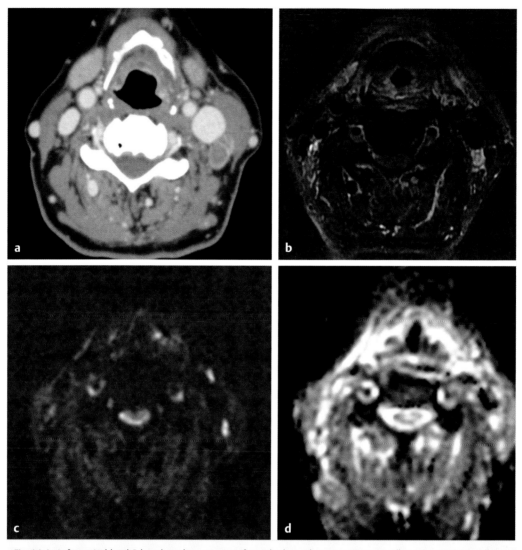

Fig. 14.4 Left cervical level 2 lymph node metastases from the hypopharynx squamous cell carcinoma. (a) Axial enhanced computed tomography shows a heterogeneous node in contact with the left internal jugular vein. (b) After 4 months of chemoradiation a reduction in size and contrast enhancement of the lymph node are observed on the enhanced axial T1-weighted image. (c) There is intermediate signal intensity on the *b* 1,000 diffusion sequence. (d) There is high signal on the apparent diffusion coefficient map, which indicates response to treatment.

values and perfusion-related parameter values of lymphomas were the smallest among all head and neck tumors[17]

14.2.3 Orbital Tumors

Orbital tumors are very heterogeneous, and it is sometimes a challenge to distinguish inflammatory lesions from neoplasms. Diffusion restriction is observed in high cellularity tumors; however,

not all malignant lesions are hypercellular, and some benign tumors, such as meningioma, fibrous histiocytoma, and dermoid cyst, have restricted diffusion.[18]

According to Sepahdari et al the optimal ADC threshold for differentiating malignant from benign lesions is 1×10^{-3} mm^2/s, and an ADC ratio of 1.2 results in a 63% sensitivity, 84% specificity, and 77% accuracy. The best results in malignant tumors are among T2-dark infiltrative lesions

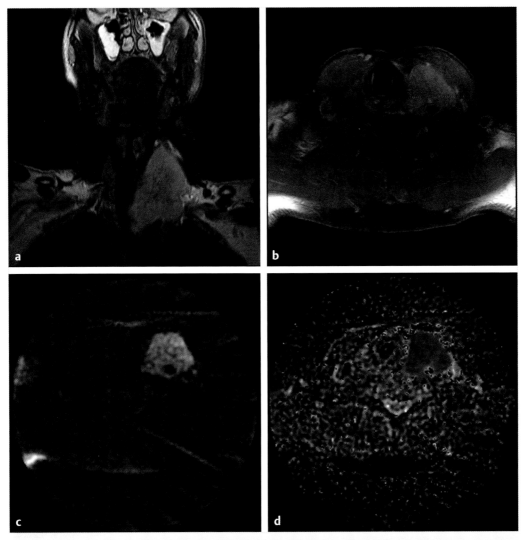

Fig. 14.5 B cell lymphoma. (a) Coronal T2-weighted imaging shows a hyperintense mass in the left cervical region. (b) Contrast enhanced T1-weighted imaging shows enhancement of the lesion. (c) The lesion is hyperintense on diffusion weighted imaging and (d) shows restricted diffusion on the apparent diffusion coefficient map.

because of their high cellularity. DWI is excellent in differentiating lymphoma, which has a low ADC from inflammatory pseudotumor that has high ADC; however, there is an overlap between benign and malignant lesions, particularly in the intermediate ones[19] (▶ Fig. 14.6). Hemangioma is composed of capillaries in a fibrous stroma. Some may grow rapidly and have a tendency to bleed. DWI shows low signal intensity, and their ADC value is higher compared to that of the brain (▶ Fig. 14.7).[20]

ADC measurements in optic pathway gliomas are controversial. According to Jost et al a mean ADC value of 1.4×10^{-3} mm^2/s did not correlate with either clinical aggressiveness or presence of Neurofibromatosis type 1 (NF1). On the other hand, Yeom et al found that optic pathway gliomas with baseline ADC > 1.4×10^{-3} mm^2/s, have higher water content and are more aggressive, requiring treatment earlier than those with lower ADC.[21,22]

MRI has an important role in the diagnosis of retinoblastoma and also in its staging and determination of prognosis depending on tumor size, invasion of the choroid and optic nerve, and presence of bilateral tumors. Moreover, neovascularization of the iris causes enhancement of the anterior eye

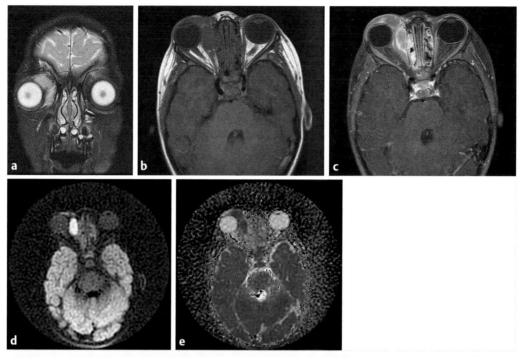

Fig. 14.6 Rhabdomyosarcoma. (a) Coronal T2-weighted imaging shows a hyperintense mass in the right orbit. (b) T1-weighted pre- and (c) postcontrast images show enhancement of the lesion. (d) The lesion is hyperintense on diffusion weighted imaging and (e) shows restricted diffusion on the apparent diffusion coefficient map.

segment and is associated with tumor recurrence and metastasis.[23] According to Razek et al the ADC value is higher in well-differentiated tumors than in undifferentiated retinoblastomas (▶ Fig. 14.8).[23] ADC is lower in larger tumors (15 mm), bilateral lesions, and instances of optic nerve invasion. Calcification is very common in retinoblastomas but does not interfere in DWI measurements.[24]

Orbital meningiomas may be classified as primary if they arise from arachnoid cap cells within the optic nerve sheath, or secondary if they correspond to extension of tumors adjacent to the orbit, which represent most of the orbital meningiomas. According to Bano et al benign meningiomas may have high cellularity and variable ADC values.[25] Filippi et al found ADC values slightly higher than those for brain parenchyma in noncalcified meningiomas. On the other hand, malignant and atypical meningiomas that have conventional MRI features of benign lesions had lower ADC values compared to truly benign meningiomas.[26]

14.2.4 Salivary Gland Tumors

Although DWI enables differentiation of pleomorphic adenomas and myoepithelial adenomas from malignant tumors, a final distinction between benign and malignant parotid gland tumors based on ADCs is not possible, owing to an overlap between values for Warthin tumors and malignant lesions. Recent studies have shown that the combined use of DWI and DCE imaging significantly improves diagnostic accuracy in salivary gland tumors.[27] Parotid MRI should include a T2-weighted sequence (without fat saturation), a DWI sequence with ADC maps, and a perfusion sequence with enhancement curve to facilitate a correct diagnosis in more than 80% of patients[27] (▶ Fig. 14.9). For malignant and benign parotid gland tumors, the value of combining results from DWI and dynamic contrast-enhanced MRI is impressive when an ADC threshold is applied to tumors that show a washout pattern on dynamic

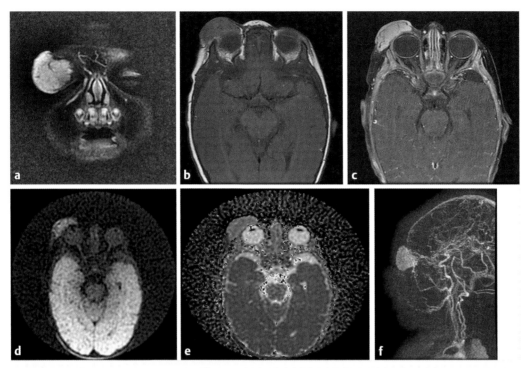

Fig. 14.7 Capillary hemangioma. (**a**) Coronal T2-weighted imaging shows a hyperintense mass in the right eyelid. (**b**) Pre- and (**c**) postcontrast T1-weighted images show enhancement of the lesion. (**d**) Diffusion weighted imaging and (**e**) apparent diffusion coefficient map shows no restricted diffusion. (**f**) Magnetic resonance venography shows vessels communicating the hemangioma and superficial and deep venous drainage systems.

contrast-enhanced images (ADC threshold of 1×10^{-3} mm^2/s distinguished Warthin tumors from carcinomas) and to tumors that show a plateau pattern (ADC threshold of 1.4×10^{-3} mm^2/s distinguished pleomorphic adenomas from carcinomas). However, there is a significant overlap in the ADC values and TIC patterns between benign and malignant salivary gland tumors. Therefore, the use of any single technique may not be effective in establishing differentiation for salivary gland tumors of different histologies.[1,4]

Another application of DWI is in patients with symptoms of xerostomia after radiation treatment when it might help to noninvasively detect the underlying cause (if it originates from the parotid gland) and provide information on parotid gland function.[28]

14.2.5 Thyroid Gland Tumors

The investigation of thyroid nodules is routinely performed with ultrasonography and fine-needle aspiration biopsy (FNAB). However, the result can be inconclusive in some patients, particularly for follicular tumors. Recent work has shown that MRI with DWI may assist in the evaluation of indeterminate nodules, especially if surgery is contemplated. Wu et al, in a recent meta-analysis, assessed the accuracy of DWI in the differentiation between benign and malignant thyroid nodules, whose cytological analysis was indeterminate. The sensitivity and specificity of DWI for detection of malignant lesions among these nodules were 91% and 93%, respectively, and the likelihood ratio was 99%.[29]

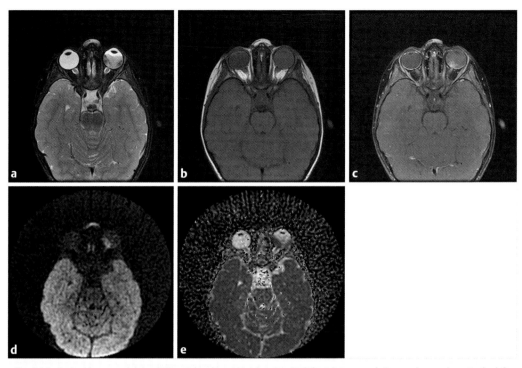

Fig. 14.8 Retinoblastoma. (**a**) Axial T2-weighted imaging shows retinal detachment and vitreous hemorrhage in the left eye. (**b**) T1-weighted images pre- and (**c**) postcontrast show tumor enhancement. (**d**) Diffusion weighted imaging and (**e**) the apparent diffusion coefficient map demonstrate restricted diffusion in the tumor.

DWI may also be helpful for select patients with an incidentally discovered thyroid nodule who require further investigation other than ultrasonography (▶ Fig. 14.10). DWI studies have shown that patients with Grave's disease have significantly higher thyroid ADC values than patients with subacute and Hashimoto thyroiditis and significantly lower ADCs than healthy volunteers.[1]

14.2.6 Paranasal Sinuses Tumors

The CT and MRI features of benign and malignant sinonasal lesions are often nonspecific and overlapping. SCCs in the maxillary sinuses are the most common sinonasal malignancies; however, small round blue cell tumors (SRBCTs), such as neuroendocrine carcinoma, olfactory neuroblastoma, malignant melanoma, and lymphoma, may be difficult to differentiate from SCCs and even from benign and inflammatory lesions. ADC maps may be an effective MRI tool for the differentiation of

benign/inflammatory lesions from malignant tumors in the sinonasal area. Sasaki et al showed that overall ADC values of malignant tumors are significantly lower than those of benign and inflammatory lesions and that there is no significant difference in ADC between benign and inflammatory lesions. On ADC maps, percentages of total tumor areas within malignant tumors having extremely low or low ADC (▶ Fig. 14.11) are significantly greater than those within benign and inflammatory lesions. ADC values also effectively discriminated lymphomas and SCCs from other malignant tumors.[30]

14.2.7 Masticator Space Tumors

Razek et al showed that ADC values of masticator space malignancies are significantly lower than those of masticator space infections, with significant differences in the ADC values between SCCs and soft tissue sarcomas as well as between

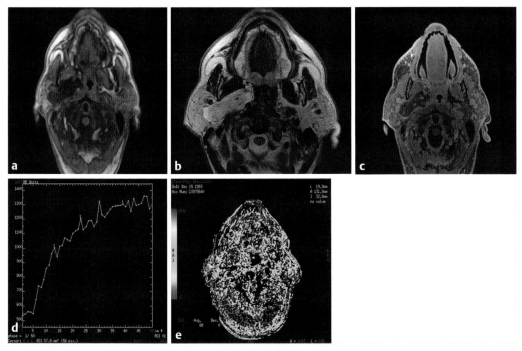

Fig. 14.9 Pleomorphic adenoma. (**a**) Axial T1-weighted imaging shows a low-intensity right parotid gland mass in the deep lobe. (**b**) T2-weighted imaging shows hyperintense lesion, (**c**) SPGR post-gadolinium shows heterogeneous contrast enhancement, (**d**) an ascending curve on the perfusion map and (**e**) color perfusion map.

bacterial and fungal infections. As soft tissue sarcomas and non-Hodgkin lymphomas are more cellular and contain more compact cells than SCC, their ADC values are lower than those of nasopharyngeal carcinoma and oral SCC that extend into masticator space. CT and MRI cannot always differentiate chronic infections or inflammatory lesions in the masticator space from malignancy, and biopsy may be needed. DWI can help in this differentiation because the ADC values of inflammatory lesions are higher than those of malignant tumors, which show hypercellularity, a high ratio of intracellular water to extracellular water content, and restricted diffusion, whereas inflammatory lesions show a low ratio of intracellular water to extracellular water and unrestricted diffusion.[31]

14.2.8 Skull Base Tumors

DWI can help in guiding clinical decisions on indeterminate skull base lesions because biopsy is associated with risks. Ginat et al showed that the average minimum ADC values in malignant tumors are lower than those found in benign tumors. No significant differences between sarcomas and carcinomas were found for the ADC values or the normalized ADC ratios. Overall, malignant skull lesions display lower ADC values than their benign counterparts. Exceptions include classic chordomas and low-grade chondrosarcomas, which show high ADC values (▶ Fig. 14.12 and ▶ Fig. 14.13), and eosinophilic granulomas, which show low ADC values.[18] Chordomas and chondrosarcomas have distinct origins and generally distinct histopathologic features and clinical behaviors, but it may be difficult to distinguish one from the other on preoperative imaging. Yeom et al showed that chondrosarcoma has the highest mean ADC values and is significantly different from classic chordoma and poorly differentiated chordoma. Poorly differentiated chordoma was characterized by low T2 signal intensity, but other conventional MRI

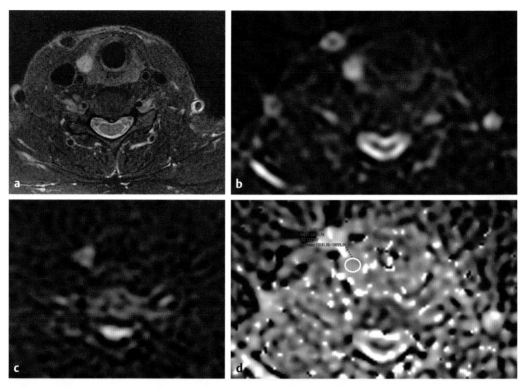

Fig. 14.10 Thyroid adenoma in the right lobe. Axial T2-weighted shows a hyperintense nodule in the right lobe (**a**), with high signal diffusion on b 0 (**b**) and *b* 1,000 (**c**), and (**d**) the apparent diffusion coefficient map without restricted diffusion in the nodule.

features did not distinguish it from other tumor types. The differences in ADC values may be attributed to the extracellular matrices of these tumors. The higher ADC values of chondrosarcomas, which have varying degrees of cellularity within a cartilaginous stroma, likely reflect relatively free extracellular water motion. In contrast, the myxoid stroma of chordomas likely impedes extracellular water motion. In the case of very low diffusion, the diagnosis of poorly differentiated chordoma may be considered because water motion is further reduced in this cellular tumor when compared with classic chordoma and chondrosarcoma. This tumor subtype, however, may be difficult to distinguish from other highly cellular neoplasms of the skull base, such as rhabdomyosarcoma and primitive neuroectodermal tumors. The chondroid variant of chordoma may show stromal features that mimic the hyaline cartilage seen in chondrosarcoma, whereas a subset of chondrosarcoma may show a myxoid matrix characteristic of chordoma. Both tumors may have areas of calcification and even ossification. Because of the close relationship

between histology and tissue water properties, ADC may fail as a sole predictor of diagnosis in such cases of histopathologic crossover and variability but can still provide worthwhile information about the presumptive diagnosis of a skull base lesion. Despite higher ADC among irradiated chordomas, the values were still lower than those of chondrosarcomas.[32]

14.3 Inflammatory Process

14.3.1 Cholesteatoma

One of the most useful applications of DWI in the head and neck is the diagnosis of cholesteatomas. CT has been considered the method of choice for imaging inflammatory process of the middle ear, including cholesteatoma.[33] However, in recent years, several studies have shown an increasing role of DWI in the evaluation of cholesteatomas, especially in their postoperative follow-up. The performance of CT is unsatisfactory in differentiating cholesteatoma from other soft tissue masses of

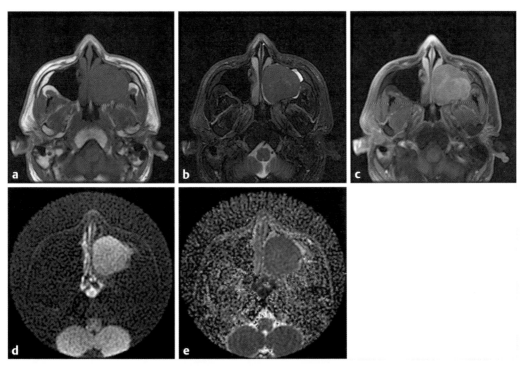

Fig. 14.11 Squamous cell carcinoma of the left maxillary sinus. Axial images show a left maxillary sinus mass which is isointense on (**a**) T1-weighted imaging and (**b**) T2-weighted imaging, (**c**) shows contrast enhancement. (**d**) Diffusion weighted imaging and (**e**) the apparent diffusion coefficient map demostrate restricted diffusion in the tumor.

the middle ear or changes in the surgical bed, such as granulation tissue, fibrous tissue, edematous mucosa, and cholesterol granulomas.

MRI protocols for diagnosis of cholesteatoma include T1- and T2-weighted sequences associated with DWI. A delayed postcontrast T1 sequence can also be included. Cholesteatoma is an avascular lesion and does not enhance, even in the delayed postcontrast sequence. Other tissues, such as granulation and fibrous tissues, enhance after gadolinium administration (► Fig. 14.14). De Foer et al reported that DWI has significantly higher sensitivity and specificity than delayed gadolinium-enhanced T1-weighted sequences in the assessment of cholesteatoma. Another advantage of DWI is that it is faster and does not require the administration of gadolinium.[33,34] It is important to evaluate all the sequences acquired, including the conventional spin-echo sequences, in order to make the correct diagnosis of cholesteatoma, because there are other causes of restricted diffusion in temporal bone, which include hemorrhage following recent surgery, cerumen in the external ear canal, Silastic sheets, bone pate, abscess, and cholesterol granuloma.[35]

Cholesteatomas are hyperintense on DWI due to both restricted diffusion and T2 shine-through. Two different DWI techniques may be used in the evaluation of cholesteatoma: Echo planar imaging (EPI) and non-EPI sequences. EPI-DWI has limited spatial resolution and susceptibility artifacts due to field inhomogeneity in the temporal bone causing a characteristic high intensity curvilinear artifact (► Fig. 14.15). These artifacts can obscure a small cholesteatoma. It is known that a size limit for detection of cholesteatoma on EPI-DWI is approximately 5 mm. Non-EPI sequences result in thinner section thickness and a higher imaging matrix and are less prone to susceptibility artifacts.[33,34]

Non-EPI sequences improve diagnostic accuracy for acquired middle ear cholesteatomas in comparison with EPI ones detecting smaller lesions, (~ 2 mm). These sequences have also been shown to have high reliability in detecting recurrent cholesteatoma with good interobserver agreement and include single-shot turbo spin- echo sequences—Half-Fourier single-shot turbo spin-echo (HASTE) (► Fig. 14.16) and periodically rotated overlapping parallel lines with enhanced reconstruction

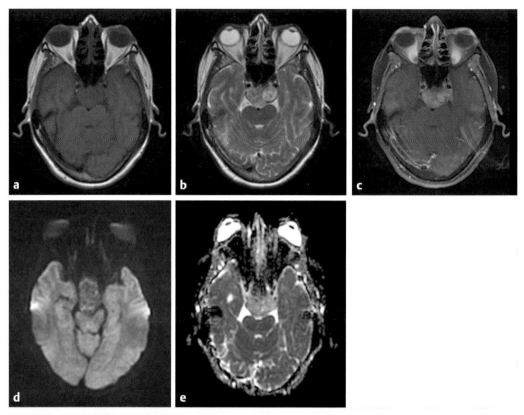

Fig. 14.12 Clival chordoma. Axial images show central skull base mass, which is (**a**) isointense on T1-weighted imaging, (**b**) hyperintense on T2-weighted imaging, and (**c**) shows contrast enhancement, without restricted diffusion in the tumor (**d**) on the diffusion weighted imaging and (**e**) the apparent diffusion coefficient map.

(PROPELLER) DWI.[36] Currently, DWI is considered an alternative to second look surgery for screening for, cholesteatoma, helping to avoid unnecessary surgeries. Recurrence of cholesteatoma after surgical excision is frequent, especially after closed mastoidectomy. Before DWI a second-look surgery was mandatory and considered a standard procedure to be performed 6 to 12 months after a closed mastoidectomy.[36]

14.4 Other Inflammatory Processes

DWI may also be used in the evaluation of other inflammatory and infectious lesions of the head and neck. Data from recent studies suggest that DWI can distinguish abscesses from cystic lesions and tumors.[6,31,37,38] The differences in ADC values

of these lesions may be explained by their viscosity. The mobility of water protons in cystic lesions and abscesses is influenced by their viscosity and protein concentrations. This water mobility will be lower in a liquid with high proteins and viscosity.[6] Razek et al reported that branchial cleft cysts have the highest ADC values of the cystic lesions due to their low protein contents, whereas thyroglossal duct cysts and Tornwaldt cysts showed slightly lower ADC values due to their higher amounts of proteins.[38]

Abscesses cause restricted diffusion of water molecules and have high signal on DWI due to several factors, such as the presence of pus with high viscosity, inflammatory cells, proteins, cellular debris, and bacteria, whereas necrotic tumors present lower signal on diffusion because the movement of water molecules is facilitated in these lesions due to the presence of fewer

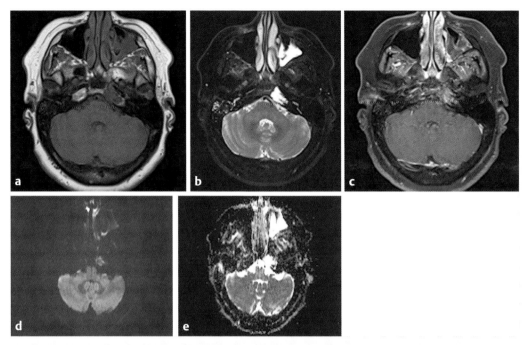

Fig. 14.13 Low-grade chondrosarcoma. Axial (**a**) T1-weighted image shows a left-sided isointense mass, (**b**) hyperintense on T2-weighted image, (**c**) enhancement post gadolinium, and no restricted diffusion on (**d**) diffusion weighted imaging and (**e**) in the apparent diffusion coefficient map.

inflammatory cells and a more serous fluid (▶ Fig. 14.17). Koc et al showed that the ADC values of abscesses and lymphadenitis were lower than those of tumor necrosis.[37]

On the contrary, bacterial infections of the masticator space in patients with necrotizing otitis externa and odontogenic infections show unrestricted diffusion with high ADC values (▶ Fig. 14.18). Fungal infections have smaller overall ADC values and greater percentages of total tumor areas with extremely low or low ADC values among all inflammatory and benign lesions.[31]

14.4.1 Sinusitis

Secretions within the sinuses may show great variability, depending on their composition. Extremely thick secretions produce signal voids on both T1 and T2 sequences and may simulate normal aerated sinuses. Normal sinonasal secretions are predominantly watery and are observed as having high signal on T2- and low signal on T1-weighted imaging. In chronically obstructed sinuses, the amount of free water decreases and protein concentration and viscosity increase, resulting in hypointensity on T2- and hyperintensity on T1-weighted imaging. There is a correlation between ADC values and the amount of the proteins in the secretions.[39] In addition to protein concentration, the ADC values are also influenced if the infection is bacterial or fungal and by the presence of hemorrhage. It is reported that fungal infections have ADC values lower than bacterial ones and are similar to hematomas. Organized and coagulated areas within a hematoma also interfere with diffusion.[30]

14.4.2 Orbital Infections

DWI can be used in evaluation of inflammatory processes of the orbit. Fluid-attenuated inversion recovery (FLAIR) and enhanced T1-weighted images are sensitive for detection of inflammatory processes in the uvea, muscles, and vitreous chamber; however, DWI is better for detecting

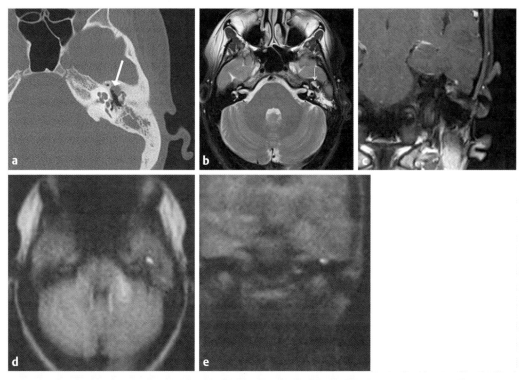

Fig. 14.14 Cholesteatoma. (a) Axial computed tomography shows a round, soft tissue mass in the anterior left epitympanum (arrow) and mild erosion of the head of the malleus. (b) Axial T2-weighted imaging shows that the lesion is hyperintense, (c) there is no contrast enhancement on enhanced coronal T1-weighted imaging, and (d) the mass is hyperintense on axial and (e) coronal half-Fourier acquisition single-shot turbo-spin-echo diffusion weighted MR (DW-HASTE).

subchoroidal and subretinal abscesses. According to Bhuta et al the ADC values of the abscesses are low compared with those of the normal vitreous[40] (▶ Fig. 14.19).

14.4.3 Optic Neuritis

Optic neuritis may be ischemic, demyelinating, or infectious. MRI is useful for diagnosing optic neuritis, which shows hyperintensity on T2, contrast enhancement, and restricted diffusion. The ADC value is low in an early phase (▶ Fig. 14.20) and high in a chronic phase.

DWI of the optic nerve is challenging because this is a small, mobile structure surrounded by fluid, and susceptibility artifacts from adjacent structures are common. Images in the coronal plane

with DTI can improve infarct detection.[41] Ischemic optic neuropathy (ION) occurs in the middle-aged and elderly population, resulting in varying degrees of blindness.

The changes of ADC in ION are theoretically similar to those seen in cerebral ischemia. The ADC is lower within 24 hours (related to cytotoxic edema), gradually increases to normal around 7 days, and remains high in the chronic phase because of vasogenic edema, axonal loss, and demyelination.[42]

14.4.4 Diffusion Tensor Imaging

A number of recently published papers have shown advancements of DTI in neuroradiology with increasing clinical importance. However,

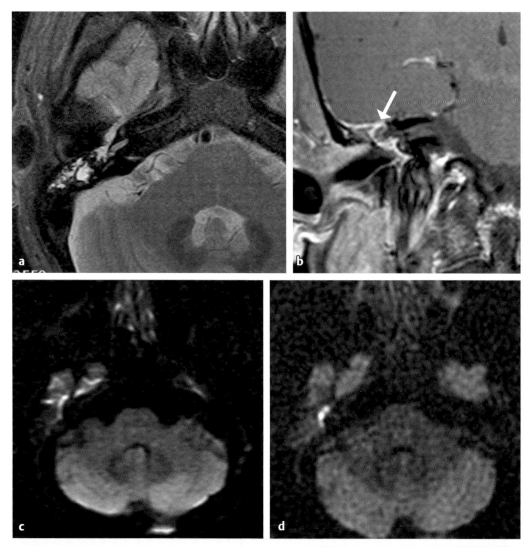

Fig. 14.15 Cholesteatoma. Axial images demonstrate a lesion in the right epitympanum with hyperintensity on (**a**) T2-weighted imaging and (**b**) no enhancement on T1-weighted imaging postcontrast (arrow). There are enhancing granulation tissues surrounding the nonenhancing cholesteatoma. (**c**) Axial echo-planar imaging diffusion weighted image (EPI-DWI) and (**d**) periodically rotated overlapping parallel lines with enhanced reconstruction (PROPELLER) DWI show restricted diffusion, which is better demonstrated on the (**d**) PROPELLER sequence. Also, notice the high-intensity curvilinear artifact in the EPI-DWI.

applications in the head are yet not well established. A feasibility study performed in 2009 on a 3 T magnet demonstrated that it was possible to define the relationship between the inferior alveolar nerves and adjacent tissues by using DTI and tractography.[43] This information can prevent injuries during surgical removal of masses.[15] Another possible application could be the use of DTI to characterize the courses of large cervical nerves, such as the vagus, the phrenic, and the sympathetic chains, for planning in the resection of cervical schwannomas and neurofibromas.

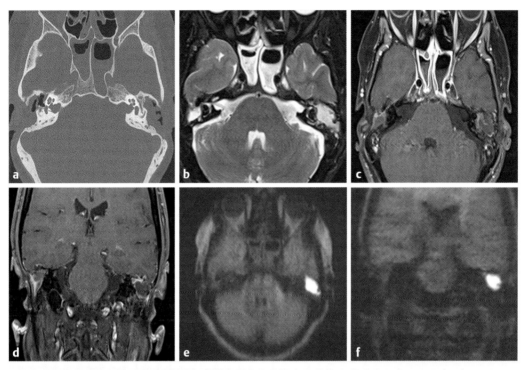

Fig. 14.16 Recurrent left cholesteatoma after bilateral mastoidectomy. (**a**) Axial computed tomography shows obliteration of both surgical cavities by soft tissue material. (**b**) Hyperintense tissues on axial T2-weighted imaging with peripheral contrast enhancement are seen (**c,d**) bilaterally, and there is hyperintensity of the lesion on the left side on the (**e**) axial and coronal (**f**) half-Fourier acquisition single-shot turbo-spin-echo diffusion weighted MR (DW-HASTE).

New applications that are beginning to be studied are the evaluation of the optic pathways in traumatic, neoplastic, and inflammatory lesions,[4, 44] as well as evaluating the auditory pathways in cases of neurosensory hearing loss and tinnitus.[14]

DTI may play a role in preoperative evaluation of patients with large vestibular schwannomas. The position of the facial nerves in cerebellopontine angles in relation to the tumors can be predicted using DTI. Knowledge of the location and course of the facial nerve is necessary to prevent its injury during the surgery.[45,46]

14.5 Summary

The use of DWI in head and neck imaging is recent, and there are few articles addressing this issue, most of them with small samples. There are also some technical difficulties, such as susceptibility artifacts and low resolution of diffusion images and ADC maps, in this complex anatomical area. The main indications for DWI in the head and neck are tissue characterization for primary tumors and nodal metastases, prediction and monitoring of treatment response, differentiation of recurrent tumor from post therapeutic changes, and evaluation of inflammatory and infectious lesions.

Head and neck malignant tumors in general have high cellularity, hence they show greater restriction of diffusion and a lower ADC compared to normal tissues and benign tumors. Of the malignant tumors, lymphomas tend to have some of the lowest ADC values, whereas SCC, the most prevalent tumor of the head and neck region, tends to have intermediated values.

One of the most useful applications of DWI in the head and neck is in the evaluation of cholesteatomas, mainly in the postoperative follow-up. The other indications are also described in this

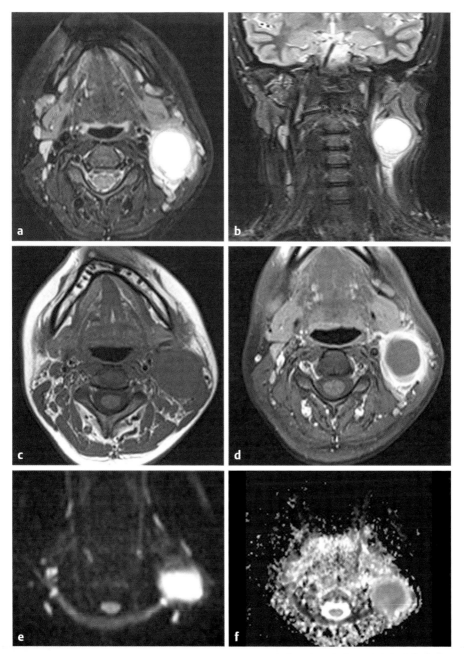

Fig. 14.17 Infected second branchial cleft cyst. (**a**) Axial and (**b**) coronal T2-weighted images show a hyperintense lesion located anterior to the left sternocleidomastoid muscle, posterior to the left submandibular gland, and anterolateral to the left carotid artery. (**c**) Axial T1-weighted images pre- and (**d**) post-gadolinium show a thick rim of enhancement surrounding the lesion secondary to acute inflammation. (**e**) Diffusion weighted imaging shows hyperintensity in the lesion. (**f**) The apparent diffusion coefficient map shows restricted diffusion due to the infectious process.

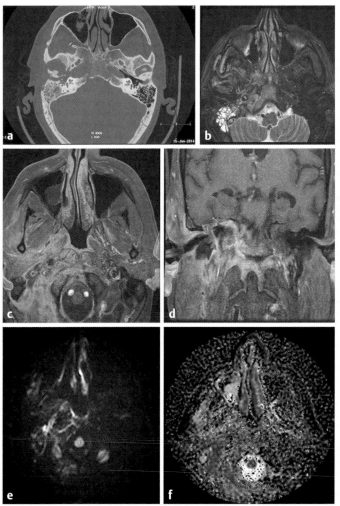

Fig. 14.18 Necrotizing external otitis complicated with skull base osteomyelitis in a diabetic patient. (a) Axial bone window computed tomography shows right-sided middle ear opacification with multiple areas of bone erosions involving the mandibular condyle, zygomatic arch, floor of the middle ear, petrous apex, and clivus. (b) Axial T2-weighted imaging and (c, d) contrast-enhanced T1-weighted imaging demonstrate an inflammatory soft tissue in the right temporal bone with extension into the temporomandibular joint. Notice the enhancing tissue extending from the right temporal bone into mastication, parapharyngeal, retropharyngeal, and prevertebral spaces. (e) Diffusion weighted imaging and (f) the apparent diffusion coefficient map show no restricted diffusion.

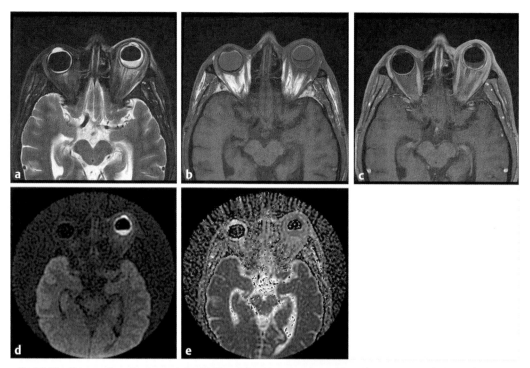

Fig. 14.19 Abscess after vitrectomy. (**a**) Axial T2-weighted imaging shows bilateral vitrectomy and surrounding hyperintensity in the left eye. (**b**) T1-weighted images pre- and (**c**) postgadolinium show contrast enhancement posteriorly in the left globe, suggesting abscess and endophthalmitis. (**d**) Diffusion weighted imaging shows hyperintensity. (**e**) The apparent diffusion coefficient map shows restricted diffusion in the abscess.

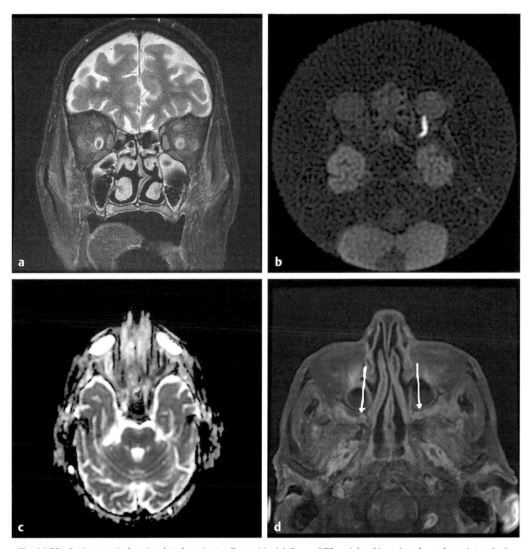

Fig. 14.20 Optic nerve ischemia related to giant cell arteritis. (**a**) Coronal T2-weighted imaging shows hyperintensity in the left optic nerve. (**b**) Diffusion weighted imaging shows hyperintensity in the left optic nerve. (**c**) The apparent diffusion coefficient map confirms restricted diffusion. (**d**) Axial T1-weighted imaging after gadolinium shows contrast enhancement of the pterygopalatine and temporal fossae with arteritis (arrows).

chapter, divided by location and type of involvement, and tumoral or inflammatory process.

References

[1] Thoeny HC, De Keyzer F, King AD. Diffusion weighted MR imaging in the head and neck. Radiology 2012; 263(1): 19–32

[2] Emonts P, Bourgeois P, Lemort M, Flamen P. Functional imaging of head and neck cancers. Curr Opin Oncol 2009; 21 (3): 212–217

[3] Purandare NC, Rangarajan V. Newer imaging techniques in head and neck cancer. Indian J Surg Oncol 2010; 1(2): 186–193

[4] Sumi M, Nakamura T. Head and neck tumours: combined MRI assessment based on IVIM and TIC analyses for the differentiation of tumors of different histological types. Eur Radiol 2014; 24(1): 223–231

[5] Chawla S, Kim S, Wang S, Poptani H. Diffusion weighted imaging in head and neck cancers. Future Oncol 2009; 5(7): 959–975

[6] Wang J, Takashima S, Takayama F, et al. Head and neck lesions: characterization with diffusion weighted echo-planar MR imaging. Radiology 2001; 220(3): 621–630

[7] Maeda M, Kato H, Sakuma H, Maier SE, Takeda K. Usefulness of the apparent diffusion coefficient in line scan diffusion weighted imaging for distinguishing between squamous cell carcinomas and malignant lymphomas of the head and neck. AJNR Am J Neuroradiol 2005; 26(5): 1186–1192

[8] Sumi M, Sakihama N, Sumi T, et al. Discrimination of metastatic cervical lymph nodes with diffusion weighted MR imaging in patients with head and neck cancer. AJNR Am J Neuroradiol 2003; 24(8): 1627–1634

[9] Surov A, Ryl I, Bartel-Friedrich S, Wienke A, Kösling S. Diffusion weighted imaging of nasopharyngeal adenoid hypertrophy. Acta Radiol 2014(May): 22

[10] Driessen JP, van Kempen PM, van der Heijden GJ, et al. Diffusion weighted imaging in head and neck squamous cell carcinomas: A systematic review. Head Neck 2013(Dec): 17

[11] Wu LM, Xu JR, Liu MJ, et al. Value of magnetic resonance imaging for nodal staging in patients with head and neck squamous cell carcinoma: a meta-analysis. Acad Radiol 2012; 19(3): 331–340

[12] Vandecaveye V, De Keyzer F, Vander Poorten V, et al. Head and neck squamous cell carcinoma: value of diffusion weighted MR imaging for nodal staging. Radiology 2009; 251(1): 134–146

[13] Tshering Vogel DW, Zbaeren P, Geretschlaeger A, Vermathen P, De Keyzer F, Thoeny HC. Diffusion weighted MR imaging including bi-exponential fitting for the detection of recurrent or residual tumour after (chemo)radiotherapy for laryngeal and hypopharyngeal cancers. Eur Radiol 2013; 23(2): 562–569

[14] Trojanowska A. Squamous cell carcinoma of the head and neck-The role of diffusion and perfusion imaging in tumor recurrence and follow-up. Rep Pract Oncol Radiother 2011; 16(6): 207–212

[15] Srinivasan A, Mohan S, Mukherji SK. Biologic imaging of head and neck cancer: the present and the future. AJNR Am J Neuroradiol 2012; 33(4): 586–594

[16] Herneth AM, Mayerhoefer M, Schernthaner R, Ba-Ssalamah A, Czerny Ch, Fruehwald-Pallamar J. Diffusion weighted imaging: lymph nodes. Eur J Radiol 2010; 76(3): 398–406

[17] Sumi M, Nakamura T. Head and neck tumors: assessment of perfusion-related parameters and diffusion coefficients based on the intravoxel incoherent motion model. AJNR Am J Neuroradiol 2013; 34(2): 410–416

[18] Ginat DT, Mangla R, Yeaney G, Johnson M, Ekholm S. Diffusion weighted imaging for differentiating benign from malignant skull lesions and correlation with cell density. AJR Am J Roentgenol 2012; 198(6): W597–601

[19] Sepahdari AR, Aakalu VK, Setabutr P, Shiehmorteza M, Naheedy JH, Mafee MF. Indeterminate orbital masses: restricted diffusion at MR imaging with echo-planar diffusion weighted imaging predicts malignancy. Radiology 2010; 256(2): 554–564

[20] Kamano H, Noguchi T, Yoshiura T, et al. Intraorbital lobular capillary hemangioma (pyogenic granuloma). Radiat Med 2008; 26(10): 609–612

[21] Jost SC, Ackerman JW, Garbow JR, Manwaring LP, Gutmann DH, McKinstry RC. Diffusion weighted and dynamic contrast-enhanced imaging as markers of clinical behavior in children with optic pathway glioma. Pediatr Radiol 2008; 38 (12): 1293–1299

[22] Yeom KW, Lober RM, Andre JB, et al. Prognostic role for diffusion weighted imaging of pediatric optic pathway glioma. J Neurooncol 2013; 113(3): 479–483

[23] Abdel Razek AA, Elkhamary S, Al-Mesfer S, Alkatan HM. Correlation of apparent diffusion coefficient at 3T with prognostic parameters of retinoblastoma. AJNR Am J Neuroradiol 2012; 33(5): 944–948

[24] Sepahdari AR, Kapur R, Aakalu VK, Villablanca JP, Mafee MF. Diffusion weighted imaging of malignant ocular masses: initial results and directions for further study. AJNR Am J Neuroradiol 2012; 33(2): 314–319

[25] Bano S, Waraich MM, Khan MA, Buzdar SA, Manzur S. Diagnostic value of apparent diffusion coefficient for the accurate assessment and differentiation of intracranial meningiomas. Acta Radiol Short Rep 2013; 2(7): 2047981613512484

[26] Filippi CG, Edgar MA, Uluğ AM, Prowda JC, Heier LA, Zimmerman RD. Appearance of meningiomas on diffusion weighted images: correlating diffusion constants with histopathologic findings. AJNR Am J Neuroradiol 2001; 22(1): 65–72

[27] Espinoza S, Halimi P. Interpretation pearls for MR imaging of parotid gland tumor. Eur Ann Otorhinolaryngol Head Neck Dis 2013; 130(1): 30–35

[28] Zhang Y, Ou D, Gu Y, et al. Diffusion weighted MR imaging of salivary glands with gustatory stimulation: comparison before and after radiotherapy. Acta Radiol 2013; 54(8): 928–933

[29] Wu LM, Chen XX, Li YL, et al. On the utility of quantitative diffusion weighted MR imaging as a tool in differentiation between malignant and benign thyroid nodules. Acad Radiol 2014; 21(3): 355–363

[30] Sasaki M, Eida S, Sumi M, Nakamura T. Apparent diffusion coefficient mapping for sinonasal diseases: differentiation of benign and malignant lesions. AJNR Am J Neuroradiol 2011; 32(6): 1100–1106

[31] Abdel Razek AA, Nada N. Role of diffusion weighted MRI in differentiation of masticator space malignancy from infection. Dentomaxillofac Radiol 2013; 42(4): 20120183

[32] Yeom KW, Lober RM, Mobley BC, et al. Diffusion weighted MRI: distinction of skull base chordoma from chondrosarcoma. AJNR Am J Neuroradiol 2013; 34(5): 1056–1061, S1

[33] De Foer B, Vercruysse JP, Spaepen M, et al. Diffusion weighted magnetic resonance imaging of the temporal bone. Neuroradiology 2010; 52(9): 785–807

[34] De Foer B, Vercruysse JP, Bernaerts A, et al. Middle ear cholesteatoma: non-echo-planar diffusion weighted MR imaging versus delayed gadolinium-enhanced T1-weighted MR imaging—value in detection. Radiology 2010; 255(3): 866–872

[35] Lingam RK, Khatri P, Hughes J, Singh A. Apparent diffusion coefficients for detection of postoperative middle ear cholesteatoma on non-echo-planar diffusion weighted images. Radiology 2013; 269(2): 504–510

[36] Li PM, Linos E, Gurgel RK, Fischbein NJ, Blevins NH. Evaluating the utility of non-echo-planar diffusion weighted imaging in the preoperative evaluation of cholesteatoma: a meta-analysis. Laryngoscope 2013; 123(5): 1247–1250

[37] Koç O, Paksoy Y, Erayman I, Kivrak AS, Arbag H. Role of diffusion weighted MR in the discrimination diagnosis of the cystic and/or necrotic head and neck lesions. Eur J Radiol 2007; 62(2): 205–213

[38] Abdel Razek AA, Gaballa G, Elhawarey G, Megahed AS, Hafez M, Nada N. Characterization of pediatric head and neck masses with diffusion weighted MR imaging. Eur Radiol 2009; 19(1): 201–208

[39] White ML, Zhang Y. Sinonasal secretions: evaluation by diffusion weighted imaging and apparent diffusion coefficients. Clin Imaging 2008; 32(5): 382–386

[40] Bhuta S, Hsu CC, Kwan GN. Scedosporium apiospermum endophthalmitis: diffusion weighted imaging in detecting subchoroidal abscess. Clin Ophthalmol 2012; 6: 1921–1924

[41] Iwasawa T, Matoba H, Ogi A, et al. Diffusion weighted imaging of the human optic nerve: a new approach to evaluate optic neuritis in multiple sclerosis. Magn Reson Med 1997; 38(3): 484–491

[42] Hickman SJ, Wheeler-Kingshott CA, Jones SJ, et al. Optic nerve diffusion measurement from diffusion weighted imaging in optic neuritis. AJNR Am J Neuroradiol 2005; 26(4): 951–956

[43] Akter M, Hirai T, Minoda R, et al. Diffusion tensor tractography in the head-and-neck region using a clinical 3-T MR scanner. Acad Radiol 2009; 16(7): 858–865

[44] Wang MY, Qi PH, Shi DP. Diffusion tensor imaging of the optic nerve in subacute anterior ischemic optic neuropathy at 3 T. AJNR Am J Neuroradiol 2011; 32(7): 1188–1194

[45] Roundy N, Delashaw JB, Cetas JS. Preoperative identification of the facial nerve in patients with large cerebellopontine angle tumors using high-density diffusion tensor imaging. J Neurosurg 2012; 116(4): 697–702

[46] Gerganov VM, Giordano M, Samii M, Samii A. Diffusion tensor imaging-based fiber tracking for prediction of the position of the facial nerve in relation to large vestibular schwannomas. J Neurosurg 2011; 115(6): 1087–1093

15 Future Applications of Diffusion Weighted Imaging: Diffusional Kurtosis and Other Nongaussian Diffusion Techniques

Maria Gisele Matheus

Key Points

- Diffusional kurtosis imaging (DKI) is a nongaussian diffusion technique that shows higher sensitivity and specificity compared with diffusion tensor imaging (DTI) in identifying white and gray matter microstructure abnormalities.
- DKI also enables more accurate WM tractography in anatomical locations of fiber crossing when compared to diffusion tensor imaging.
- Diffusion spectrum imaging (DSI) and Q-ball imaging are high b value diffusion techniques that are being developed, but still should be validated for clinical use.

15.1 Introduction

Diffusional kurtosis imaging (DKI) is a technique that shows higher sensitivity and specificity compared with diffusion tensor imaging (DTI) in identifying abnormalities in tissue microstructure.[1] DKI complements DTI by assessing measures of nongaussian distribution in diffusion.[2] To analyze gaussian versus nongaussian diffusion let's remember that water molecule diffusion is a random process and may be depicted by a probability distribution. For homogeneous solutions, molecular diffusion follows a gaussian curve form of distribution, with the width of the distribution curve proportional to the diffusion coefficient (▶ Fig. 15.1a). This is the assumption used by DTI, resembling the classical diffusion example of a drop of ink in a bucket of still water (▶ Fig. 15.1b).

Data from water molecules diffusing in the brain can be used to probe tissue microstructure noninvasively with diffusion magnetic resonance imaging (MRI) techniques. Diffusion MRI is most sensitive to the microstructural spaces of 10 µm, which is the typical distance that a water molecule diffuses during approximately 100 ms (the interval of time needed to acquire an individual diffusion signal). Thus diffusion MRI is ideal for investigating cell-sized microstructural features and represents a unique ability to noninvasively assess the microstructure of human brain tissue *in vivo*. Using the gaussian model approximation, DTI can be used,

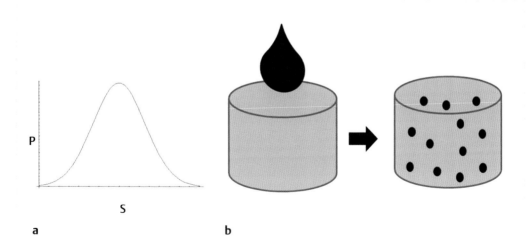

Fig. 15.1 (a) Graphic shows diffusion displacement (S) probability (P). (b) Diagram shows random diffusion displacement in a homogeneous solution, which resembles a drop of ink in a still bucket of water.

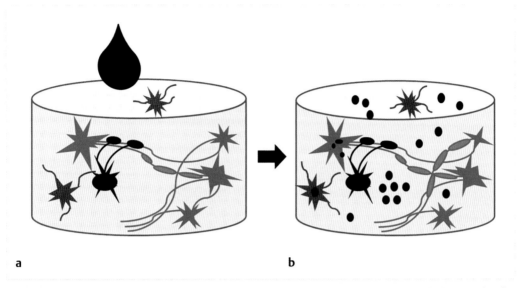

Fig. 15.2 (a) Diagram shows a heterogeneous medium that resembles brain tissue, before a drop of ink is introduced. (b) Diagram shows the uneven diffusivity of a drop of ink in the heterogeneous medium.

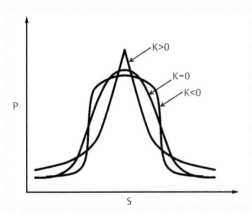

Fig. 15.3 Diagram shows displacement (S) probability (P). K = 0 curve shows a purely gaussian distribution. K > 0 curve shows more weight in the center when compared to the gaussian form. K < 0 curve shows less weight in the center.

for example, to measure the anisotropic properties of white matter by exploring the coherent diffusion along axonal fibers. However, the human brain does not resemble a homogeneous solution; it has a variety of compartments, including different types of cells with variable degrees of membrane permeability (depending on channels and membrane properties), and distinct intra- and extracellular contents. This is quite different from the example of a drop of ink in a bucket of still water (▶ Fig. 15.2). Therefore, the gaussian distribution assumption does not truly reflect the probabilistic distribution of water molecules diffusing in brain tissue.[3,4,5]

More specifically, there are two critical issues for which DTI is limited. The first one involves fiber tractography; the DTI model is incapable of resolving multiple fiber orientations (i.e., crossing fibers). The second issue is that DTI samples only a fraction of the information contained in the dynamics of molecular water diffusion; it does not denote multiple distinct intravoxel compartments and is therefore not capable of depicting intravoxel heterogeneity.[6,7,8,9,10] Interestingly, these two limitations are closely related to each other, so that addressing the second leads to a resolution of the first.

Several strategies have been studied to solve these problems; DKI is one of them and it opens the opportunity for further microstructural assessment. The origin of the word *kurtosis* comes from the Greek word *kyrtos*, meaning curved or arching. In probabilistic theory and statistics, kurtosis is a description of a dimensionless metric of "peakedness" (width of peak) for a probability distribution of a random value. Excess of kurtosis, measured by DKI, denotes the deviation of a probability distribution from a gaussian form (▶ Fig. 15.3). DKI is not a distinctly new way of acquiring diffusion images, but it is a different way to investigate the information that is contained within the diffusion data.[2,3,4,5,11]

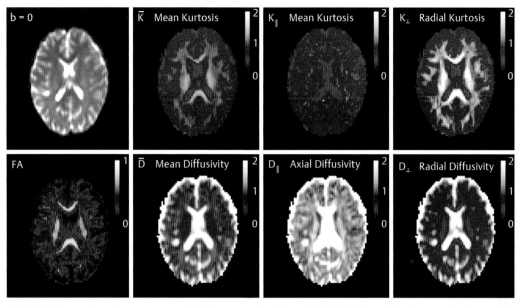

Fig. 15.4 Images show the postprocessed diffusion tensor imaging and diffusional kurtosis imaging metrics of a normal patient. FA, fractional anisotropy. (With permission from Jensen JH, Helpern JA. MRI quantification of non-Gaussian water diffusion by kurtosis analysis. NMR Biomed 2010; 23(7): page 707.)

15.2 DKI Acquisition

DKI can be obtained on modern clinical MRI systems within a clinically acceptable timeframe of 6 to 7 minutes. DKI data are acquired in a similar fashion compared with conventional DTI, but require at least three b values (up to 2,000 s/mm^2), which is somewhat higher than typically used in DTI (1,000 s/mm^2). DKI is related to q-space imaging methods, but it is relatively less demanding in terms of imaging time, hardware requirement, and postprocessing effort compared with other techniques.

In order to obtain the DKI with a reasonable degree of precision, b values somewhat larger than those employed in DTI are necessary so that the departure from linearity is measurable. In the brain, b values of ~ 2,000 s/mm^2 are sufficient. The precision of DKI estimates decreases rapidly if the maximum b values are reduced substantially below 2,000 s/mm^2.[1]

Additionally, the DKI sequence is acquired with at least 15 diffusion gradient directions. Although this is the minimum number of diffusion directions required, we typically acquire 30 directions for two reasons: first, oversampling of the diffusion directions makes the final estimates for the DKI metrics less sensitive to motion artifacts, such as those caused by cardiac-induced brain pulsations; second, by using more directions one effectively averages some of the higher angular frequencies. In addition, 30 directions is a particularly convenient choice because the diffusion directions can be chosen to lie on the vertices of a truncated icosahedron.

Finally, DKI maintains the ability to estimate all standard DTI metrics, including mean, axial, and radial diffusivity (respectively denoted as MD, $D\parallel$, $D\perp$) and fractional anisotropy (FA), and one can also generate kurtosis metrics, such as mean, axial, and radial kurtosis (similarly, denoted as MK, $K\parallel$, $K\perp$)[2,3,4,11,12,13,14] (▶ Fig. 15.4).

15.2.1 Postprocessing

In the conventional analysis of DTI data, the logarithm of the signal intensity is fit to a linear function of the b value, and an estimate for the diffusion coefficient is extracted. In the DKI calculation the data are fitted to a quadratic function, which allows for estimates of both the diffusion and kurtosis tensors. From these tensors, DTI and DKI metrics are then calculated. Most scanner consoles provide DWI and FA calculations, as well as DTI tractography automatically (▶ Fig. 15.5). The resolution is somewhat inferior to that of conventional clinical DWI, but it maintains diagnostic quality (▶ Fig. 15.5a). Postprocessing also

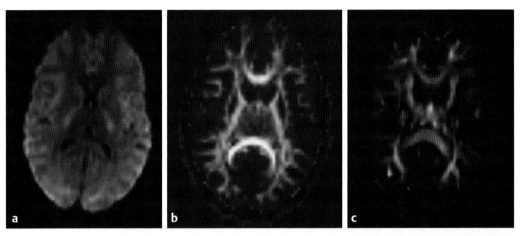

Fig. 15.5 Three diffusion weighted images (DWIs) acquired with multiple *b* values, maximum *b* value of 2,000 s/mm². **(a)** DWI *b* 1,000 s/mm², **(b)** fractional anisotropy map, **(c)** tractography with color orientation. The images were generated automatically by the scanner software.

includes coregistration, averaging, and (optionally) smoothing.

Noise, motion, and imaging artifacts can introduce errors into the estimated tensors, and sufficiently large errors can cause the tensor estimates to be physically and/or biologically erroneous. Typically, it is required that the diffusion coefficients be positive and that the kurtosis lie between a predefined minimum value, Kmin, and a predefined maximum value, Kmax. Any outlier values are systematically brought into this range. For example, if the diffusion coefficient is calculated to be less than zero, then both the diffusion coefficient and the kurtosis are reset to zero. In this manner, the extrinsic and intrinsic artifacts effects on the final diffusion metric maps can be substantially reduced.

There are a number of factors that can lead to errors in DKI values. These include regions with short T2 relaxation (e.g., regions with high iron content leading to poor signal:noise), gradient pulse duration effects, motion, inaccuracies of the fitting model, not fully accounting for imaging gradient contributions to *b* values, and system noise. However, the reproducibility of DKI measures of nongaussianity is similar to that for standard DTI metrics.[4,11,13,15]

15.3 DKI Metrics Interpretation: Applications in the Human Brain

Here we review the accumulating evidence that DKI can be a powerful and feasible investigational tool to assess microstructural changes in several developmental and pathological processes. Kurtosis metrics may act as the earliest biomarker to identify some of these pathological processes. The principal advantage of DKI metrics compared with other diffusion metrics is that they are sensitive measures of tissue structure organization and complexity at a micrometer scale believed to arise from diffusion barriers, such as cell membranes, organelles, and water compartments (e.g., extracellular and intracellular). Another advantage is that DKI is sensitive not only to white matter (WM) microstructural changes but also to gray matter (GM) abnormalities.[2,14] DKI also enables more accurate WM tractography in anatomical locations of fiber crossing when compared to DTI (see ▶ Fig. 15.6).

One typical example of DTI metrics interpretation is increased mean diffusivity (MD) and decreased FA, indicating loss of WM integrity. Increased $D^\perp$ is believed to be derived from an increase in axonal membrane permeability and loss of myelin integrity, and decreased $D\parallel$ is believed to reflect axonal damage. Mean kurtosis (MK) is the kurtosis counterpart of MD, and an increase in MK appears to be related to an increase in complexity of the medium due to various factors, possibly including an increase in organelles, cell membrane layers, and cell packing, among others. $K^\perp$ and $K\parallel$ resemble directional $D^\perp$ and $D\parallel$ and correspond to directional kurtosis. The combination of these parameters ensures a more sensitive characterization than fitting the signal decay to a monoexponential model only.[16]

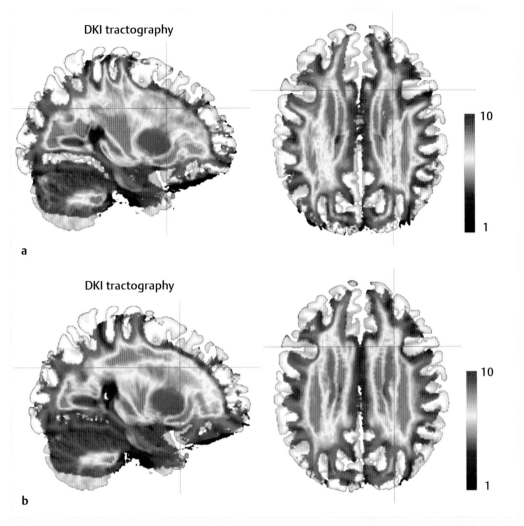

Fig. 15.6 (a) Conventional diffusion tensor imaging (DTI) tractography is limited by its ability to resolve fiber tracking in locations of white matter fiber crossing. (b) Conversely diffusional kurtosis imaging (DKI) is more sensitive to the orientation distribution of water diffusion. The panel shows the voxelwise count of tractography streamlines. Note the count drop in the corona radiata in DTI tractography compared to DKI. (Courtesy of Dr. Leonardo Bonilha with permission.)

15.3.1 Aging Process

MK can be regarded as a general index of tissue microstructural complexity, and, already mentioned it refers to tissue structure length scales compared to or larger than the water molecule diffusion length (typically 5–30 µm) but smaller than the voxel size. The MK length covers cell membranes, axon sheaths, and myelin layers that act as barriers to free diffusion in each voxel. More specifically, MK is a sensitive indicator of diffusional heterogeneity. Falangola et al[14] has demonstrated changes in kurtosis metrics in the human frontal lobes with aging. The WM MK showed a rapid shift to higher values until age 18 years, likely reflecting the intense and continuous myelination and fiber organization that occurs at this time, with a shift to lower values with aging, probably related to degenerative changes, including a decrease of myelin density and myelinated fibers. MK in GM showed a shift to higher values until age 18, which is consistent with the known increase of cortical cell–packing density. This sequence of change in MK with age is in agreement with postmortem studies sensitive for evaluation of the microstructural complexity of both GM and WM.[14,16] More recently, Coutu et al[17] analyzed DTI and DKI metrics in 111 healthy adults between the ages of 33 and 91 years and concluded that DKI metrics provide additional unique complementary information of microstructural changes in the context of healthy aging when used in combination with DTI metrics.

15.3.2 Alzheimer Disease

In a study of Alzheimer disease (AD), Fieremans et al[13] demonstrated that WM tract integrity (WMTI) metrics (derived from DKI using a white matter microstructural model that relates DKI-derived metrics directly to WM microstructure) provide unique information regarding the specific underlying mechanism of WM alterations. The WMTI metrics reported were axonal water fraction (AWF), a marker of axonal density; $D\ axon$, the intrinsic diffusivity inside the axon; and $D_{e,\parallel}$ and $D_{e,\perp}$, the axial and radial diffusivity, respectively, in the extra-axonal space. They proposed that a decrease in AWF may act as a specific marker of axonal density loss, and as a biomarker of AD progression. They also observed increased $D_{e,\perp}$ in the splenium of the corpus callosum from amnestic mild cognitive impairment (aMCI) patients. The analyses of the WMTI metrics also corroborate with previously reported abnormalities in the WM occurring early in the course of AD, including decreased myelin and axonal attenuation, loss of oligodendrocytes, and activation of glial cells.[18] Additionally, kurtosis metrics illustrate the distinct pathophysiologies underlying WM microstructural changes in AD as seen in previous diffusion MRI studies of the largest cerebral WM tract, corpus callosum (CC), which showed that the anterior part of the CC appears to degenerate due to myelin breakdown, whereas decline in the posterior part of the CC is attributed to wallerian degeneration secondary to distal GM pathology in the temporoparietal areas.[19]

15.3.3 Brain Development

MRI diffusion analysis of brain maturation in the last decade has used DTI and DKI in animal and human models, revealing that DKI provides additional microstructural information in brain development when compared to DTI.[1] A progressive increase in FA throughout all WM regions reflects an increase in anisotropy and myelination progression. This trend is most evident in the first 2 years of life when myelination is the dominant contributor to the increase in the microstructural complexity of the WM. The FA peaks relatively earlier in the splenium than in the genu of the corpus callosum in keeping with its well-known caudorostral pattern of myelination. Paydar et al[20] recently demonstrated that MK, like FA, increases in all WM regions, likely also as a function of myelination. However, unlike FA, MK continues to rise beyond 2 years of life and plateaus at later ages in all WM locations. It is speculated that this MK pattern represents continued development of the WM as a result of an increase in the complexity of intrinsic cellular processes and extracellular matrices, axonal pruning, and functional reorganization of myelin to allow the progressive increase in axonal conduction velocities, all of which continue during later stages of development. This later MK peak and plateau pattern may also represent the continued maturation of crossing fibers in WM during late childhood. DTI is limited in the evaluation of both anisotropy and directionality of crossing fibers because the diffusion tensor can resolve only a single fiber orientation within each voxel. Although FA is diminished inside voxels containing crossing fibers, MK can better define the multidirectional environment inside these voxels. Therefore, as isotropic diffusion barriers and more complex fiber patterns continue to materialize in the WM after myelination has been established, a nongaussian diffusion approach may better characterize these delayed developmental changes.

15.3.4 Trauma

Previous studies of brain injury have observed reactive astrogliosis activity to peak at 4 to 7 days postinjury. Animal models show that the combined effect of increased glial cell activity and neuronal pruning may essentially offset any changes in DTI parameters, including MD and FA. However, this complex scenario of microstructural changes appears to be reflected in MK. This observation agrees with histopathological findings where significant increases in reactive astrocytosis and microglial response at 7 days were observed.[21] Furthermore, this increased reactive astrogliosis corresponds directly to the increased MK seen *in vivo* at the subacute stage when DTI parameters, such as FA and MD, return to baseline, indicating that MK is sensitive to changes in tissue microstructure in response to the injury. Taken together, the results from DKI and histology support the idea that MK is sensitive to the changes in tissue microstructural complexity in response to brain injury. In addition, a well-designed, complex study of mild traumatic brain injury (TBI) in humans reported by Grossman et al[22] showed that, when cognitively impaired patients were compared with cognitively unimpaired patients at baseline visits, they showed significantly lower MK and FA in the thalamus and optic radiations. Furthermore, patients showed associations between MK in the thalamus and neuropsychological performance on tests of attention, concentration, and information processing, as well as associations between MK and MD in various WM regions measured and neuropsychological performance on the same tests previously mentioned. Because these results were observed in patients only at baseline and not at follow-up visits, they may be viewed as suggesting that repair had occurred and was consistent with the longitudinal changes observed in DTI and DKI. Nevertheless, it appears that neuropsychological performance in mild TBI may be complex and involve global interaction among many brain regions.

15.3.5 Epilepsy

DKI may be an exquisite tool to investigate structural abnormalities associated with epileptogenesis, notably in patients where macromorphological abnormalities are not identified or their full extent cannot be ascertained. Examples include malformations of cortical development and medial temporal lobe sclerosis. Moreover, DKI may disclose abnormalities associated with forms of epilepsy typically considered to be "MRI-negative." For example, Lee et al[23] investigated patients with idiopathic generalized epilepsy (IGE), which is believed to arise from paroxysmal thalamocortical dysfunction. The authors noted DKI-based complex microstructural abnormalities despite a normal MRI scan on visual inspection. They observed that conventional microstructural measures (MD and FA) revealed WM abnormalities in thalamocortical projections, whereas MK disclosed a broader pattern of WM abnormalities involving thalamocortical and cortical-cortical projections. The authors concluded that, even though IGE is traditionally considered a nonlesional form of epilepsy, microstructural abnormalities may be located within thalamocortical and cortical-cortical WM connections. Particularly, WM abnormalities shown by MK extended into cortical-cortical projections, which suggests that the extent of microstructural abnormalities in IGE may be better assessed with DKI metrics.[23]

15.3.6 Other Applications

In stroke, Hui et al[24] reported that WM metrics revealed an increase in axonal density and a large decrease in intra-axonal diffusion compared to the extra-axonal diffusion microenvironment of ischemic WM lesions. The well-known decrease in the apparent diffusion coefficients of WM after ischemia was found to be driven mainly by a significant drop in the intra-axonal diffusion microenvironment. The results suggested that ischemia preferentially alters the intra-axonal environment, consistent with a proposed mechanism of focal enlargement of axons kwon as axonal swelling or beading.

In gliomas, Raab et al[25] reported changes in MK values among gliomas of different World Health Organization grades. Low-grade tumors are different from normal tissue, and higher-grade tumors demonstrated MK values relatively similar to normal WM. The results showed that structural complexity, reflected in MK values, is higher in high-grade gliomas than in low-grade gliomas but does not reach the complexity of normal WM. Baek et al[26] reported being able to distinguish early tumor progression from pseudoprogression on treated gliomas using histogram analyses of skewness and kurtosis in a normalized cerebral blood volume perfusion map.

DKI is still in an early stage of development, and its practical applications are being explored; however, it is natural to speculate that DKI will be useful for many of the same applications as DTI. The potential advantage of DKI over DTI is that the added metrics quantifying diffusional nongaussianity may supply new information to better characterize both normal and pathological brain tissue. This may be particularly important in GM because its water diffusion is nearly isotropic (on the length scales of diffusion MRI), which limits the value of FA and other metrics of diffusional anisotropy obtainable with DTI.

Diffusional kurtosis metrics may complement more conventional diffusion metrics in at least two ways. First, diffusional kurtosis can potentially be more sensitive to some tissue properties, such as microstructural heterogeneity. Second, diffusional kurtosis may be less sensitive to certain confounding effects and thereby serve as a more robust biomarker. One study has found that the MK in GM is altered substantially less by cerebrospinal fluid contamination than either the MD or the FA.[27] A few studies have shown encouraging, if preliminary, results for applications of DKI to attention deficit hyperactivity disorder.[28] It has also been recently reported[29] that the additional information provided by DKI can be used to resolve intravoxel fiber crossings, which is not possible with DTI. As a consequence, DKI may be used to improve standard DTI-based fiber tracking (see ▶ Fig. 15.6). Key advantages of DKI relative to other methods of quantifying diffusional nongaussianity are that its diffusion metrics can be readily obtained from routine clinical scanning.

15.4 Parei Aqui Faltam Key Points

Diffusion spectrum imaging (DSI) is a q-space method with the ability to fully characterize the diffusion process.[30] To perform DSI, however, one needs to acquire hundreds of diffusion attenuated images with variable directions and very high strengths of diffusion sensitizing gradients. This high sampling of q-space prolongs scan time, and the high b values required pose a challenge to the gradient performance in current clinical systems. In addition, these high b values in current clinical scanners result in low signal-to-noise ratio (SNR) due to prolonged echo time (TE) and substantial diffusion induced signal decay. One approach to overcoming these limitations is to reduce the number of the diffusion encoding gradients as well as the $b$max of DSI. For example, by reducing the number of diffusion encoding gradients from 515 to 203, the scan time can be reduced from 1 h to 30 min. By lowering $b$max, the maximum diffusion gradient strength can be reduced to provide better gradient stability. Moreover, diffusion time and TE can be reduced to provide better SNR for the diffusion weighted images.

Q-ball imaging (QBI) is a high angular resolution diffusion imaging (HARDI) method that is capable of resolving complex subvoxel WM architecture. It samples data of a constant b value in q-space.[31] Typically, its $b$max and number of gradient encodings are approximately two- to threefold lower than those of DSI; thus it is considered more feasible for clinical applications. In QBI the orientation distribution function (ODF) along each radial direction is derived, and the local fiber orientation can be inferred by the local maximum ODF in each voxel. Although QBI and DSI with reduced $b$max and encoding numbers are potentially advantageous for reducing scan time and improving gradient stability, insufficient sampling and inadequate $b$max over the q-space may lead to inaccuracies in estimating fiber orientations.[32]

15.5 Summary

DKI is a robust and promising investigational tool to detect changes in microstructural environments. It is a clinically feasible extension of DTI that allows for quantification of diffusional nongaussianity. With DKI, one obtains all the usual DTI diffusion metrics plus additional metrics related to diffusional kurtosis. These new metrics help to better characterize water diffusion properties in brain tissues and, in particular, are sensitive to diffusional heterogeneity. Implementation of DKI is similar to that of DTI, except that at least three distinct b values (usually 0, 1,000, and 2,000 s/mm^2) and at least 15 distinct diffusion directions are needed; however, they are usually oversampled with 30 directions for improved imaging quality. A whole brain DKI data set with isotropic voxels can be acquired with clinical 3 T MRI scanners in < 7 min.

15.6 Acknowledgments

The author would like to thank Dr. Joseph A. Helpern, Dr. Jens H. Jensen, and Dr. Leonardo Bonilha for their help with concepts and illustration of kurtosis metrics and tractography.

References

[1] Cheung MM, Hui ES, Chan KC, Helpern JA, Qi L, Wu EX. Does diffusion kurtosis imaging lead to better neural tissue characterization? A rodent brain maturation study. Neuroimage 2009; 45(2): 386–392

[2] Jensen JH, Helpern JA, Ramani A, Lu H, Kaczynski K. Diffusional kurtosis imaging: the quantification of non-gaussian water diffusion by means of magnetic resonance imaging. Magn Reson Med 2005; 53(6): 1432–1440

[3] Lu H, Jensen JH, Ramani A, Helpern JA. Three-dimensional characterization of non-gaussian water diffusion in humans using diffusion kurtosis imaging. NMR Biomed 2006; 19(2): 236–247

[4] Jensen JH, Helpern JA. MRI quantification of non-Gaussian water diffusion by kurtosis analysis. NMR Biomed 2010; 23 (7): 698–710

[5] Steven AJ, Zhuo J, Melhem ER. Diffusion kurtosis imaging: an emerging technique for evaluating the microstructural environment of the brain. AJR Am J Roentgenol 2014; 202 (1): W26–33

[6] Mukherjee P, Berman JI, Chung SW, Hess CP, Henry RG. Diffusion tensor MR imaging and fiber tractography: theoretic underpinnings. AJNR Am J Neuroradiol 2008; 29(4): 632–641

[7] Mukherjee P, Chung SW, Berman JI, Hess CP, Henry RG. Diffusion tensor MR imaging and fiber tractography: technical considerations. AJNR Am J Neuroradiol 2008; 29(5): 843–852

[8] Chung HW, Chou MC, Chen CY. Principles and limitations of computational algorithms in clinical diffusion tensor MR tractography. AJNR Am J Neuroradiol 2011; 32(1): 3–13

[9] Basser PJ, Pajevic S, Pierpaoli C, Duda J, Aldroubi A. In vivo fiber tractography using DT-MRI data. Magn Reson Med 2000; 44(4): 625–632

[10] Mori S, van Zijl PC. Fiber tracking: principles and strategies - a technical review. NMR Biomed 2002; 15(7–8): 468–480

[11] Tabesh A, Jensen JH, Ardekani BA, Helpern JA. Estimation of tensors and tensor-derived measures in diffusional kurtosis imaging. Magn Reson Med 2011; 65(3): 823–836

[12] Fieremans E, Jensen JH, Helpern JA. White matter characterization with diffusional kurtosis imaging. Neuroimage 2011; 58(1): 177–188

[13] Fieremans E, Benitez A, Jensen JH, et al. Novel white matter tract integrity metrics sensitive to Alzheimer disease progression. AJNR Am J Neuroradiol 2013; 34(11): 2105–2112

[14] Falangola MF, Jensen JH, Babb JS, et al. Age-related non-Gaussian diffusion patterns in the prefrontal brain. J Magn Reson Imaging 2008; 28(6): 1345–1350

[15] André ED, Grinberg F, Farrher E, et al. Influence of noise correction on intra- and inter-subject variability of quantitative metrics in diffusion kurtosis imaging. PLoS ONE 2014; 9(4): e94531

[16] Falangola MF, Jensen JH, Tabesh A, et al. Non-Gaussian diffusion MRI assessment of brain microstructure in mild cognitive impairment and Alzheimer's disease. Magn Reson Imaging 2013; 31(6): 840–846

[17] Coutu JP, Chen JJ, Rosas HD, Salat DH. Non-Gaussian water diffusion in aging white matter. Neurobiol Aging 2014; 35(6): 1412–1421

[18] Gouw AA, Seewann A, Vrenken H, et al. Heterogeneity of white matter hyperintensities in Alzheimer's disease: postmortem quantitative MRI and neuropathology. Brain 2008; 131(Pt 12): 3286–3298

[19] Clerx L, Visser PJ, Verhey F, Aalten P. New MRI markers for Alzheimer's disease: a meta-analysis of diffusion tensor imaging and a comparison with medial temporal lobe measurements. J Alzheimers Dis 2012; 29(2): 405–429

[20] Paydar A, Fieremans E, Nwankwo JI, et al. Diffusional kurtosis imaging of the developing brain. AJNR Am J Neuroradiol 2014; 35(4): 808–814

[21] Zhuo J, Xu S, Proctor JL, et al. Diffusion kurtosis as an in vivo imaging marker for reactive astrogliosis in traumatic brain injury. Neuroimage 2012; 59(1): 467–477

[22] Grossman EJ, Jensen JH, Babb JS, et al. Cognitive impairment in mild traumatic brain injury: a longitudinal diffusional kurtosis and perfusion imaging study. AJNR Am J Neuroradiol 2013; 34(5): 951–957, S1–S3

[23] Lee CY, Tabesh A, Spampinato MV, Helpern JA, Jensen JH, Bonilha L. Diffusional kurtosis imaging reveals a distinctive pattern of microstructural alternations in idiopathic generalized epilepsy. Acta Neurol Scand 2014; 130(3): 148–155

[24] Hui ES, Fieremans E, Jensen JH, et al. Stroke assessment with diffusional kurtosis imaging. Stroke 2012; 43(11): 2968–2973

[25] Raab P, Hattingen E, Franz K, Zanella FE, Lanfermann H. Cerebral gliomas: diffusional kurtosis imaging analysis of microstructural differences. Radiology 2010; 254(3): 876–881

[26] Baek HJ, Kim HS, Kim N, Choi YJ, Kim YJ. Percent change of perfusion skewness and kurtosis: a potential imaging biomarker for early treatment response in patients with newly diagnosed glioblastomas. Radiology 2012; 264(3): 834–843

[27] Yang AW, Jensen JH, Hu CC, Tabesh A, Falangola MF, Helpern JA. Effect of cerebral spinal fluid suppression for diffusional kurtosis imaging. J Magn Reson Imaging 2013; 37(2): 365–371

[28] Adisetiyo V, Tabesh A, Di Martino A, et al. Attention-deficit/hyperactivity disorder without comorbidity is associated with distinct atypical patterns of cerebral microstructural development. Hum Brain Mapp 2014; 35(5): 2148–2162

[29] Jensen JH, Helpern JA, Tabesh A. Leading non-Gaussian corrections for diffusion orientation distribution function. NMR Biomed 2014; 27(2): 202–211

[30] Wedeen VJ, Wang RP, Schmahmann JD, et al. Diffusion spectrum magnetic resonance imaging (DSI) tractography of crossing fibers. Neuroimage 2008; 41(4): 1267–1277

[31] Tuch DS, Reese TG, Wiegell MR, Wedeen VJ. Diffusion MRI of complex neural architecture. Neuron 2003; 40(5): 885–895

[32] Van AT, Granziera C, Bammer R. An introduction to model-independent diffusion magnetic resonance imaging. Top Magn Reson Imaging 2010; 21(6): 339–354

Index

Note: Page numbers set **bold**
or *italic* indicate headings or
figures, respectively.

A

abscesses
- Aspergillus 123, *127*
- brain tumors 99, *100*
- differential diagnosis 94,
  130, 173
- fungal 112, 122, *125–126*
- head and neck 228, *233*
- post-victrectomy *235*
- pyogenic 112–114, *116–
  118*, 122, *126*
- toxoplasmosis 126
- tuberculous 112
active inflammatory demyelination **155**, *167*
acute disseminated encephalomyelitis **133**, *137*, *157*, **157**
aging
- Alzheimer disease 64, *65*,
  66, **69**, *72–73*, 74, 76
- association fibers *68*
- axial diffusivity 66, *70*
- balance, gait 69, *71*
- cognitive impairment
  (mild) **66**, *70*, 71
- cognitive impairment spectrum *65*
- cognitive performance 63–
  64, *65*, 67, *68*
- corpus callosum 67, 71, *72*
- dementia *65*, 69
- dementia with Lewy
  bodies **73**, *75*
- diffusion based imaging
  strategies 63
- executive function 63
- fractional anisotropy
  changes 66, *67–68*, *70*, 75
- frontotemporal demen-
  tia *73*, **73**
- function-change associations *67*
- hippocampus 71
- imaging physics *63*
- imaging techniques *63*, **63**
- mean diffusivity
  changes 66, *67–68*, *70*, 71
- memory 63–64, 69, 71
- myelination 53, 66, *69*
- normal *65*, **66**, *67*
- pathophysiology **66**
- posterior cortical atrophy 74, *77*
- progressive supranuclear
  palsy **74**, *76*
- radial diffusivity 66, *70*
- tractography 71

- vascular dementia **74**
- Wallerian degeneration 70
- white matter degenera-
  tion 63, 71, *72*, 76
- white matter indices 63
AIDS 115, 119, *123*
alcoholism 69, *71*
Alzheimer disease 64, *65*, 66,
  69, *72–73*, 74, 76, **244**
anterior commissure *45*, **45**
apolipoprotein E (ApoE4) 71
apparent diffusion coefficient **3**
- as marker *4*, **4**
- astrocytoma 99
- brain tumors 99–101, 108,
  110
- epidermoid **105**, *106*
- head and neck diseases 215,
  216
- hematoma **193**
- lymphoma 105, *216*
- meningitis *113*, **115**
- pediatric DWI, DTI 154
- physics 1
- principles *82*
- rFOV sequences 203
- stroke 83–84, *87*
- TBI 172, 174, *174*, *177*
- ventriculitis 118
aquaporin-4 (AQP-4) 136, *138*
arcuate fasciculus **40**, *41*
arterial infarction *20*, *23*
Aspergillus 122–123, *127*
astrocytoma
- anaplastic *22*
- apparent diffusion coefficient 99
- edema *21–22*
- fractional anisotropy 204
- pilocytic *21*, 204, *208*
- spinal cord 204, *207–208*
Atlas, S. W. 193
autism spectrum disorders 59,
  60
axial diffusivity
- aging 66, *70*
- brain tumors 101–102
- demyelinating lesions 133
- heritability 56, *56*
- metrics, correlates 64, *65*
- white matter tract imaging 51, *51–52*, *54–55*

B

b factor *2*, *3*, **4**, *5*, 11
b factor selection **5**
Baek, H. J. 245
Baló concentric sclerosis **138**,
  140
bevacizumab 108
brain tumors

- abscesses 99, *100*
- apparent diffusion coefficient 99–101, 108, 110
- astrocytomas 99
- axial diffusivity 101–102
- biomarkers 99
- cystic lesion differentiation **99**, *100*
- differential diagnosis 137,
  183
- diffusion kurtosis (DK)
  imaging 110
- drop metastases, in children 204
- DWI benefits 99
- epidermoid **105**, *106*
- FLAIR *101*, *103*, 105, *105*,
  107
- fractional anisotropy 101–
  102
- functional diffusion maps
  (fDMs) 110
- germinoma 107
- glioblastoma multi-
  forme 99, *100*, 105
- glioma 100–101, *101*, *102*,
  108, 137, 245
- grading **100**, *101*
- high b value DWI
  (HBDWI) **109**
- infiltration **100**, *101*
- Ki-67 expression 99, 103
- lymphoma (CNS), *see* lymphoma
- medulloblastoma *107*
- meningioma 99, **102**, *104*
- pediatric intracranial 106
- peritumoral white matter
  tract patterns **102**, *103*
- pineal masses 107
- pinealoblastomas 107
- post treatment evalua-
  tion **107**
- postoperative evalua-
  tion **107**
- primitive neuroectodermal
  tumor (PNET) 106, *107*
- prognosis 107
- pseudoprogression **108**
- pseudoresponse **108**, *109*
- radial diffusivity 101–102
- recurrence 108
- tractography 102, *103*, **110**
breast cancer *208*
Brownian motion *1*, *2*
Buckle, C. 119

C

Canavan disease 163, *164*, *167*
Candida 122
capillary leak syndromes **92**

carbon monoxide 147, *150–
  151*
carotid endarterectomy **92**
Castillo, M. 119
central pontine, extrapontine
  myelinolysis **164**, *165*, *167*
cerebral venous thrombo-
  sis 79, **93**, *94*
chasing the dragon syn-
  drome 144, *146*
Chavez, S. 17
chemotherapy **141**, *151*, **159**,
  161, *167*
- *See also* specific drugs
Chen, Y. 53, 100, 119
childhood ataxia with diffuse
  CNS hypomyelination
  (CACH) *165*, *166*
cholesteatoma 215, **226**, *230–
  232*
chondrosarcoma 229
Chung, S. P. 197
cingulum bundle **39**, *40*
clival chordoma 228
cocaine **144**, *151*
commissural pathways 39, **43**
conduction aphasia 40
corpus callosum
- aging 67, 71, *72*
- anatomy **43**, *44*
- splenium *27*, *33*, 52, 55
corticobasal degeneration syndrome *76*
Coutu, J. P. 244
Creutzfeldt-Jakob Disease *23*,
  26, 94, 128, 130, *130*
Crohn's disease 145
Cryptococcus 122, *125–127*
cyclosporine **144**, *147*, *151*
cystic lesions, tumors 228
cytomegalovirus 118, *122*

D

delayed myelination 155
dementia *65*, 69
dementia with Lewy
  bodies **73**, *75*
demyelinating lesions
- acute disseminated encephalomyelitis **133**, *137*
- axial diffusivity 133
- Baló concentric sclero-
  sis *138*, *140*
- DTI benefits 132–133
- fractional anisotropy 132
- mean diffusivity *133*
- multiple sclerosis, *see* multiple sclerosis
- neuromyelitis optica 132,
  134, *136*, *138*, **207**, **209**

– osmotic myelinolysis **138**, *141*
– overview 132, **132**, 149
– pediatric 155
– radial diffusivity 133
– tumefactive **136**, *139*
diffuse axonal injury 28, *34*, 171
diffusion kurtosis imaging (DKI)
– advantages *243*, 245
– aging process 243
– Alzheimer disease 244
– brain development **244**
– brain tumors 110
– clinical applications **242**, *243*
– epilepsy **245**
– errors 242
– glioma 245
– image acquisition *241*, **241**
– postprocessing **241**, *242*
– principles 239, *239*, 240, *240*
– stroke 245
– TBI 175, **244**
diffusion MRI 239
diffusion sensitized MRI (dMRI) 170, 184
diffusion spectrum imaging (DSI) 37, 246
diffusion tensor imaging (DTI), *see* specific diseases and conditions, white matter tract imaging
– clinical applications 58, *59–60*, 64, *65*, 239
– data analysis 64, *64*
– infectious diseases 112
– limitations 240
– metrics, correlates 64, *65*
– multiple sclerosis 132
– principles 37, 50, *63*, **63**
diffusion weighted imaging (DWI), *see* specific diseases and conditions
– acquisition matrix 11
– CSF pulsation effects 15
– eddy current artifacts **15**, 16
– motion artifacts 15
– Nyquist ghosts 12, 15, **15**
– parameters **11**, *14*
– perfusion effects **13**, *14*
– phase-encoding errors 11
– physics, *see* physics
– principles *63*, **63**, 79, *82*
– schematic *82*
– SENSE artifacts *17*, **17**
– spike artifacts *16*, **16**
– techniques, *see* techniques
Does, M. D. 195
Dubios, J. 57
dysmyelination 155

E

edema
– acute stroke *88*
–– *See also* stroke
– arterial infarction **20**, *23*
– cellular 19
– cerebral, diseases associated 20
– cytotoxic **20**, 79, 94, 121, 154, 171, *177*
– diffuse *175–176*
– excitotoxic brain injury **19–20**
– extracellular 19
– neoplasm-related vasogenic **20**, *21–22*
– pathophysiology 19
– vasogenic **19–20**, 83, *84*, 101, 154
– venous infarction **22**, *24*
Einstein, Albert 1
end-stage demyelination **165**, *167*
ependymoma *204*, *206*
epidermoid tumors *105*, *106*
epidural hematoma *198*, *201*
epilepsy
– corpus callosum splenium focal lesions *27*, *33*
– DKI **245**
– reversible splenial lesions *148*, *151*
Epstein-Barr virus 119
Escolar, M. L. 58
excitotoxic brain injury **19–20**

F

Falangola, M. F. 244
fiber density mapping (FDM) 64, 66
Filippi, C. G. 222
FLAIR techniques **11**, *13*, 15
florbetapir 69
fludarabine *143*, *145*, *151*
fluorouracil *142*, *143*, *151*
fractional anisotropy
– aging changes 66, *67–68*, 70, 75
– Alzheimer disease *75*
– astrocytoma 204
– brain tumors 101–102
– dementia with Lewy bodies *75*
– demyelinating lesions 132
– diffusivity heritability 55, *56*
– measurement standardization 178
– metrics, correlates 64, *65*
– multiple sclerosis *136*
– spatial standardization *179*, **180**

– TBI 174, 176–178, *178*, 179, *181*, 183
– white matter tract anatomy 36–37, *38–39*
– white matter tract imaging 51, *51–52*
fronto-occipital fasciculus *43*, **43**, *44*
frontotemporal dementia *73*, **73**
functional diffusion maps (fDMs) **110**

G

Gao, W. 51–53
Geng, X. 53, 55, 57
germinoma 107
glioblastoma multiforme 99, *100*, 105
glioma 100–101, *101*, 102, 108, 137, 245
global neonatal hypoxic injury **157**, *159*, *167*
GRE imaging 84
Grossman, E. J. 245
Grydeland, H. 117
Gupta, R. K. 114

H

HARDI 37, 110, 175, 246
HASTE 227
Haynes, R. L. 52
head and neck diseases
– abscesses 228, *233*
– apparent diffusion coefficient 215, *216*
– cholesteatoma 215, **226**, *230–232*
– cystic lesions, tumors 228
– DTI **230**
– DWI benefits 215
– DWI indications 215
– infection 229, *234*
– IVIM-MRI 215, 219
– lymph nodes, malignant 218–219, *220*
– lymphoma, *see* lymphoma
– masticator space tumors **224**
– optic neuritis 230, *236*
– orbital infections 229, *235*
– orbital tumors 220, *222–224*
– overview **215**
– paranasal sinus tumors 224, *227*
– salivary gland tumors 222, *225*
– sinusitis 229
– skull base tumors 225, *228–229*
– squamous cell carcinoma, *see* squamous cell carcinoma

– thyroid gland tumors **223**, *226*
hemangioma 221, *223*
hematoma
– acute **191**, *193*
– acute basal ganglia *196*
– apparent diffusion coefficient **193**
– chronic stage **193**, *196*
– clinical studies 193, 195
– CT 189
– DWI 189, *189*, 190, *191–194*
– epidural *198*, *201*
– extra-axial 197
– hyperacute **190**, 191, *191–192*, 196
– MRI 189, *189*, 190
– overview **189**
– subacute (early) 191, **191**, *194*
– subacute (late) 191, *195*
– subdural 197, *200*
hemorrhage
– DWI 189, *189*, 190
– hyperacute 197
– infarctions **197**, *198–199*
– small intracranial *197*, **197**
– subacute microhemorrhages (late) 197
– subarachnoid **198**
– venous sinus thrombus 197, *200*
heroin **144**, *146*, *151*
herpes encephalitis **25**, *29*, 94, *95*, **95**, 112, 117, *121*, 130
high b value DWI (HBDWI) **109**
HIV *23*, 119
Hui, E. S. 245
hydrocephalus 58
hyperperfusion syndrome *92*
hypoglycemia *95*
hypomyelination 155, **162**
hypothyroidism, congenital *162*, *167*
hypoxic ischemic encephalopathy *24*, *27–28*

I

infectious diseases
– abscesses (fungal) 112, 122, *125–126*
– abscesses (pyogenic) 112–114, *116–118*, 122, 126
– abscesses (tuberculous) 112
– AIDS 115, 119, *123*
– Aspergillus 122–123, *127*
– bacterial **112**, *116*
– Candida 122
– Creutzfeldt-Jakob Disease *23*, *26*, 94, 128, 130, *130*
– Cryptococcus 122, *125–127*
– cytomegalovirus 118, *122*

- DWI benefits 112
- effusion/hygroma *116*
- empyema *116*
- Epstein-Barr virus 119
- fungal 121, *124*
- granulomas, fungal 122
- herpes encephalitis 112, 117, *121*, 130
- influenza 119
- meningitis (bacterial) 112–113, *113–114*, 115, *115–116*, *118–119*
- meningitis (fungal) 122, *125*
- mucormycosis *124*
- neurocysticercosis 123, *128–129*
- neurotuberculosis (neurotb) 115, *120*
- parasitic *123*
- prion **128**
- progressive multifocal leukoencephalopathy (PML) 112, 119, *123*, 130
- subacute sclerosing panencephalitis (SSPE) 121
- toxoplasmosis 126, *129*
- venous thrombosis 115, *119*
- ventriculitis 114, *116, 118*
- viral **115**
influenza 119
intra-axial isotropic diffusion restriction **173**

K

Kang, B. K. 193
Khedr, S. A. 193
Koc, O. 229
Krabbe disease 58, *59*, **161**, *162, 167*

L

lacunar infarction 79, **89**, *91*
Le Bihan, D. 11
Lee, C. Y. 245
leukodystrophy, metachromatic **161**, *162, 167*
leukoencephalopathy
- spongiform 144, *146, 151*
- subacute 141, *142, 151*
- toxic 139–140
limbic encephalitis 26, *30*
lymphoma
- apparent diffusion coefficient 105, *216*
- B cell *221*
- cerebral 95, *96*
- characterization **219**, *221*
- CNS 99, **103**, *105*
- differential diagnosis 94, 220
- pediatric 154

M

Maeda, M. 217, 219
Maldjian, J. A. 195
malnutrition **162**, *167*
maple syrup urine disease **159**, *160, 167*
masticator space tumors **224**
mean diffusivity
- aging 66, *67–68, 70*, 71
- clinical applications 242
- demyelinating lesions *133*
- herpes encephalitis *117*
- metrics, correlates 64, *65*
- TBI 175–176
mean kurtosis 242–243
medulloblastoma *107*
megalencephalic leukoencephalopathy with subcortical cysts 163, *164, 167*
memedulloblastoma 154
meningioma 99, **102**, *104*
meningioma, orbital 222
meningitis
- bacterial 112–113, *113–114*, 115, *115–116, 118–119*
- fungal 122, *125*
methanol 148, *150–151*
methotrexate 142, *144, 151*, **159**, *161, 167*
metronidazole 145, *148, 151*
mitochondrial respiratory chain deficiency 157, *158*
mucormycosis *124*
multiple sclerosis
- characterization 96, *97*, **133**
- cytotoxic edema 22, *25*
- differential diagnosis 97, 173, 183
- DTI imaging 132, *133–136*, **206, 209**
- pediatric 157, *167*

N

necrotizing external otitis 229, *234*
neurocysticercosis 123, *128–129*
neurofibromatosis type 1 221
neuromyelitis optica 132, 134, **136, 138, 207, 209**
neurosurgical planning 47, *48*
neurotuberculosis (neurotb) 115, *120*
nuclear magnetic resonance (NMR) 1–2, *2*
Nyquist ghosts *12, 15*, **15**

O

oligoastrocytoma (anaplastic) *24*
oligodendroglioma *103*
Oppenheim, C. 84

optic neuritis **230**, *236*
orbital infections 229, *235*
orbital tumors **220**, *222–224*
osmotic demyelination syndrome 164, *165, 167*
osmotic myelinolysis 26, *31*, **138, 141**
outlier detection basedde-spiking (ODD) 17
ovarian cancer *30*

P

paranasal sinus tumors **224**, *227*
pediatric DWI, DTI
- active inflammatory demyelination **155**, *167*
- acute disseminated encephalomyelitis **157**, *157*
- apparent diffusion coefficient 154
- brain tumors drop metastases 204
- Canavan disease 163, *164, 167*
- clinical applications **155**
- cystic degeneration **165**
- end-stage demyelination **165**, *167*
- global neonatal hypoxic injury **157**, *159, 167*
- hypomyelination 155, **162**
- hypothyroidism, congenital **162**, *167*
- Krabbe disease **161**, *162, 167*
- malnutrition **162**, *167*
- maple syrup urine disease **159**, *160, 167*
- megalencephalic leukoencephalopathy with subcortical cysts 163, *164, 167*
- methotrexate **159**, *161, 167*
- mitochondrial respiratory chain deficiency 157, *158*
- multiple sclerosis **157**, *167*
- myelin rarefaction **165**
- neurotoxicity **159**
- osmotic demyelination syndrome 164, *165, 167*
- Pelizaeus-Merzbacher disease **162**, *163, 167*
- physics **154**
- spine, spinal cord diseases 203–204
- vanishing white matter disease 165, *166–167*
- water mobility **154**
- X-linked adrenoleukodystrophy 155, *156, 167*
pediatric intracranial tumors 106
Pelizaeus-Merzbacher disease **162**, *163, 167*

physics
- apparent diffusion coefficient 1
- apparent diffusion coefficient as marker 4, *4*
- apparent diffusion coefficient map 3
- axial diffusion 7, *9*
- b factor 2, *3*, **4**, *5*, 11
- b factor selection **5**
- brain water diffusion 1, *4*, **4**, 36
- brain water diffusion anisotropy 6, **6**, 7, *7*, 8, *8–9*
- Brownian motion **1**, *2*
- fractional anisotropy 7–8, *9*
- pediatric DWI, DTI **154**
- radial diffusion 7
- relative anisotropy 7–8, *9*
- Stejskal and Tanner pulse sequence **1**, *2–3*
- T2 shine-through effect *3*
- tensor model 1, **6**, *8–9*
- tissue compartment size 4, *4*
- tractography 9, *10*
pineal masses 107
pinealoblastomas 107
posterior cortical atrophy 74, *77*
posterior reversible encephalopathy syndrome (PRES) 92, *93*
primitive neuroectodermal tumor (PNET) 106, *107*
progressive multifocal leukoencephalopathy (PML) 112, 119, *123*, 130
progressive supranuclear palsy 74, *76*
PROPELLER 11, *12–13*, 227
punctate cortical infarctions 90, *91*
pyramidal tracts 45, *46*

Q

Q-ball imaging (QBI) 246

R

Raab, P. 245
radial diffusivity
- aging 66, *70*
- brain tumors 101–102
- demyelinating lesions *133*
- heritability 56, *56*
- herpes encephalitis 117
- metrics, correlates 64, *65*
- TBI 174
- white matter tract imaging 51, *51–52, 54–55*
radiation therapy **141**, *142, 151*
Razek, A. A. 222, 224

recreational drugs **144**, *151*
retinoblastoma 221, *224*
reversible splenial lesions **148**, *151*
rFOV sequences 203
rhabdomyosarcoma *222*

S

salivary gland tumors 222, *225*
Schaefer, P. W. 195
SE-EPI **11**, *12*
Sepahdari, A. R. 220
septic infarction **94**
Short, S. J. 57
sinusitis **229**
skull base tumors 225, *228–229*
spine, spinal cord diseases
– clinical rationale **206**
– degenerative changes **210**
– differential diagnosis 206
– DWI/DTI benefits 203
– ischemia **204**, *205*
– multiple sclerosis, *see* multiple sclerosis
– neuromyelitis optica, *see* neuromyelitis optica
– pediatric 203–204
– rFOV sequences 203
– spondylodiskitis **210**, *212–213*
– technical considerations 203
– transverse myelitis **209**
– trauma **209**
– tumors 204, *206–208*
– vertebral body fracture **209**, *210–211*
spondylodiskitis **210**, *212–213*
squamous cell carcinoma
– cancer recurrence 218
– DWI benefits, limitations 219
– lymph nodes, malignant 218, *220*
– overview *217*, **217**
– paranasal sinus tumors 224, *227*
– treatment response 218, *218–219*
– TSE MRI 218
status epilepticus **27**, *32*
stroke
– acute stage **82**
– apparent diffusion coefficient 83–84, *87*
– cell death **81**
– chronic stage **83**
– differential diagnosis 183
– diffusion changes time course **83**, *85–88*
– DKI 245
– DWI imaging benefits 79
– DWI reliability **84**
– hemorrhagic transformation **84**, *88*
– hyperacute stage *82*, **82**, *83*
– large vessel acute **82**
– metabolic changes *80*, **80**, *81*
– operationally defined penumbra *82*, *83*
– overview **79**
– pathophysiology **80**
– pump failures *80*, **80**, *81*
– subacute stage **83**, *84*
subacute sclerosing panencephalitis 121
subarachnoid hemorrhage **198**
subdural hematoma 197, *200*
Sumi, M. 219
susceptibility-weighted images (SWI) 84

T

techniques
– FLAIR **11**, *13*, 15
– PROPELLER **11**, *12–13*, 227
– SE-EPI **11**, *12*
tensor model 1, 6, *8–9*
thyroid gland tumors 223, *226*
tissue plasminogen activator (tPA) 84
toxic leukoencephalopathy 139–141
toxicity (CNS), *see* specific drugs
– chemotherapy **141**, *151*, **159**, *161*, *167*
– environmental toxins **147**, *151*
– imaging findings 132
– leukoencephalopathy (subacute) 141, *142*, *151*
– overview **138**, 149
– radiation therapy **141**, *142*, *151*
– recreational drugs **144**, *151*
– reversible splenial lesions **148**, *151*
– toxic leukoencephalopathy 139–141
toxoplasmosis 126, *129*
tract-based spatial statistics 64
tractography
– aging 71
– brain tumors 102, *103*, **110**
– clinical applications *243*
– TBI 176, *178–181*, 182, *183*, *186*
– technique *9*, *10*
– white matter tract anatomy 37
transient global amnesia **96**
transient ischemic attack 79, **90**
traumatic axonal injury **171**, 173, *173*, *175*, 176, *178–179*, *181*, 182, *184–185*
traumatic brain injury (TBI)
– abnormalities **176**
– apparent diffusion coefficient *172*, *174*, *174*, *177*
– clinical context **170**
– concussion 170
– contrecoup contusion 171
– contusion *171–172*, *173*, *180*
– coup contusion 171
– diagnostic criteria **170**
– differential diagnosis *172–173*, *175–176*, 179, *181*, **182**, 183, *183–187*
– diffuse injury **171**
– diffusion kurtosis imaging (DKI) 175, **244**
– diffusion sensitized MRI (dMRI) 170, 184
– DTI abnormalities biophysical basis *174*, *177*
– DTI abnormalities detection **176**
– DWI abnormalities detection *172*, *173–174*
– DWI abnormalities pathophysiology **171**
– focal injury **171**
– fractional anisotropy 174, *176–178*, *178*, *179*, *181*, 183
– HARDI 175
– intra-axial isotropic diffusion restriction **173**
– mean diffusivity *175–176*
– measurement standardization 178, *179*
– pathology, pathophysiology **171**, *172*
– radial diffusivity 174
– regions of interest analysis 180, 182
– spatial standardization 179, **180**
– tractography 176, *178–181*, 182, *183*, 186
– visual assessment *183–184*
– voxelwise analysis 182
– Wallerian degeneration *185*
– white matter injury 176, *181*
tumefactive demyelinating lesions **136**, *139*
tumors, *see* brain tumors

U

uncinate fasciculus *42*, **42**

V

vanishing white matter disease **165**, *166–167*
vascular dementia **74**
vascular pathology
– capillary leak syndromes **92**
– cerebral venous thrombosis 79, *93*, *94*
– DWI applications 79
– edema, *see* edema
– hyperperfusion syndrome **92**
– lacunar infarction 79, *89*, *91*
– lesion mimics **94**
– posterior reversible encephalopathy syndrome (PRES) *92*, *93*
– punctate cortical infarctions *90*, *91*
– septic infarction **94**
– stroke, *see* stroke
– transient global amnesia **96**
– transient ischemic attack 79, **90**
– watershed infarcts 79, **85**, *89–90*
venous thrombosis 115, *119*
ventriculitis 114, *116*, *118*
vertebral body fracture **209**, *210–211*
vigabatrin **146**, *149*, *151*

W

Wang, J. 217
Wang, L. H. 130
watershed infarcts 79, **85**, *89–90*
white matter tract anatomy
– anterior commissure *45*, **45**
– arcuate fasciculus **40**, *41*
– association tracts 38, **39**
– brain water diffusion 36
– categorization **38**
– cingulum bundle **39**, *40*
– commissural pathways 39, **43**
– corpus callosum **43**, *44*
– dorsal bundle 46
– FACT 37
– fiber-tracking algorithms 37
– fractional anisotropy *36–37*, *38–39*
– fronto-occipital fasciculus **43**, *43*, *44*
– functions 36
– imaging *36–37*
– inferior longitudinal fasciculus **41**, *42*
– optic radiation 46, *47*
– overview **36**
– projection tracts 39, **45**
– pyramidal tracts **45**, *46*

- streamlines 37
- superior fronto-occipital fasciculus 43, *44*
- superior longitudinal fasciculus 40, *41*
- technical considerations **36**
- tractography 37
- uncinate fasciculus *42*, **42**
- ventral bundle 46
white matter tract imaging
- axial diffusivity 51, *51–52*, *54–55*
- axial diffusivity heritability 56, *56*
- corpus callosum splenium 52, 55, *55*
- diffusion cognition correlations 50, **57**

- diffusion-cognition correlations *58*
- diffusivity heritability 56, *56*
- early brain development 50
- environmental effects **55**, *56*
- fractional anisotropy 51, *51–52*, 53, *54–55*
- fractional anisotropy heritability 56
- GAP43 staining 52
- gender effects **57**
- genetic control 50, **55**, *56*
- handedness 57
- interneuron connection development 50
- language 57

- lateralization 50
- lateralization effects **57**
- linear anisotropy 53
- maturation 50
- myelination 53, 66, *69*
- planar anisotropy 53
- radial diffusivity 51, *51–52*, *54–55*
- radial diffusivity heritability 56, *56*
- region of interest approach 51–52
- spatial growth patterns **53**
- temporal growth patterns *51*, **51**, *52*
- tract-based approach 53, *54*
- working memory correlations 57, *58*

Wintermark, M. 195
Wolff, J. J. 59

X

X-linked adrenoleukodystrophy **155**, *156*, *167*

Y

Yuan, W. 58

Z

Zhai, G. 53